Study Guide for

Maternal Child Nursing Care

Study Guide for

Maternal Child Nursing Care

Seventh Edition

Maternity

Megan Ross, MSN, RNC-MNN
Clinical Instructor
School of Nursing
University of North Carolina at Chapel Hill
Chapel Hill, North Carolina

Pediatrics

Debbie Stayer, PhD, CPN, RN-BC, CCRN-K
Assistant Professor
Bloomsburg University
Bloomsburg, Pennsylvania

ELSEVIER

ELSEVIER
3251 Riverport Lane
St. Louis, Missouri 63043

STUDY GUIDE FOR MATERNAL CHILD NURSING CARE,
SEVENTH EDITION

ISBN: 978-0-323-80909-2

Previous editions copyrighted 2018, 2014, 2011, 2010, 2006, 2002, and 1998

Senior Content Strategist: Sandra Clark
Senior Content Development Specialist: Maria Broeker
Senior Content Development Manager: Luke Held
Publishing Services Manager: Shereen Jameel
Project Manager: Vishnu T Jiji

Printed in India

Last digit is the print number: 9 8 7 6 5 4 3 2 1

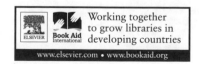

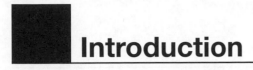

Introduction

Maternal Child Nursing Care, seventh edition, is a comprehensive textbook of maternity and pediatric nursing. This *Study Guide* is designed to help students use the textbook more effectively. In addition to reviewing the content of the text, this *Study Guide* encourages students to think critically in applying their knowledge.

ORGANIZATION

Each chapter in this *Study Guide* is designed to incorporate learning activities that will help students meet the objectives of the corresponding textbook chapter. The content is organized as follows:

- **Learning Key Terms**—Matching or fill-in-the-blank questions give students the opportunity to test their ability to define all key terms in the corresponding textbook chapter.
- **Reviewing Key Concepts**—A variety of questions (matching, fill-in-the-blank, true/false, short answer, and multiple choice) are used to provide students with ample opportunity to assess their knowledge and comprehension of the information covered in the text. These activities are specifically designed to help students identify the important content of the chapter and test their level of knowledge and understanding after reading the chapter.
- **Clinical Judgment And Next-Generation NCLEX® Examination-Style Questions**—A variety of questions enable students to sharpen clinical judgment skills in preparation NCLEX® Exam
- **Answer Key**—Answers to all questions are provided at the end of this *Study Guide*.

Contents

1 21st Century Maternity Nursing

I. LEARNING KEY TERMS

MATCHING: Match each term with its corresponding description.

1. _____ Number of live births in 1 year per 1000 population.

2. _____ All deaths during pregnancy and within 1 year following the end of pregnancy.

3. _____ Number of maternal deaths from births and complications of pregnancy, childbirth, and puerperium (the first 42 days after termination of the pregnancy) per 100,000 live births.

4. _____ An infant who, at birth, demonstrates no signs of life, such as breathing, heartbeat, or voluntary muscle movements.

5. _____ Number of stillbirths and number of neonatal deaths per 1000 live births.

6. _____ Number of births per 1000 women between the ages of 15 and 44 years (inclusive), calculated on an annual basis.

7. _____ An embryo or fetus that is removed or expelled from the uterus at 20 weeks of gestation or less, weighs 500 g or less, or measures 25 cm or less.

8. _____ Number of deaths of infants younger than 1 year of age per 1000 live births.

9. _____ Number of deaths of infants younger than 28 days of age per 1000 live births.

10. _____ Deaths that are a complication of pregnancy, an aggravation of an unrelated condition by the physiology of pregnancy, or a chain of events initiated by the pregnancy.

a. Fertility rate

b. Infant mortality rate

c. Birth rate

d. Maternal mortality rate

e. Neonatal mortality rate

f. Perinatal mortality rate

g. Pregnancy-associated deaths

h. Pregnancy-related deaths

i. Stillbirth

j. Abortus

FILL IN THE BLANKS: Insert the term that corresponds to each of the following definitions or descriptions.

1. _____ Specialty area of nursing practice that focuses on the care of childbearing women and their families through all stages of pregnancy and childbirth, as well as the first 4 weeks after birth.

2. _____ A set of goals based on assessments of major risks to health and wellness, changes in public health priorities, and issues related to the health preparedness and prevention of our nation.

3. _____ A set of 17 goals to be achieved by 2030 that respond to the world's main development challenges and are replacing the previous Millennium Development Goals.

4. _____ Approach to health care that encompasses complementary and alternative therapies in combination with conventional Western modalities of treatment.

5. _____ An umbrella term for the use of communication technologies and electronic information to provide or support health care when the participants are separated by distance.

6. _____ This percentage of maternal deaths are preventable, primarily through the access to and the use of prenatal care services.

7. _____ Term that refers to a spectrum of abilities, ranging from reading an appointment slip to interpreting medication instructions.

8. _____ Nonbiologic factors which have profound influences on health.

9. _____ Guidelines for nursing practice that reflect current knowledge, represent levels of practice agreed on by leaders in the specialty, and can be used for clinical benchmarking.

10. _____ A list of abbreviations, acronyms, and symbols developed by The Joint Commission to decrease the risk of errors in the administration of medications.

11. _____ Term used by The Joint Commission to describe an unexpected occurrence involving death or serious physical or psychological injury, or risk thereof that is not due to underlying conditions.

12. _____ Failure to recognize or act on early signs of distress. Key components include careful surveillance and identification of complications and quick action to initiate appropriate interventions and activate a team response.

13. _____ Level of practice that a reasonably prudent nurse would provide in the same or similar circumstances.

14. _____ When faculty and students from two or more health professions create and foster a collaborative learning environment.

15. _____ A teamwork system for health professionals to provide higher quality, safer patient care. It provides an evidence base to improve communication and teamwork skills.

II. REVIEWING KEY CONCEPTS

1. When assessing pregnant women, what factors would you recognize as having the potential to contribute to the rate of maternal mortality in the United States?

2. Briefly discuss the impact of technology on the growing number of ethical concerns and debates related to perinatal nursing and women's health care.

3. An integrative health care approach implies which of the following? (Circle all that apply.)
   a. The focus is on the whole person.
   b. Conventional Western modalities of treatment are not included.
   c. The beliefs, values, and desires of the patient in terms of health and health care are respected.
   d. Patient autonomy is limited in terms of choosing alternative therapies.
   e. The patient's disease complex is the primary consideration when choosing treatment approaches.

4. A nurse manager of a prenatal clinic should recognize that the most significant barrier encountered by pregnant women in accessing health care would be which of the following?
   a. Lack of transportation to the clinic
   b. Child care responsibilities
   c. Inability to pay
   d. Deficient knowledge related to the benefits of prenatal care

5. In the United States, one of the leading causes of maternal mortality is which one of the following?
   a. Unsafe abortion
   b. Acute renal failure
   c. Cardiovascular disease
   d. Diabetes

6. Pregnant women who are obese are more likely to develop one or both of the two most frequently reported maternal risk factors. These factors include which of the following combinations?
   a. Premature labor and infection
   b. Hemorrhage and hypertension associated with pregnancy
   c. Infection and diabetes
   d. Diabetes and hypertension associated with pregnancy

III. CLINICAL JUDGMENT AND NEXT-GENERATION NCLEX® EXAMINATION-STYLE QUESTIONS

1. *NGN Item Type: Extended multiple response exercise*
   You are the nursing director of a prenatal clinic that primarily serves Black and Hispanic women. The clinic cares for a large number of mothers who are younger than 20 years of age. Which of the following are critical factors to consider when caring for this population?
   Select all that apply.
   a. Social determinants of health play a minimal role in maternal and infant outcomes
   b. The focus in this population should only be on the immediate pregnancy
   c. Racial disparities contribute to a significant increase in maternal mortality
   d. There is a minimal need to address income concerns as a prenatal clinic
   e. Clients should be assessed for financial barriers to care
   f. Transportation access can be a barrier to prenatal appointments
   g. Education materials should address cultural and linguistically competent care
   h. Early risk assessments are a critical part of prenatal care to improve outcomes

2. Support the accuracy of the following statement: An emphasis on high-technology medical care and lifesaving techniques will not reduce the rate of preterm and low-birth-weight infants in the United States.

3. Explain how a nurse could use social media to improve the health care provided to pregnant women and their families. Identify the precautions the nurse must take to ensure that patient confidentiality and privacy are respected.

4. Many barriers interfere with a woman's participation in early and ongoing prenatal care. Describe incentives and services that you would offer to pregnant women to encourage their participation in prenatal care. State the rationale for your proposals. Your answer should reflect an understanding of the barriers.

5. Discuss community-based care as it relates to pregnancy and women's health care.

6. Discuss measures that can be taken to ensure that the health literacy needs of patients are met.

7. Medical errors are a leading cause of death in the United States. Explain the process that you will use as a student to prevent medical errors.

8. Discuss two international concerns that have serious detrimental effects on the health and safety of women. Explain how nurses can address these concerns.

2 The Family, Culture, Spirituality, and Home Care

LEARNING KEY TERMS

MATCHING: Match the family described with the appropriate family category.

1. _____ A single mother lives with her 4-year-old adopted daughter.

2. _____ Anne and Duane are married and live with their daughter and Duane's aunt and uncle.

3. _____ Gloria and Andy are a married couple living with their new baby.

4. _____ Jane and Dillion are unmarried and live with their two children.

5. _____ A family consists of Jim; his second wife, Jane; and Jim's two daughters by a previous marriage.

6. _____ Tammy and Joseph live with their grandmother Irene who has been caring for them since their mother died.

7. _____ Ruth lives with her son, Peter, his wife Anne, and their twin sons.

a. Multigenerational family
b. Single-parent family
c. Cohabitating-parent family
d. Nuclear family
e. Extended family
f. Married-blended family
g. Non-biologic parent family

MATCHING: Match the description with the appropriate cultural concept.

8. _____ Maria is Mexican-American and just gave birth, tells the nurse not to include certain foods on her meal tray because her mother told her to avoid those foods while breastfeeding. The nurse tells her that she doesn't have to avoid any foods and should eat whatever she desires.

9. _____ Thanh, an immigrant from Vietnam, has lived in the United States for 1 year. She tells you that while she enjoys the comfort of wearing blue jeans and sneakers for casual occasions, like shopping, she still wears traditional or "conservative" clothing for family gatherings.

10. _____ A Cambodian family immigrated to the United States and has been living in Denver for over 5 years. The parents express concern about their children, ages 10, 13, and 16, stating, "The children act so differently now. They are less respectful to us, they only want to eat American food, and go to rock concerts. It's hard to believe they are our children."

11. _____ The nurse is preparing a healthy diet plan for her client. In doing so, she takes the time to learn about her preferred foods, and include the Polish foods that she enjoys in her diet plan.

a. Cultural relativism
b. Ethnocentrism
c. Assimilation
d. Acculturation

FILL IN THE BLANKS: Insert the cultural concept that corresponds to each of the following definitions.

12. _____ An ongoing process that influences a person throughout his or her life. It provides an individual with beliefs and values about each facet of life that are passed from one generation to the next.

13. _____ Recognizing that people from different cultural backgrounds comprehend the same objects and situations differently; that a culture determines a person's viewpoint.

14. _____ Changes that occur within one group or among several groups when people from different cultures come in contact with one another and exchange and adopt each other's mannerisms, styles, and practices.

15. _____ Process in which one cultural group loses its identity and becomes a part of the dominant culture.

16. _____ A belief that one's cultural way of doing things is the right way, supporting the notion that "My group is the best."

17. _____ Approach that involves the ability to think, feel, and act in ways that acknowledge, respect, and build upon ethnic, cultural, and linguistic diversity; to act in ways that meet the needs of the patient and are respectful of ways and traditions that may be different from one's own.

18. _____ Type of time orientation that maintains a focus on achieving long-term goals; families or people who practice this time orientation are more likely to return for follow-up visits related to health care and to participate in primary prevention activities.

19. _____ Type of time orientation of families or people who are more likely to strive to maintain tradition or the status quo and have little motivation for formulating future goals.

20. _____ Type of time orientation of families or people who may have difficulty adhering to strict schedules and are often described as living for the moment.

21. _____ Cultural concept that reflects dimensions of personal comfort zones. Actions such as touching, placing the woman in proximity to others, taking away personal possessions, and making decisions for the woman can decrease personal security and heighten anxiety.

22. _____ A unit of socialization and nurturing within a community that preserves and transmits culture. It is a social network that acts as a potent support system for its members.

23. _____ Family category in which husband and wife and their children live as an independent unit, sharing roles, responsibilities, and economic resources.

24. _____ Family category that includes the nuclear family and other people related by blood (kin) such as grandparents, aunts, uncles, and cousins.

25. _____ Family category in which an unmarried biologic or adoptive parent heads the household; it is becoming an increasingly recognized structure in our society. These families tend to be vulnerable both socially and economically.

26. _____ Family category that forms as a result of divorce and remarriage. It includes stepparents, stepchildren, and stepsiblings who join to create a new household.

27. _____ Family category consisting of grandparents, children, and grandchildren. This family form is becoming increasingly common.

28. _____ Family category in which children live independently in foster or kinship care such as living with a grandparent.

29. _____ Family category in which children live with two unmarried biologic parents or two adoptive parents.

30. _____ Term for the family tree format that depicts relationships of family members over at least three generations; it provides valuable information about a family and its health.

31. _____ Term for a graphic portrayal of social relationships of the patient and family including school, work, religious affiliations, and club memberships.

32. _____ Groups within the community who are more likely to experience health status problems and negative health outcomes as a result of a variety of sociocultural, economic, and environmental risk factors that contribute to disparities in health.

II. REVIEWING KEY CONCEPTS

1. Discuss why the nurse should take each of the following "products of culture" into consideration when providing care within a cultural context:

   a. Communication

   b. Personal space

   c. Time orientation

   d. Family roles

2. State the rationale for the increasing emphasis on home- and community-based health care. How has this trend changed the demands placed on the community-based nurse?

3. Community health promotion requires the collaborative efforts of many individuals and groups within a community. Cite several programs that could be established to promote the health of a community's child-bearing families.

4. Explain why each of the groups listed below have been identified as vulnerable populations:

   ■ Women in general

   ■ Adolescent girls

   ■ Older women

   ■ Racial and ethnic people of color

   ■ Incarcerated women

   ■ Immigrant, refugee, and migrant women

5. Describe the ways that nurses can provide care to perinatal patients using the telephone.

6. Which one of the following nursing actions is most likely to reduce a patient's anxiety and enhance the patient's personal security as it relates to the concept of personal space needs?
   a. Touching the patient before and during procedures
   b. Providing explanations when performing tasks
   c. Making eye contact as much as possible
   d. Reducing the need for the patient to make decisions

7. Which of the following strategies are used to deliver culturally competent care. Select all that apply.
   a. Maintain appropriate personal space during interactions.
   b. Ask about woman's fears and those of her family regarding an unfamiliar care setting
   c. Provide hospital menu for meals and let the patient know the set meals
   d. Be sensitive regarding interpreters and language barriers
   e. Ask about group practices and beliefs

1. A nurse has been providing care to a family who experienced the birth of twin girls at 38 weeks of gestation. It is the first birth experience for both parents and the first grandchildren for the extended family. Both newborns are healthy and living at home. The newborn's parents and grandparents all live in the same house with another aunt. Describe considerations the nurse may take when caring for an extended family.

2. The nurse-midwife at a prenatal clinic has been assigned to care for a refugee couple who recently immigrated to the United States. The woman just found out she 2 months pregnant. Neither she nor her husband speaks English. Outline the process that this nurse should use when working with a translator to facilitate communication with this couple to enhance care management.

3. Imagine that you are a nurse who has just been hired to provide in-home health care. Before you begin seeing your patients, you realize that it would be helpful for you to become familiar with the neighborhood and resources in the community where your patients live. You decide to conduct a walking survey of this community.

   a. Describe how you would go about conducting this survey and gathering data.

   b. List the data you believe it would be essential to gather.

   c. Discuss how you would use the findings from your walking survey when providing health care to the patients you will be visiting.

4. Marie is a single parent of two young children ages 4 years and 1 year. She and her children have been homeless for 3 months because her husband abandoned her, and she lost her job because she had no one to help her care for her children.

   a. Discuss the basis for the types of health problems to which Marie and her children are most vulnerable.

   b. What factors related to being homeless could increase Marie's risk for becoming pregnant? If she did become pregnant, explain why it would be considered a high risk pregnancy.

   c. How would you, as a nurse, provide health care services to Marie and her children?

5. You are caring for the wife of a migrant laborer. She and her husband, along with their two children, have been working on a California farm for 2 weeks. She has arrived at a health center established for migrant laborers. She states that she is 4 months pregnant. As the women's health nurse practitioner assigned to care for her, what approaches would you use to ensure that she obtains quality health care that addresses her unique health risks as a migrant worker?

6. Write a series of questions that you would ask when making a postpartum follow-up call to a woman who gave birth 3 days ago.

7. Eileen gave birth to a son 36 hours ago. A home care nurse has been assigned to visit Eileen and her husband in their home to assess the progress of her recovery after birth, the health status of her newborn son, and the adaptation of family processes to the responsibilities of newborn care.

    a. Outline the approach the nurse should take in preparing for this visit.

    b. Describe the nurse's actions during the visit using the care management process as a format.

    c. Discuss how the nurse should end the visit.

    d. Identify interventions the nurse should implement at the conclusion of the visit with Eileen and her husband.

    e. Specify how the nurse should protect her personal safety both outside and inside Eileen's home.

    f. Cite the infection control measures the nurse should use when conducting the visit and providing care in Eileen's home.

8. Angela has recently been diagnosed with hyperemesis gravidarum and has been hospitalized to stabilize her fluid and electrolyte balance. The hospital-based nurse must evaluate Angela for referral to home care.

    a. State the criteria that this nurse should follow to determine Angela's readiness for discharge from hospital to home care.

9

b. Angela has been discharged and will be receiving parenteral nutrition in her home. Discuss the additional information required related to high technology home care.

c. Identify specific home environment criteria that must be met to ensure the safety and effectiveness of Angela's treatment.

9. A nurse is seeking funding to start a home care agency designed to provide home visits to postpartum women and their families within 1 week of birth and follow-up visits as indicated. State the points the nurse should emphasize as a rationale for the importance of this health care service and the cost-effectiveness of funding such a service.

10. A nurse is caring for a postpartum woman whose preferred language is French. The nurse will be using a video interpreter to communicate with planning to communicate with her postpartum client. **Use an X to indicate whether the nursing actions listed below are Indicated (appropriate or necessary) or Not Indicated (not appropriate or contraindicated) when using an interpreter for the client's care at this time**.

Nursing Action	Indicated	Not Indicated
Chooses a female interpreter from the woman's country of origin.		
Uses a quiet location free from interruptions.		
Emphasizes that this is an introductory session, and the client can ask questions at a later time.		
Asks questions while looking at the interpreter.		
Gathers culturally appropriate reading materials to use during the interaction.		
Speaks loudly to enhance understanding		

3 Assessment and Health Promotion

I. LEARNING KEY TERMS

FILL IN THE BLANKS: Insert the term that corresponds to each of the following definitions related to the female reproductive system and breasts. Use the anatomic drawings (Figs. 3-1, 3-2, 3–4, 3–5, and 3–6 in your textbook) to visualize each of the structures as you are inserting the terms

1. _____ Fatty pad that lies over the anterior surface of the symphysis pubis.

2. _____ Two rounded folds of fatty tissue covered with skin that extend downward and backward from the mons pubis; their purpose is to protect the inner vulvar structures.

3. _____ Two flat, reddish folds composed of connective tissue and smooth muscle, which are supplied with nerve endings that are extremely sensitive.

4. _____ Hood-like covering of the clitoris.

5. _____ Fold of tissue under the clitoris.

6. _____ Thin flat tissue formed by the joining of the labia minora; it lies underneath the vaginal opening at the midline.

7. _____ Small structure underneath the prepuce composed of erectile tissue with numerous sensory nerve endings; it increases in size during sexual arousal.

8. _____ Almond-shaped area enclosed by the labia minora that contains openings to the urethra, Skene's glands, vagina, and Bartholin's glands.

9. _____ Bladder opening found between the clitoris and the vagina.

10. _____ Skin-covered muscular area between the fourchette and the anus that covers the pelvic structures.

11. _____ Fibromuscular, collapsible tubular structure that extends from the vulva to the uterus and lies between the bladder and rectum. Its mucosal lining is arranged in transverse folds called _____, _____ glands (located on each side of the urethra), and _____ glands (located on each side of the vagina) secrete mucus that lubricates the vagina. The _____ is a connective tissue membrane that surrounds the vaginal opening and can be perforated during strenuous exercise, insertion of tampons, masturbation, and vaginal intercourse.

12. _____ Anterior, posterior, and lateral pockets that surround the cervix.

13. _____ Muscular pelvic organ located between the bladder and the rectum and just above the vagina. The _____ is a deep pouch, or recess, posterior to the cervix formed by the posterior ligament.

14. _____ Upper triangular portion of the uterus.

15. _____ Also known as the lower uterine segment, it is the short, constricted portion that separates the corpus of the uterus from the cervix.

16. _____ Dome-shaped top of the uterus.

17. _____ Highly vascular lining of the uterus.

18. _____ Layer of the uterus composed of smooth muscles that extend in three different directions.

19. _____ Lower cylindric portion of the uterus composed of fibrous connective tissue and elastic tissue.

20. _____ Canal connecting the uterine cavity to the vagina. The opening between the uterus and this canal is the

_____. The opening between

the canal and the vagina is the _____.

21. _____ Location in the cervix where the squamous and columnar epithelium meet; it is also known as the

_____ zone; it is the most common site for neoplastic changes; cells from this site are scraped for the Pap smear.

22. _____ Passageways between the ovaries and the uterus; they are attached at each side of the dome-shaped uterine fundus.

23. _____Almond-shaped organs located on each side of the uterus; their two

functions are _____ and the

production of the hormones _____,

_____, and _____.

24. _____ Structure that protects the bladder, uterus, and rectum; accommodates the growing fetus during pregnancy; and anchors support structures.

25. _____ The paired mammary glands.

26. _____ Segment of mammary tissue that extends into the axilla.

27. _____ Mammary papilla.

28. _____Pigmented section of the breast that surrounds the nipple.

29. _____ Sebaceous glands that secrete a fatty substance to lubricate the nipple and cause the areola to appear rough.

FILL IN THE BLANKS: Insert the term that corresponds to each of the following definitions related to the menstrual cycle. Use the illustration of the Menstrual Cycle (Figs. 3–7 in your textbook) to visualize the cycle as you are inserting the terms.

30. _____ The first menstruation.

31. _____Transitional stage between childhood and sexual maturity.

32. _____Transitional phase during which ovarian function and hormone production decline.

33. _____ The last menstrual period dated with certainty once one year has passed after menstruation ceases.

34. _____ Period preceding the last menstrual period that lasts about 4 years; during this time ovarian function declines, ova diminish, more menstrual cycles become anovulatory, and irregular bleeding occurs.

35. _____ Periodic uterine bleeding that begins approximately 14 days after ovulation. It is controlled by the feedback system of

three cycles, namely _____,

_____, and _____.
The average length of each menstrual cycle is

_____ but variations are normal. The

first day of bleeding is considered to be _____ of the menstrual cycle. The average duration of

menstrual flow is _____ with a range

of _____ .

36. _____ Cycle that involves cyclic changes in the lining of the uterus.

It consists of four phases, namely _____,

_____, _____,

and _____.

37. _____ Cycle that involves secretion of hormones required to stimulate ovulation.

38. _____ Cycle that involves the changes in the ovary leading to ovulation.

It consists of two phases, namely _____

and _____.

39. _____ Hormone secreted by the hypothalamus when ovarian hormones are reduced to a low level. It stimulates the pituitary gland to secrete two critical hormones for the

menstrual cycle, namely _____

and _____.

40. _____ Pituitary hormone that stimulates the development of graafian follicles in the ovary.

41. _____ Pituitary hormone that stimulates the expulsion of the ovum from the graafian follicle and formation of the corpus luteum.

42. _____ Ovarian hormone that stimulates the thickening of the endometrium that occurs after menstruation and prior to ovulation; it is also responsible for changes in the cervix and the stretchable quality of the cervical mucus called _____.

43. _____ Ovarian hormone that is responsible for the changes in the endometrium that occur after ovulation to facilitate implantation should fertilization occur; it is also responsible for the rise in _____ temperature that occurs after ovulation.

44. _____ Localized, lower abdominal pain that coincides with ovulation. Some vaginal spotting may occur.

45. _____ Oxygenated fatty acids classified as hormones. They are thought to play an essential role in ovulation, transport of sperm, regression of the corpus luteum, and menstruation. By increasing the myometrial response to oxytocin, they also play a role in labor and dysmenorrhea.

FILL IN THE BLANKS: Insert the term that corresponds to each of the following definitions or descriptions related to women's health care.

46. _____ Type of health care that provides women and their partners with information that is needed to make decisions about their reproductive future.

47. _____ Term that describes a body mass index (BMI) of 30 or greater.

48. _____ Term that describes a chronic eating disorder in which women undertake strict and severe diets and rigorous, extreme exercise as a result of a distorted view of their bodies as being much too heavy.

49. _____ Term that describes an eating disorder characterized by secret, uncontrolled binge eating alternating with practices that prevent weight gain, which can include self-induced vomiting, laxatives or diuretics, strict diets, fasting, and rigorous exercise.

50. _____, _____, and _____ Terms that describe the intentional removal of all or part of the external female genitalia.

51. _____, _____, _____, and _____ or _____ violence are terms applied to a pattern of assaultive and coercive behaviors inflicted by a male partner in a marriage or other heterosexual, significant, intimate relationship.

52. _____ According to the cycle of violence theory, battering occurs in cycles. The three-phase cyclic pattern that occurs begins with a period of _____ leading to the _____, which is then followed by a period of _____ and _____ known as the _____ phase.

II. REVIEWING KEY CONCEPTS

1. It is essential that guidelines for laboratory and diagnostic procedures be followed exactly in order to ensure the accuracy of the results obtained. Outline the guidelines that should be followed when performing a Papanicolaou test in terms of each of the following:

   a. Patient preparation

   b. Timing during examination when the specimen is obtained

   c. Sites for specimen collection

   d. Handling of specimens

   e. Frequency of performance

2. Although women may recognize the need for reproductive health care, they may encounter barriers to accessing this type of care. Identify one barrier

represented by each of the following issues and describe a solution you would propose for helping women overcome the barrier identified.

- Financial issues

- Cultural issues

- Gender issues

- Sexual orientation issues

3. A nurse is preparing a pamphlet designed to alert adolescents to the dangers of sexually transmitted infections and what they can do to prevent their transmission.

a. Describe what information the pamphlet should provide about STI transmission prevention.

b. As an impetus to motivate adolescents to use prevention measures, the nurse decides to include a section on the consequences of sexually transmitted infections. Discuss the points that should be emphasized in this section of the pamphlet.

4. What are the essential questions that should be asked when providing health care to women to assess them for abuse?

5. Eating disorder screening tools can be used to determine whether a woman is experiencing an eating disorder and to what degree. Explain the SCOFF tool and how you would use it when providing well woman care.

6. Using and abusing some substances while pregnant can increase the risk for adverse outcomes for the woman and her fetus-newborn. Identify the maternal effects for each of the substances listed below.

- Alcohol

- Tobacco

- Caffeine

- Cocaine

- Marijuana

- Opiates

- Methamphetamines

- Phencyclidine

7. A women's health nurse practitioner is preparing an education presentation on the topic of intimate partner violence (IPV) to a group of women who come to the clinic where she practices. As part of the presentation, she plans to dispel commonly held myths regarding IPV. Which of the following statements represent the facts related to IPV? Select all that apply.
a. Battering almost always affects women who are poor.
b. Of women who experience battering, 25% are battered by an intimate partner.
c. Women usually are safe from battering while they are pregnant.
d. Women tend to leave the relationship if the battering is bad.
e. Pregnant adolescents are abused at higher rates than pregnant adults.
f. Battering tends to occur in a cyclical pattern instead of random acts of violence.

8. A nurse instructed a female patient regarding vulvar self-examination (VSE). Which of the statements made by the patient will require further instruction?
a. "I will perform this examination at least once a month, especially if I change sexual partners or am sexually active."
b. "I will become familiar with how my genitalia look and feel so that I will be able to detect changes."
c. "I will use the examination to determine when I should get medications at the pharmacy for infections."
d. "I will wash my hands thoroughly before and after I examine myself."

9. A women's health nurse practitioner is going to perform a pelvic examination on a female patient. Which of the following nursing actions would be least effective in enhancing the patient's comfort and relaxation during the examination?
   a. Encourage the patient to ask questions and express feelings and concerns before and after the examination.
   b. Use a chilled speculum to minimize the pain response.
   c. Allow the patient to keep her shoes and socks on when placing her feet in the stirrups.
   d. Instruct the patient to place her hands over her diaphragm and take deep, slow breaths.

10. To enhance the accuracy of the Papanicolaou (Pap) test, the nurse should instruct the patient to do which of the following?
    a. Schedule the test just prior to the onset of menses.
    b. Stop taking birth control pills for 2 days before the test.
    c. Avoid intercourse for 24–48 hours before the test.
    d. Douche with a specially prepared antiseptic solution the night before the test.

11. When assessing women, it is important for the nurse to keep in mind the possibility that they are victims of violence. The nurse should:
    a. use an abuse assessment screen during the assessment of every woman.
    b. recognize that abuse rarely occurs during pregnancy.
    c. assess a woman's legs and back as the most commonly injured areas.
    d. notify the police immediately if abuse is suspected.

12. A 52-year-old woman asks the nurse practitioner about how often she should be assessed for the common health problems women of her age could experience. The nurse would recommend which of the following screening measures? Select all that apply.
    a. An endometrial biopsy every 2–3 years
    b. A fecal occult blood test every year
    c. A mammogram every other year
    d. Clinical breast examination every year
    e. Bone mineral density testing every year beginning when she is 55
    f. Vision examination every 2–4 years

13. Which of the following group descriptions is most accurate regarding those persons who should participate in preconception counseling?
    a. All women and their partners as they make decisions about their reproductive future, including becoming parents
    b. All women during their childbearing years
    c. Sexually active women who do not use birth control
    d. Women with chronic illnesses such as diabetes who are planning to get pregnant

14. A newly married 25-year-old woman has been smoking since she was a teenager. She has come to the women's health clinic for a checkup before she begins trying to get pregnant. The woman demonstrates a need for further instruction about the effects of smoking on reproduction and health when she makes which of the following statements? Select all that apply.
    a. "Smoking can interfere with my ability to get pregnant."
    b. "My husband also needs to stop smoking because secondhand smoke can have an adverse effect on my pregnancy and the development of the baby."
    c. "Smoking can make my pregnancy last longer than it should."
    d. "Smoking can reduce the amount of calcium in my bones."
    e. "Smoking will mean I will experience menopause at an older age than my friends who do not smoke."

15. A pregnant woman in her first trimester tells her nurse midwife that although she does drink alcohol during pregnancy, she does so only on the weekend and only a little bit. What should the nurse's initial response be to this woman's comment?
    a. "You need to realize that use of alcohol, in any amount, will result in your child being mentally retarded."
    b. "I am going to refer you to a counseling center for women with alcohol problems."
    c. "Tell me what you mean by drinking a little on the weekend."
    d. "Antioxidants can reduce the effect of alcohol exposure for your baby. I will tell you what you can take."

16. When communicating with an abused woman, which of the following statements should be avoided? Select all that apply.
    a. "Why do you think your husband hits you even though you are pregnant?"
    b. "I cannot believe how terrible your husband is being to you."
    c. "The violence you are experiencing now is likely to continue and to get even worse as your pregnancy progresses."
    d. "Tell me why you did not go to the shelter I recommended to you; they are very helpful and you would have avoided this beating if you had gone."
    e. "Next time you come in for care, I want you to be sure to bring your husband so I can talk to him myself."
    f. "I am afraid for your safety and the safety of your other children."

1. An inner-city women's health clinic serves a diverse population in terms of age, ethnic background, and health problems. Describe how each of the following factors should influence a women's health nurse practitioner's approach when assessing the health of the women who come to the clinic for care.

    a. Culture

    b. Age

    c. Disabilities

    d. Abuse

    e. Gender identify

2. Imagine that you are a nurse working at a clinic that provides health care to women. Describe how you would respond to each of the following concerns or questions of women who have come to the clinic for care.

    a. Jane, a newly married woman, is concerned that she did not bleed during her first coital experience with her husband. She states, "I was a virgin and always thought you had to bleed when you had sex for the first time. Do you think my husband will still believe I was a virgin on our wedding night?"

    b. Serena, a 17-year-old woman, has just been scheduled for her first women's health checkup, which will include a pelvic examination and Pap smear. She nervously asks if there is anything she needs to do to get ready for the examination.

    c. Andrea is trying to get pregnant. She wonders if there are signs she could observe in her body that would indicate that she is ovulating and therefore able to conceive a baby with her partner.

3. Julie, a 21-year-old woman, has come to the women's health clinic for a women's health checkup. During the health history interview she becomes very anxious and states, "I have to tell you this is my first examination. I am very scared; my friends told me that it hurts a lot to have this examination." Describe how the nurse should respond in an effort to reduce Julie's anxiety.

4. As a nurse working in a women's health clinic, you have been assigned to interview Angie, a 25-year-old new patient, to obtain her health history.

   a. List the components that should be emphasized in gathering Angie's history.

   b. Write a series of questions that you would ask to obtain data related to Angie's reproductive and sexual health and practices.

   c. Give an example of how you would use each of the following therapeutic communication techniques to develop trust, to facilitate the collection of data, and to provide support during the assessment process.

      Facilitation

      Reflection

      Clarification

      Empathy

      Confrontation

      Interpretation

      Open-ended questions and statements

5. If a woman chooses to do self-examination of the breasts and would also like to be taught how to perform a vulvar self-examination, outline the procedure that you would use to teach each technique to one of your patients. Include the teaching methodologies that you would use to enhance learning.

6. Lu is a 25-year-old exchange student from China who has been living in the United States for 3 months. This is the first time that she is away from home. She comes to the university women's health clinic for a checkup and to obtain birth control. Describe how the nurse assigned to Lu would approach and communicate with her in a culturally sensitive manner.

Chapter **3** **Assessment and Health Promotion**

7. Nurses working in women's health care must be aware of the growing problem of violence against women. All women should be screened when being assessed during health care for the possibility of abuse.

   a. Describe how you as a nurse would adjust the environment and your communication style when conducting the health history interview and physical examination in order to elicit a woman's confidence and trust.

   b. Identify indicators of possible abuse that you would look for before the appointment and then during the health history interview and physical examination.

   c. State the questions you would ask to screen for abuse.

   d. Discuss the approach you would take if abuse is confirmed during the assessment.

8. As a student you may be assigned to assist a health care provider during the performance of a pelvic examination for one of your patients.

   a. Describe how you would do each of the following:

      i. Prepare your patient for the examination

      ii. Support your patient during the examination

      iii. Assist your patient after the examination

   b. Describe how you would assist the health care provider who is performing the examination.

9. A nurse is teaching a group of young adult women about health promotion activities. As part of the discussion, the nurse identifies preconception care and counseling as an important health promotion activity. One woman in the class asks, "I know you need to go for checkups once you are pregnant, but why would you need to see a doctor before you get pregnant? Isn't that a big waste of time and money?" Explain how the nurse should respond to this woman's question.

10. During a routine checkup for her annual Pap smear, Julie, a 26-year-old woman, asks the nurse for advice regarding nutrition and exercise. She is considered to be overweight with a body mass index (BMI) of 27.4 and wants to lose weight sensibly. Discuss the advice the nurse should give to Julie.

11. You are a nurse midwife working in a prenatal clinic. As part of your role, you need to teach newly diagnosed pregnant women about the importance of coming for their prenatal care visits. What would you tell them?

12. A 30-year-old woman comes to the women's health clinic complaining of fatigue, insomnia, headaches, and feeling anxious. She works as a stockbroker for a major Wall Street brokerage firm. She states that, although she enjoys the challenge of her job, she never can seem to find time for herself or to socialize with her friends. She tells the nurse that she has been drinking more and started to smoke again to help her relax. She is glad that she has lost some weight, attributing this occurrence to her diminished appetite. **Highlight or place a check mark next to the assessment findings that require further assessment by the nurse**.

13. Laura is a 28-year-old pregnant woman at 8 weeks of gestation. This is her first pregnancy. During the health history interview she reveals that she smokes at least 2 packs of cigarettes each day. When discussing this practice with the nurse, Laura states, "My friends smoked when they were pregnant and their babies are okay. In fact, two of them had pregnancies that were a little shorter than expected and they had nice small babies." Describe how the nurse should respond to Laura's comments.

14. As a nurse working in a prenatal health clinic you must be alert to cues indicative of battery committed against women when they are pregnant.

    a. Describe the activities in which the nurse can become involved in order to prevent the escalating incidence of violence against women.

    b. Carol, a 24-year-old married woman, comes to the clinic to confirm her belief that she is pregnant. During the assessment phase of the visit, you note cues that lead you to suspect that Carol is being abused by her husband. Discuss the approach you would take to confirm your suspicion that Carol is being abused.

    c. Carol admits to you that her husband "beats her sometimes and it has been increasing." Now she is afraid it will get worse since she "was not supposed to get pregnant." Discuss the nursing actions that you could take to help Carol.

    d. List the possible reasons why Carol, now that she is pregnant, is experiencing an escalation of battering/abuse from her husband.

    e. Discuss how Carol's pregnancy could be adversely affected by the abuse she is experiencing.

4 Reproductive System Concerns

I. LEARNING KEY TERMS

FILL IN THE BLANKS: Insert the term that corresponds to each of the following descriptions related to menstrual problems.

1. _____ Absence of menstrual flow.

2. _____ Cessation of menstruation related to a problem in the central hypothalamic–pituitary axis.

3. _____ Syndrome characterized by the interrelation of disordered eating, absence of menstrual flow, and premature osteoporosis.

4. _____ Painful menstruation; one of the most common gynecologic problems for women during their childbearing years.

5. _____ Type of painful menstruation associated with ovulatory cycles; it has a biochemical basis arising from the release of prostaglandins.

6. _____ Type of painful menstruation that occurs later in life, typically after age 25, and is associated with pelvic pathology.

7. _____ A cluster of physical and psychological symptoms that begins in the luteal phase of the menstrual cycle and is followed by a symptom-free follicular phase.

8. _____ Diagnostic term for a disorder that affects a smaller percentage of women who suffer from severe PMS with an emphasis on symptoms related to mood disturbances.

9. _____ A concept that includes dysmenorrhea, premenstrual syndrome (PMS), and premenstrual dysphoric disorder (PMDD) as well as symptom clusters that occur before and after the menstrual flow starts. Symptoms occur cyclically and can include mood swings as well as pelvic pain and physical discomforts.

10. _____ A menstrual disorder that is characterized by the presence and growth of endometrial tissue outside of the uterus.

11. _____ Infrequent menstrual periods.

12. _____ Scanty menstruation at normal intervals.

13. _____ Excessive bleeding during menstruation.

14. _____ Bleeding between menstrual periods.

15. _____ Any form of uterine bleeding that is irregular in amount, duration, or timing and is not related to regular menstrual bleeding; it can have organic causes such as systemic or reproductive tract disease.

16. _____ Benign tumors of the smooth muscle of the uterus.

FILL IN THE BLANKS: Insert the term that corresponds to each of the following descriptions related to infection.

17. _____ Infections or infectious disease syndromes primarily transmitted by intimate contact.

18. _____ The physical barrier promoted for the prevention of sexual transmission of human immunodeficiency virus (HIV) and other sexually transmitted infections (STIs).

19. _____ Bacterial infection that is the most frequently reported infectious disease in the United States. This infection is often asymptomatic and highly destructive to the female reproductive tract.

20. _____ The oldest communicable disease in the United States. Because it is a reportable communicable disease, health care providers are legally responsible for reporting all cases to health authorities.

21. _____ One of the earliest described sexually transmitted infections (STIs). It is caused by *Treponema pallidum*, a spirochete. During the primary stage, a characteristic lesion called a

_____ appears 5–90 days after infection. During the second stage, a widespread

_____ appears on the palms and soles

along with generalized _____.

_____ (broad, painless, pink-gray, wart-like infectious lesions) may develop on the vulva, perineum, or anus.

22. _____ Infectious process that most commonly involves the uterine tubes, uterus, and more rarely, ovaries and peritoneal surfaces.

23. _____ Infection also known as genital warts. It is now the most common viral STI seen in ambulatory health care settings.

24. _____ A viral infection that is transmitted sexually and is characterized by painful, recurrent ulcers.

25. _____ Viral infection involving the liver that is acquired primarily through a fecal–oral route by ingestion of contaminated food and fluids and through person-to-person contact.

26. _____ Viral infection involving the liver that is transmitted parenterally, perinatally, and through intimate contact. A vaccine is available to protect infants, children, and adults.

27. _____ The most common chronic bloodborne infection in the United States. It is a disease of the liver that is transmitted parenterally and through intimate contact. No vaccine is available to provide protection against this infection.

28. _____ A virus that is transmitted primarily through exchange of body fluids. _____ is the severe depression of the cellular immune system associated with this infection.

29. _____ Vaginal infection formerly called *nonspecific vaginitis, Haemophilus vaginitis*, or *Gardnerella*; it is the most common type of symptomatic vaginitis and is characterized by a profuse, thin, and white, gray, or milky discharge that has a characteristic "fishy" odor.

30. _____ Yeast infection that is the second most common type of vaginal infection in the United States. It is characterized by a thick, white, lumpy discharge.

31. _____ A vaginal infection caused by an anaerobic one-celled protozoan with characteristic flagella. The typically copious discharge is yellowish- green, frothy, mucopurulent, and malodorous. It is almost always sexually transmitted.

32. _____ A normal vaginal flora that is present in 25% of healthy pregnant women. Infection associated with this bacteria is associated with poor pregnancy outcomes. Vertical transmission to the newborn during birth has been implicated as an important factor in perinatal and neonatal morbidity and mortality.

II. REVIEWING KEY CONCEPTS

MATCHING: Match the description with the appropriate breast disorder.

1. _____ Lumpiness with or without tenderness in both breasts; simple cysts can occur; symptoms are often cyclical.

2. _____ Fatty unilateral breast tumor that is soft, nontender, and mobile with discrete borders; no nipple discharge occurs.

3. _____ Unilateral, firm, occasional tenderness, discrete benign breast mass; it increases in size during pregnancy but decreases in size with aging.

4. _____ Rare, benign condition that develops in the terminal nipple ducts and is usually too small to palpate; a unilateral spontaneous serous, serosanguineous, or bloody nipple discharge can also occur.

5. _____ Spontaneous, bilateral milky sticky breast discharge unrelated to malignancy.

6. _____ Benign lesion in the breast characterized by dilated ducts and acquired nipple inversion. Burning pain, itching, and greenish nipple discharge may be experienced. A mass may be palpated behind the nipple.

a. Fibroadenoma

b. Fibrocystic changes

c. Mammary duct ectasia

d. Lipoma

e. Galactorrhea

f. Intraductal papilloma

7. Cite several common risk factors for sexually transmitted infections.

8. Describe one implementation measure for each of the following Standard Precautions categories.

   Hand hygiene

   Use of personal protective equipment (PPE)

   Respiratory hygiene and cough etiquette

   Safe injection practices

9. Heterosexual transmission is the most common means of infecting women with HIV.

   a. What behaviors increase a woman's risk for HIV infection?

   b. List the clinical manifestations that may be exhibited during seroconversion to HIV positivity.

   c. Outline counseling tips associated with HIV testing.

   d. Discuss the anticipated intrapartum care for a woman infected with HIV

10. Describe the how the Zika virus is transmitted.

    a. List information that should be given to women regarding the risks during pregnancy.

11. Breast cancer is a major health problem facing women in the United States. Nurses are often responsible for educating women about breast cancer.

    a. Outline the information the nurse should give women about the risk factors associated with breast cancer.

    b. List the clinical manifestations that are strongly suggestive of breast cancer.

12. Describe how each of the following approaches are used in the diagnosis and care of women with breast cancer.

    a. Lumpectomy

    b. Mastectomy

    c. Breast reconstruction

    d. Radiation

    e. Adjuvant therapy

    f. Chemotherapy

    g. Testing for BRCA1 and BRCA2 genes

    h. Mammography

    i. Sonography

    j. Biopsy (fine needle, core needle, needle localization)

13. Which of the following women is at greatest risk for developing hypogonadotropic amenorrhea?
    a. 48-year-old woman experiencing perimenopausal changes
    b. 13-year-old underweight, competitive figure skater
    c. 18-year-old softball player with a BMI of 22
    d. 30-year-old (G3 P3003) breastfeeding woman

14. Pharmacologic preparations can be used to treat primary dysmenorrhea. Which preparation would be least effective in relieving the symptoms of primary dysmenorrhea?
    a. Oral contraceptive pill (OCP)
    b. Naproxen sodium (Anaprox)
    c. Acetaminophen (Tylenol)
    d. Ibuprofen (Motrin)

15. Women experiencing PMS should be advised to avoid the use of which of the following?
    a. Chamomile tea
    b. Coffee
    c. Whole-grain cereals
    d. Parsley to season food

16. The nurse counseling a 30-year-old woman regarding effective measures to use to relieve the discomfort associated with dysmenorrhea could suggest which of the following? Select all that apply.
    a. Decrease intake of fruits, especially peaches and watermelon.
    b. Use back massages and heat application to abdomen to enhance relaxation and circulation.
    c. Avoid exercise just before and during menstruation when discomfort is at its peak.
    d. Add vegetables such as asparagus to the diet.
    e. Perform guided imagery for relaxation and distraction.
    f. Limit intake of salty and fatty foods.

17. A 28-year-old woman has been diagnosed with endometriosis. She has been placed on a course of treatment with danazol (Danocrine). The woman exhibits understanding of this treatment when she says which of the following? Select all that apply.
    a. "Because this medication stops ovulation, I do not need to use birth control."
    b. "I will experience more frequent and heavier menstrual periods when I take this medication."
    c. "I will monitor my diet because this medication can increase the level of cholesterol in my blood."
    d. "I can experience a decrease in my breast size, oily skin, and hair growth on my face as a result of taking this medication."
    e. "I may experience hot flashes while taking this medication."
    f. "I may need to use a lubricant during intercourse to reduce discomfort."

18. A 55-year-old woman tells the nurse that she has started to experience pain when she and her husband have intercourse. The nurse would record that this woman is experiencing:
    a. dyspareunia.
    b. dysmenorrhea.
    c. dysuria.
    d. dyspnea.

19. Infections of the female reproductive tract, such as chlamydia, are dangerous primarily because these infections:
    a. are asymptomatic.
    b. cause primary infertility.
    c. lead to HBV.
    d. are difficult to treat.

20. A finding associated with HPV infection would include which of the following?
    a. White, curd-like, adherent discharge
    b. Soft papillary swelling occurring singly or in clusters
    c. Vesicles progressing to pustules and then to ulcers
    d. Yellow to green frothy malodorous discharge

21. A recommended medication effective in the treatment of vulvovaginal candidiases would be which of the following?
    a. Metronidazole (Flagyl)
    b. Miconazole (Monistat)
    c. Ampicillin
    d. Acyclovir

22. A woman is determined to be Group B streptococcus (GBS) positive at the onset of her labor. The nurse should prepare this woman for which of the following?
    a. The need for a cesarean birth
    b. Intravenous administration of an antibiotic during labor
    c. Transplacental infection of her newborn with GBS
    d. Application of acyclovir to her labial lesions

23. When providing a woman recovering from primary genital herpes with information regarding the recurrence of herpes infection of the genital tract, the nurse would tell her which of the following?
    a. Fever and flulike symptoms will precede each recurrent infection.
    b. Little can be done to control the recurrence of infection.
    c. Cortisone-based ointments should be used to decrease discomfort.
    d. Itching and tingling often occur before the appearance of vesicles.

24. When teaching women about breast cancer, the nurse should emphasize which of the following facts? Select all that apply.
    a. The incidence of breast cancer is highest among African-American women.
    b. One in ten American women will develop breast cancer in her lifetime.
    c. The mortality rate from breast cancer decreases with early detection.
    d. Most women diagnosed with breast cancer report a family history of breast cancer.
    e. Reducing heavy alcohol intake could reduce a woman's chances of developing breast cancer.
    f. The majority of breast lumps found by women are not malignant.

25. When providing discharge instructions to a woman who had a modified right radical mastectomy, the nurse should emphasize the importance of which of the following?
    a. Reporting any tingling or numbness in her incisional site or right arm immediately
    b. Telling health care providers not to take a blood pressure or draw blood from her right arm
    c. Learning how to use her left arm to write and accomplish the activities of daily living such as brushing her hair
    d. Wearing clothing that snugly supports her right arm

26. A 26-year-old woman has just been diagnosed with fibrocystic change in her breasts. Which of the following nursing diagnoses would be a priority for this woman?
    a. Acute pain related to cyclical enlargement of breast cysts or lumps
    b. Risk for infection related to altered integrity of the areola associated with accumulation of thick, sticky discharge from nipples
    c. Anxiety related to anticipated surgery to remove the cysts in her breasts
    d. Fear related to high risk for breast cancer

27. When assessing a woman with a diagnosis of fibroadenoma, the nurse would expect to find which of the following characteristics?
    a. Bilateral tender lumps behind the nipple
    b. Milky discharge from one or both nipples
    c. Soft and nonmobile lumps
    d. Well-delineated, firm moveable lump in one breast

28. A 40-year-old woman at risk for breast cancer has elected chemoprevention as an approach to reduce her risk. She will be receiving tamoxifen (Nolvadex). The nurse will recognize that this woman understood instructions given to her regarding this medication if she makes which of the following statements?
    a. "This medication helps prevent breast cancer by helping my body use estrogen efficiently."
    b. "I may need to wear a sweater to keep me warm when I experience chills that can occur when I am taking this medication."
    c. "I can take this medication on an empty stomach or with food."
    d. "I should use an oral contraceptive pill to ensure that I do not get pregnant."

III. CLINICAL JUDGMENT AND NEXT-GENERATION NCLEX® EXAMINATION-STYLE QUESTIONS

1. Odette is a 16-year-old gymnast who has been training vigorously for a placement on the US Olympic team. She has been experiencing amenorrhea, and the development of her secondary sexual characteristics has been limited. Odette expresses concern because her nonathletic friends have all been menstruating for at least 1 year and have well-developed breasts. After a health assessment, Odette was diagnosed with hypogonadotropic amenorrhea.

    a. State the risk factors and assessment findings for this disorder that Odette most likely exhibited during the assessment process.

    b. State one nursing diagnosis reflective of Odette's concern.

    c. Outline a typical care management plan for Odette that will address the issues associated with hypogonadotropic amenorrhea.

d. At Odette's all female high school there is a large athletic department that emphasizes participation and excellence in a wide variety of sports. As the school nurse, you are concerned that there are other students like Odette who may be exhibiting signs of the female athlete triad. The nurse has decided to institute an education program aimed at prevention and early detection of the triad.

   (1) What is the meaning of the female athlete triad?

   (2) Which sports should the nurse emphasize with her program?

   (3) What measures should this nurse include in her program as a means of prevention and early detection of the female athlete triad?

2. Mary, a 17-year-old who experienced menarche at age 16, comes to the women's health clinic for a routine checkup. She complains to the nurse that her last few periods have been very painful. "I have missed a few days of school because of it. What can I do to reduce the pain that I feel during my periods?" Physical examination and testing reveal normal structure and function of Mary's reproductive system. A medical diagnosis of primary dysmenorrhea is made.

   a. What questions should the nurse ask Mary to get a full description of her pain?

   b. What should the nurse tell Mary about the likely cause for the type of pain she is experiencing?

   c. Identify appropriate relief measures for primary dysmenorrhea that the nurse could suggest to Mary.

   d. What alternative therapies could the nurse suggest to Mary to help relieve her discomfort?

3. Maya experiences physical and psychologic signs and symptoms associated with PMS during every ovulatory menstrual cycle.

   a. List the signs and symptoms most likely described by Maya that led to the diagnosis of PMS.

   b. Identify one nursing diagnosis that may be appropriate for Maya when she is experiencing the signs and symptoms of PMS.

   c. Describe the approach the nurse would use in helping Maya deal with this menstrual disorder.

25

d. What symptoms would Maya describe that would indicate she is also experiencing PMDD?

4. Annika is 26 years old and has been diagnosed recently with endometriosis.

   a. List the signs and symptoms Annika most likely exhibited that led to this medical diagnosis.

   b. Annika asks, "What is happening to my body as a result of this disease?" Describe the nurse's response.

   c. Annika asks about her treatment options. "Are there medications I can take to make me feel better?" Describe the action/effect and potential side effects for each of the following pharmacologic approaches to treatment.

      i. Oral contraceptive pills

      ii. Gonadotropin-releasing hormone agonists

      iii. Androgenic synthetic steroids

   d. Identify support measures the nurse can suggest to assist Annika to cope with the effects of endometriosis.

5. Terry, a 20-year-old woman, comes to a women's health clinic for her first visit.

   a. During the health history interview, it is imperative that the nurse practitioner determine Terry's risk for contracting an STI, including HIV. Write one question for each of the following risk categories.

      i. Sexual risk

      ii. Drug use–related risk

      iii. Blood-related risk

      HIV concerns

b. Terry asks the nurse about measures she could use to protect herself from STIs. Cite the major points that the nurse practitioner should emphasize when teaching Terry about prevention measures.

c. Terry tells the nurse that she does not know if she could ever tell a partner that he must wear a condom. Describe the approach the nurse can take to enhance Terry's assertiveness and communication skills.

6. Ada is 4 weeks pregnant. As part of her prenatal assessment, it was discovered that she was HIV positive. Identify the measures that can be used to reduce the risk of transmission of HIV from Ada to her baby.

7. Karina, a 20-year-old woman, is admitted for suspected severe, acute PID.

a. Identify the risk factors for PID that the nurse would be looking for in Karina's health history.

b. A complete physical examination is performed to determine whether the criteria for PID are met. Specify the criteria that Karina's health care provider would be alert for during the examination.

c. Karina is hospitalized when the diagnosis of PID secondary to chlamydial infection is confirmed. Intravenous antibiotics will be used as the primary medical treatment followed by oral antibiotics at the time of discharge. State three priority nursing diagnoses that are likely to be present during the acute stage of Karina's infection and treatment.

d. Outline a nursing management plan for Karina in terms of each of the following:

i. Position and activity

ii. Comfort measures

iii. Support measures

iv. Health education in preparation for discharge

27

e. List the recommendations for Karina's self-care during the recovery phase.

f. Identify the reproductive health risks that Karina may face as a result of the pelvic infection she experienced.

8. Laura has just been diagnosed with gonorrhea, a sexually transmitted disease.

a. Laura, who is very upset by the diagnosis, states, "This is just awful. What kind of sex life can I have now?" Write a nursing diagnosis that reflects Laura's concern.

b. Outline a management plan that will assist Laura in taking control of her self-care and prevent future infections.

9. Cheryl, a 27-year-old woman, is being treated for HPV. A primary diagnosis identified for Cheryl is "pain related to lesions on the vulva and around the anus secondary to HPV infection." State the measures the nurse could suggest to Cheryl to reduce the pain from the condylomata and enhance their healing.

10. Francesca, a 20-year-old woman, has just been diagnosed with a primary herpes simplex 2 infection. In addition to the typical systemic symptoms, Francesca exhibits multiple painful genital lesions.

a. Relief of pain and healing without the development of a secondary infection are two expected outcomes for care. Identify several measures that the nurse can suggest to Francesca in an effort to help her achieve the expected outcomes of care.

b. Francesca asks the nurse if there is anything she can do so that this infection does not return. Discuss what the nurse should tell Francesca about the recurrence of HSV-2 infection and the influence of self-care measures.

11. Sonya is concerned that she has been exposed to HIV and has come to the women's health clinic for testing.

a. During the health history the nurse questions Sonya about behaviors that could have placed her at risk for HIV transmission. Cite the behaviors that the nurse would be looking for.

b. Explain the testing procedure that will most likely be followed to determine Sonya's HIV status.

c. Outline the counseling protocol that should guide the nurse when caring for Sonya before and after the test.

d. Sonya's test result is negative. Discuss the instructions the nurse should give Sonya regarding guidelines she should follow to reduce her risk for the transmission of HIV with future sexual partners.

12. Mary Anne comes to the women's health clinic complaining that her breasts feel lumpy.

   a. Outline the assessment process that should be used to determine the basis for Mary Anne's complaint.

   b. A diagnosis of fibrocystic breast changes is made. Describe the signs and symptoms Mary Anne most likely exhibited to support this diagnosis.

   c. State one nursing diagnosis that the nurse would identify as a priority when preparing a plan of care for Mary Anne.

   d. Identify measures the nurse could suggest to Mary Anne for lessening the symptoms she experiences related to fibrocystic changes.

13. Alma, a 50-year-old woman, found a lump in her left breast during a breast self-examination. She comes to the women's health clinic for help.

   a. Describe the diagnostic protocol that should be followed to determine the basis for the lump Alma found in her breast.

   b. Alma elects to have a simple mastectomy based on the information provided by her health care providers and in consultation with her husband. Identify two priority postoperative nursing diagnoses and outline the nursing care management for the postoperative phase of Alma's treatment.

      i. Nursing diagnoses

      ii. Postoperative phase care measures

   c. Alma will be discharged within 48 hours after her surgery. Describe the instructions that the nurse should give Alma to prepare her for self-care at home.

d. Discuss support measures the nurse should use to address the concerns that Alma and her husband will most likely experience and express.

14. As a nurse working in a woman's health clinic, you have been given the task of developing a breast cancer screening program. You plan to emphasize the importance of women engaging in a self-management program regarding breast health. Describe the types of obstacles you are likely to encounter from women as they attempt to implement their program and the measures you will implement to overcome the obstacles.

15. Gretchen is a 67-year-old Caucasian female who is being seen at her primary care provider's office after finding a small lump in her breast. Gretchen's assessment and health history are as follows:

■ High breast tissue density

■ Started her period at 11 years of age

■ Started menopause at 48 years of age

■ Consumes 1 glass of wine per week

■ Current BMI of 32

■ Had her first child at 36

■ Exclusively breastfed her children

Highlight or place a check mark next to the findings that increase Gretchen's risk for breast cancer.

5 Infertility, Contraception, and Abortion

I. LEARNING KEY TERMS

FILL IN THE BLANKS: Insert the term that corresponds to each of the following descriptions related to alterations in fertility.

1. _____ Diagnosis made when a couple has not achieved pregnancy after 1 year of regular, unprotected intercourse when the woman is less than 35 years of age or after 6 months when the woman is older than 35.

2. _____ Term used to describe the ability to carry a pregnancy to a live birth.

3. _____ Fertility treatments in which both eggs and sperm are handled.

4. _____ Assisted reproductive therapy that involves collection of a woman's eggs, then fertilizing them in the laboratory with sperm, and transferring the resultant embryo into her uterus.

5. _____ Assisted reproductive therapy that involves selection of one sperm cell that is injected directly into the egg to achieve fertilization; it is used with in vitro fertilization (IVF).

6. _____ Assisted reproductive therapy that involves retrieval of oocytes from the ovary, placing them in a catheter with washed motile sperm, and immediately transferring the gametes into the fimbriated end of the uterine tube. Fertilization occurs in the uterine tube.

7. _____ Assisted reproductive therapy that involves placing ova after IVF into one uterine tube during the zygote stage.

8. _____ Assisted reproductive therapy that involves using sperm from a person other than the male partner to inseminate the female partner.

9. _____ Assisted reproductive therapy that involves transferring IVF embryo(s) from one couple into the uterus of another woman who has contracted with the couple to carry the baby to term. This woman has no genetic connection with the child.

10. _____ Assisted reproductive therapy that involves inseminating a woman with the semen from the infertile woman's partner; she then carries the baby until birth.

11. _____ Assisted reproductive therapy that involves penetrating the zona pellucida chemically or manually to create an opening for the dividing embryo to hatch and to implant into the uterine wall.

12. _____ Assisted reproductive therapy that involves donating eggs by an IVF procedure; the eggs are then inseminated and transferred into the recipient's uterus, which has been hormonally prepared with estrogen–progesterone therapy.

13. _____ Assisted reproductive therapy that involves transferring another woman's embryo into the uterus of an infertile woman at the appropriate time.

14. _____ Using the sperm of a donor to inseminate the woman.

15. _____ Procedure used to freeze embryos for later implantation.

16. _____ Early genetic testing designed to eliminate embryos with serious genetic diseases before placing them into the uterus through one of the assisted reproductive therapies and to avoid future termination of the pregnancy for genetic reasons.

17. _____ Basic test for male infertility; detects ability of sperm to fertilize an ovum.

18. _____ Examination of uterine cavity and tubes using radiopaque contrast material instilled through the cervix. It is often used to determine tubal patency and to release a blockage if present.

19. _____ Test used to detect the timing of lutein hormone surge before ovulation.

20. _____ Test performed to evaluate tubal patency, uterine cavity, and myometrium; it will not disrupt a fertilized ovum.

FILL IN THE BLANKS: Insert the term that corresponds to each of the following descriptions regarding methods to prevent or plan pregnancy.

21. _____ Intentional prevention of pregnancy during sexual intercourse.

22. _____ Device and/or practice used to decrease the risk of conceiving or bearing offspring.

23. _____ Conscious decision regarding when to conceive or to avoid pregnancy throughout the reproductive years.

24. _____ Term that refers to the percentage of contraceptive users expected to have an unplanned pregnancy during the first year of using a birth control method even when they use the method consistently and correctly.

25. _____ The most effective reversible contraceptive methods used to prevent pregnancy. They include contraceptive implants and intrauterine contraception.

26. _____ Contraceptive method that requires the male partner to withdraw his penis from the woman's vagina before ejaculation.

27. _____ Group of contraceptive methods that rely on identifying the beginning and end of the fertile period of the menstrual cycle.

28. _____ Method that relies on avoiding intercourse during fertile days.

29. _____ Method based on the number of days in each cycle counting from the first day of menses. The fertile period is determined after accurately recording lengths of menstrual cycles for 6 months.

30. _____ A modified form of the calendar rhythm method that has a "fixed" number of days of fertility for each cycle; CycleBeads can be used to track fertility, with day 1 of the menstrual flow as the first day to begin counting.

31. _____ Method based on variations in a woman's lowest body temperature, which is determined after waking and before getting out of bed.

32. _____ Method that requires the woman to recognize and interpret the cyclical changes in the amount and consistency of cervical mucus that characterize her own unique pattern of changes.

33. _____ Term that refers to the stretchiness of cervical mucus.

34. _____ Method that uses the physiologic and psychologic changes that occur during each phase of the menstrual cycle to determine the occurrence of ovulation and the fertile period.

35. _____ Method that requires the woman to ask herself two questions every day: (1) "Did I note secretions today?" and (2) "Did I note secretions yesterday?" An answer of "yes" requires the use of a backup method of birth control or avoidance of coitus.

36. _____ Temporary method of birth control that is based on the suppression of ovulation, which occurs with breastfeeding.

37. _____ Chemical that destroys or limits the mobility of sperm. When inserted into the vagina it acts as both a chemical and a physical barrier to sperm.

38. _____ Thin, stretchable sheath that covers the penis or is inserted into the vagina.

39. _____ Shallow, dome-shaped rubber device with a flexible rim that covers the cervix.

40. _____ A soft natural rubber dome with a firm but pliable rim that fits snugly around the base of the cervix close to the junction of the cervix and vaginal fornices.

41. _____ A small round polyurethane device that contains a spermicide. It fits over the cervix and has a woven polyester loop to facilitate its removal.

42. _____ Birth control method that is taken orally; it contains a combination of estrogen and progesterone that inhibits the maturation of follicles and ovulation.

43. _____ Combined estrogen–progesterone birth control method that involves application of the hormones to the skin of the lower abdomen, upper outer arms, buttocks, or upper torso where the hormones are absorbed; it is applied once a week for 3 weeks.

44. _____ Combined estrogen–progesterone birth control method that

involves insertion of the hormones into the vagina for 3 weeks.

45. _____ Form of hormonal contraception in which a single-rod implant containing progestin is inserted subdermally into the inner aspect of the upper arm.

46. _____ Brand name of form of emergency contraception that involves administration of a single progestin-only pill, which should be taken as soon as possible after but within 72 hours of unprotected intercourse or birth control mishap to prevent unintended pregnancy.

_____ Brand name of form of emergency contraception that involves taking two progestin-only pills together or 12 hours apart.

47. _____ Small, T-shaped object inserted into the uterine cavity. It can be loaded with copper or a progestational agent such as levonorgestrel.

48. _____ Surgical procedures intended to render the person infertile.

_____ Method used to render a female infertile. _____ Method that is the easiest and most commonly used method for male sterilization; it involves ligating and then severing the vas deferens of each testicle.

49. _____ Purposeful interruption of a pregnancy before 20 weeks of gestation. If it is performed at the woman's request, it is termed an _____. If it is performed for reasons of maternal or fetal health or disease, it is termed a _____.

II. REVIEWING KEY CONCEPTS

1. A woman is a little uncomfortable about checking her cervical mucus and asks the nurse what she could possibly find out about doing this assessment. State the useful purpose of self-evaluation of cervical mucus.

2. Cite four factors that can contribute to a woman's decision to seek an induced abortion.

3. Joyce has chosen the diaphragm as her method of contraception. Which of the following actions would indicate that Joyce is using the diaphragm effectively? Select all that apply.
   a. Joyce came to be refitted after healing was complete following the term vaginal birth of her son.
   b. Joyce applies a spermicide only to the rim of the diaphragm just before insertion because she dislikes the stickiness of the spermicide.
   c. Joyce empties her bladder before inserting the diaphragm.
   d. Joyce inserts the diaphragm about 3–4 hours before intercourse to increase spontaneity.
   e. Joyce applies more spermicide for each act of intercourse.
   f. Joyce removes the diaphragm within 1 hour of intercourse.
   g. After removal, Joyce washes the diaphragm with warm water and an antiseptic-type soap, dries it, and then applies baby powder.
   h. Joyce carefully inspects the diaphragm before each use for puckering and holes.

4. A woman must assess herself for signs that ovulation is occurring. Which of the following is a sign associated with ovulation?
   a. Reduction in level of LH in the urine 12–24 hours before ovulation
   b. Spinnbarkeit
   c. Drop in BBT during the luteal phase of her menstrual cycle
   d. Increase in amount and thickness of cervical mucus

5. The most common, and for some women the most distressing, side effect of progestin-only contraceptives such as the minipill would be which of the following?
   a. Irregular vaginal bleeding
   b. Headache
   c. Nervousness
   d. Nausea

6. Women using Depo-Provera should be carefully screened for which of the following possible adverse reactions to its use?
   a. Diabetes mellitus—type 2
   b. Reproductive tract infection
   c. Decrease in bone mineral density
   d. Weight loss

7. A woman has had a ParaGard IUD inserted. The nurse should recognize that the woman needs further teaching if she makes which of the following statements? Select all that apply.
   a. "I should check the string before each menstrual period."
   b. "The IUD remains effective for 10 years."
   c. "It is normal to experience an increase in bleeding and cramping within the first year after it has been inserted."
   d. "My IUD works by releasing progesterone."

e. "I should avoid using NSAIDs like Motrin if I have cramping."
f. "I must use safer sex measures including maintaining a monogamous relationship to prevent infections in my uterus."

8. A woman experiencing infertility will begin taking clomiphene citrate. In order to ensure she takes this medication safely and effectively, the nurse should do which of the following?

a. Teach the patient's husband how to give his wife an IM injection.
b. Show the woman how to spray the medication into one of her nostrils, emphasizing that she use a different nostril for each dose.
c. Tell her to inject one dose of human chorionic gonadotropin subcutaneously the day after she takes the last does of the clomiphene citrate.
d. Tell her to begin taking her tablet daily beginning on the 5th day of menstruation.

III. CLINICAL JUDGMENT AND NEXT-GENERATION NCLEX® EXAMINATION-STYLE QUESTIONS

1. Miguel and his wife, Sara, are undergoing testing for impaired fertility.

   a. Describe the nursing support measures that should be used when working with this couple.

   b. Miguel must provide a specimen of semen for analysis. Describe the procedure he should follow to ensure accuracy of the test.

   c. State the semen characteristics that will be assessed.

   d. Miguel and Sara tell the nurse that they would like to solve their problem by getting pregnant using nonmedical measures if possible and ask the nurse about the use of alternative measures including the use of herbs to promote fertility. What types of measures could the nurse suggest they try?

2. Assisted reproductive therapies (ARTs) are being developed and perfected, creating a variety of ethical, legal, financial, and psychosocial concerns. Discuss the issues and concerns engendered by these technologies.

3. Fatima, an 18-year-old, has come to Planned Parenthood for information on birth control methods and assistance with making her choice. She tells the nurse that she is planning to become sexually active with her boyfriend of 6 months and is worried about getting pregnant. "I know I should know more about all of this, but I just don't."

   a. State the nursing diagnosis that reflects Fatima's concern.

   b. Outline the approach the nurse should use to help Fatima make an informed decision in choosing contraception that is right for her.

4. June plans to use a combination estrogen–progestin oral contraceptive.

   a. Describe the mode of action for this type of contraception.

   b. List the advantages of using oral contraception.

   c. Using the acronym ACHES, identify the signs and symptoms that would require June to stop taking the pill and notify her health care provider.

      A

      C

      H

      E

      S

   d. Specify the instructions the nurse should give June about taking the pill to ensure maximum effectiveness.

5. Anita has just had a levonorgestrel intrauterine device (IUD) inserted as her contraceptive method of choice. Specify the instructions that the nurse should give Anita before she leaves the women's health clinic after the insertion.

6. Judy (6-4-0–2-4) and Allen, both age 36, are contemplating sterilization now that their family is complete. They are seeking counseling regarding this decision.

   a. Describe the approach a nurse should use in helping Judy and Allen make the right decision for them.

   b. They decide that Allen will have a vasectomy. Discuss the preoperative and postoperative care and instructions required by Allen.

7. Ayra and her husband, Ian, will be using the symptothermal method of fertility awareness.

    a. List the assessment components of this method that would indicate that ovulation is occurring, and a period of fertility is present requiring abstinence or protected intercourse if pregnancy is not desired.

    b. Outline the points the nurse should emphasize when teaching Ayra and Ian to ensure that they will accurately perform the following:

       i. Measure BBT

       ii. Assess urine for LH

       iii. Evaluate cervical mucus characteristics

    c. State the effectiveness of the symptothermal fertility awareness method of contraception.

8. Edna is a 20-year-old unmarried woman. She is 9 weeks pregnant and is unsure about what to do. She comes to the women's health clinic and asks for the nurse's help in making her decision, stating, "I just cannot support a baby right now. I am alone and trying to finish my education. What can I do?"

    a. Cite the nursing diagnosis reflective of Edna's current dilemma.

    b. Describe the approach the nurse should take in helping Edna make a decision that is right for her.

    c. Edna elects to have an abortion. A vacuum aspiration will be performed in the morning. Edna asks what will happen to her as part of the abortion procedure. Describe how the nurse should respond to Edna's question.

    d. Identify the nursing measures related to the physical care and emotional support that Edna will require as part of this procedure.

    e. Outline the discharge instructions that Edna should receive.

9. Felicia is 7 weeks pregnant and is scheduled for a medically induced abortion using mifepristone and misoprostol. What should the nurse tell Felicia about how these drugs work, the method of their administration, and what adverse reactions she could experience?

10. Marlee comes to the women's health clinic to report that she had unprotected intercourse last night. She is worried about getting pregnant because she is at midcycle and has already noticed signs of ovulation. Marlee tells the nurse that she hardly knows her partner and that her emotions just got the best of her. She is very anxious and asks the nurse what her options are. Describe the approach this nurse should use to assist Marlee with her concerns.

11. The nurse is teaching Jaqueline about contraceptive methods. Jaqueline is 17 years old, single, and sexually active with males. She has previously just used condoms for birth control but is interested in learning about other options. Jaqueline makes the following statements regarding contraceptive use.

Use an X to indicate whether the statements made by Jaqueline below indicate that the health teaching by the nurse was Effective or Not Effective.

Health Teaching	Effective	Not Effective
"I can stop asking my partners to use condoms."		
"With oral contraceptives, my menstrual periods should be shorter with decreased blood loss."		
"I will need to take the oral pills at the same time each day."		
"If I try the calendar rhythm method, I will need track my body temperature daily."		
"I can tell I am ovulating if my cervical mucus is thick and white."		
"If I miss more than two pills, I will need to use a barrier method for birth control."		

6 Genetics, Conception, and Fetal Development

I. LEARNING KEY TERMS

FILL IN THE BLANKS: Insert the term that corresponds to each of the following descriptions related to conception and fetal development.

1. _____ Union of a single egg and sperm. It marks the beginning of a pregnancy.

2. _____ Male and female germ cells. The male germ cell is a _____ and the female germ cell is an _____.

3. _____ Process whereby gametes are formed and mature. For the male, the process is called _____ and for the female, the process is called _____ _____.

4. _____ Process of penetration of the membrane surrounding the ovum by a sperm. It takes place in the _____ _____ of the uterine tube. The membrane becomes impenetrable to other sperm, a process termed the _____. The _____ number of chromosomes is restored when this union of sperm and ovum occurs.

5. _____ The first cell of the new individual. Within 3 days, it becomes a 16-cell solid ball of cells called a _____ _____. This developing structure becomes known as the _____ when a cavity becomes recognizable within it. The outer layer of cells surrounding this cavity is called the _____.

6. _____ Attachment process whereby the blastocyst burrows into the endometrium. _____ or finger-like projections develop out of the trophoblast and extend into the blood-filled spaces of the uterine lining. The uterine lining is now called the _____. The portion of this lining directly under the blastocyst is called the _____ and the portion of this lining that covers the blastocyst is called the _____.

7. _____ The term that refers to the developing baby from day 15 until about 8 weeks after conception.

8. _____ The term that refers to the developing baby from 9 weeks of gestation to the end of pregnancy.

9. _____ Membranes that surround the developing baby and the fluid. The _____ is the outer layer of these membranes and becomes the covering of the fetal side of the placenta. The _____ is the inner layer.

10. _____ Fluid that surrounds the developing baby in the amniotic cavity.

11. Structure that connects the developing baby to the placenta. It contains three vessels, namely two _____ and one _____.

12. _____ The connective tissue that prevents compression of the blood vessels ensuring continued nourishment of the developing baby.

13. _____ Structure composed of 15–20 lobes called cotyledons. It produces _____ essential to

maintain the pregnancy, supplies the _____ _____ and _____ needed by the developing baby for survival and growth, and removes _____ and _____.

14. _____ Capability of fetus to survive outside the uterus.

15. _____ Surface-active phospholipid that needs to be present in fetal/newborn lungs to facilitate breathing after birth. A _____ ratio can be performed using amniotic fluid as one means of determining the degree to which this phospholipid is present in fetal lungs.

16. _____ Special circulatory pathway that allows fetal blood to bypass the lungs.

17. _____ Shunt that allows most of the fetal blood to bypass the liver and pass into the inferior vena cava.

18. _____ Opening between the fetal atria.

19. _____ Formation of blood that occurs in the _____ beginning in the third week.

20. _____ Dark green to black tarry substance that contains fetal waste products. It accumulates in the fetal intestines.

21. _____ Twins that are formed from two zygotes. They are also called _____ twins.

22. _____ Twins that are formed from one fertilized ovum that then divides. They are also called _____ twins.

MATCHING: Match the description with the appropriate genetic concept.

1. _____ The hereditary material carried in the nucleus of each somatic (body) cell; it determines an individual's characteristics.

2. _____ The process by which germ cells divide, producing gametes that each contain 23 chromosomes.

3. _____ Failure of a pair of chromosomes to separate.

4. _____ Basic physical units of inheritance that are passed from parents to offspring and contain the information needed to specify traits.

5. _____ Abnormality in chromosome number; the numeric deviation is not an exact multiple of the haploid number of chromosomes.

6. _____ Cells that contain half of the genetic material of a normal somatic cell.

7. _____ Union of a normal gamete with a gamete containing an extra chromosome resulting in a cell with 47 chromosomes.

8. _____ X, Y.

9. _____ Genes at corresponding loci on homologous chromosomes that code for different forms or variations of the same trait.

10. _____ Process whereby body (somatic) cells replicate to yield two cells with the same genetic makeup as the parent cell.

11. _____ Term that denotes a cell with the correct number of chromosomes.

12. _____ The complete set of genetic instructions in the nucleus of each human cell.

a. Mitosis

b. Meiosis

c. Haploid

d. Diploid

e. Teratogen

f. Human genome

g. Chromosome

h. Genes

i. Sex chromosomes

j. DNA

k. Aneuploidy

l. Trisomy

m. Nondisjunction

n. Monosomy

o. Translocation

p. Mutation

q. Alleles

r. Euploid

s. Polyploidy

t. Mosaicism

13. _____ Process by which genetic material is exchanged between two chromosomes.

14. _____ Thread-like packages of genes and other DNA in the nucleus of a cell.

15. _____ Abnormality in chromosome number in which the deviation is an exact multiple of the haploid number of chromosomes.

16. _____ Somatic cell containing the full number of 46 chromosomes.

17. _____ Union of a normal gamete with a gamete missing a chromosome, resulting in a cell with only 45 chromosomes.

18. _____ A spontaneous and permanent change in normal gene structure.

19. _____ A mixture of cells, some with the normal number of chromosomes and others either missing a chromosome or containing an extra chromosome.

20. _____ Environmental substance or exposure that results in functional or structural disability of the embryo/fetus.

FILL IN THE BLANKS: Insert the term that corresponds to each of the following descriptions related to genetics.

1. _____ Analysis of human DNA, ribonucleic acid (RNA), chromosomes, or proteins to detect abnormalities related to an inherited condition.

2. _____ Direct examination of the DNA and RNA that make up a gene.

3. _____ Examination of the markers that are coinherited with a gene that causes a genetic condition.

4. _____ Examination of the protein products of genes.

5. _____ Examination of chromosomes.

6. _____ Genetic testing that is used to clarify the genetic status of asymptomatic family members. _____ Genetic testing used to detect a disorder that is certain to appear if the defective gene is present and the individual lives long enough. _____ Genetic testing used to detect susceptibility to a disorder if the defective gene is present.

7. _____ Test used to identify individuals who have a gene mutation for a genetic condition but do not show symptoms of the condition because it is a condition that is inherited in an autosomal recessive form.

8. _____ Use of genetic information to individualize drug therapy.

9. _____ Therapy used to correct defective genes that are responsible for disease development; the most common technique is to insert a normal gene in a location within the genome to replace a gene that is nonfunctional.

10. _____ Matched chromosomes.

11. _____ Term that denotes an individual with two copies of the same allele for a given trait. If the two alleles are different, the person is said to be _____ for the trait.

12. _____ The genetic makeup of an individual; an individual's entire genetic makeup or all the genes that the person can pass on to future generations.

13. _____ Observable expression of an individual's genetic makeup.

14. _____ Pictorial analysis of the number, form, and size of an individual's chromosomes.

15. _____ Pattern of inheritance involving a combination of genetic and environmental factors.

16. _____ Pattern of inheritance in which a single gene controls a particular trait, disorder, or defect.

17. _____ Genetic disorder in which only one copy of a variant allele is needed for phenotypic expression.

18. _____ Genetic disorder in which both genes of a pair must be abnormal for the disorder to be expressed.

19. _____ Disorder reflecting absent or defective enzymes leading to abnormal metabolism.

II. REVIEWING KEY CONCEPTS

1. Each of the following structures plays a critical role in fetal growth and development. List the functions of each of the structures listed.

   a. Yolk sac

   b. Amnion, chorion, and amniotic fluid

   c. Umbilical cord

   d. Placenta

2. Identify the tissues or organs that develop from each of the following primary germ layers.

   a. Ectoderm

   b. Mesoderm

   c. Endoderm

3. Sofia has come for her first prenatal visit. Identify the questions the nurse should ask during the health history interview to determine whether factors are present that would place Sofia at risk for giving birth to a baby with an inheritable disorder.

4. Couples referred for genetic counseling receive an estimation of risk for the genetic disorder of concern. Explain the difference between an estimate of occurrence risk and an estimation of recurrence risk.

5. Explain the ethical issues that must be considered regarding the Human Genome Project.

6. Based on genetic testing of a newborn, a diagnosis of achondroplasia (dwarfism) was made. The parents ask the nurse if this could happen to future children. Because this is an example of autosomal dominant inheritance, the nurse would tell the parents:
   a. "For each pregnancy, there is a 50–50 chance the child will be affected by dwarfism."
   b. "This will not happen again because the dwarfism was caused by the harmful genetic effects of the infection you had during pregnancy."
   c. "For each pregnancy, there is a 25% chance the child will be a carrier of the defective gene but unaffected by the disorder."
   d. "Because you already have had an affected child, there is a decreased chance for this to happen in future pregnancies."

7. A female carries the gene for hemophilia on one of her X chromosomes. Now that she is pregnant, she asks the nurse how this might affect her baby. The nurse should tell her:
   a. "A female baby has a 50% chance of being a carrier."
   b. "Hemophilia is always expressed if a male inherits the defective gene."
   c. "Female babies are never affected by this disorder."
   d. "A male baby can be a carrier or have hemophilia."

8. A pregnant woman carries a single gene for cystic fibrosis. The father of her baby does not. Which of the following is true concerning the genetic pattern of cystic fibrosis as it applies to this family?
   a. The pregnant woman has cystic fibrosis herself.
   b. There is a 50% chance her baby will have the disorder.
   c. There is a 25% chance her baby will be a carrier.
   d. There is no chance her baby will be affected by the disorder.

III. CLINICAL JUDGMENT AND NEXT-GENERATION NCLEX® EXAMINATION-STYLE QUESTIONS

1. Imagine that you are a nurse-midwife working in partnership with an obstetrician. Formulate a response to each of the following concerns or questions directed to you from some of your prenatal patients.

   a. Valentina (2 months pregnant), Prisha (5 months pregnant), and Alice (7 months pregnant) all ask for descriptions of their fetuses at the present time.

      i. Valentina

      ii. Prisha

      iii. Alice

   b. Lina states that a friend told her that babies born after about 35 weeks have a better chance to survive because they can breathe easier. She asks if this is true.

   c. Saanvi, who is 1 month pregnant, is concerned because she hasn't felt her baby move yet.

   d. Susan, who is 6 months pregnant, states that she read in a magazine that a fetus can actually hear and see. She feels that this is totally unbelievable.

   e. Renata is 2 months pregnant. She asks how the sex of her baby was determined and whether a sonogram could tell whether she is having a boy or a girl.

   f. Karen is pregnant for the first time. She reveals that she has a history of twins in her family. She wants to know what causes twin pregnancies to occur and what the difference is between identical and fraternal twins.

2. A Jewish couple, who are newly married and are planning for pregnancy express their concerns to the nurse about a maternal a history of Tay-Sachs disease in her family. They are not sure about paternal family history.

   a. Describe the nurse's role in the process of assisting them. to determine their genetic risk.

   b. Both partners are found to be carriers of the disorder. Discuss the estimation of risk and interpretation of risk as it applies to the couple for giving birth to a child who is unaffected, is a carrier, or is affected by the disorder.

   c. Outline the nurse's role in the education and emotional support of the couple now that a diagnosis and estimation of risk have been made.

3. *NGN Item Type: Extended multiple response exercise*
The nurse is teaching a class of pregnant women about fetal development. Which of the following statements will the nurse include about fetal development? Select all that apply.

a. "The sex of your baby is determined by the 9th week of pregnancy."

b. "The baby's heart begins to pump blood during the 10th week of your pregnancy."

c. "You should be able to feel your baby move by weeks 16 to 20 of pregnancy."

d. "We will begin to hear your baby's heartbeat using an ultrasound stethoscope by the 18th week of your pregnancy."

e. "Your baby will be able to suck, swallow, and hiccup while in your uterus."

f. "By the 24th week of your pregnancy, you will notice your baby responding to sounds in the environment such as your voice and music."

g. "Prenatal genetic testing will ensure that your baby does not develop any gene mutations."

h. "The amniotic fluid allows your baby to move and develop its musculoskeletal system."

Chapter **6 Genetics, Conception, and Fetal Development**

7 Anatomy and Physiology of Pregnancy

I. LEARNING KEY CONCEPTS

FILL IN THE BLANKS: Insert the term that corresponds to each of the following descriptions related to pregnancy.

1. _____ This type of breathing replaces abdominal breathing as pregnancy progresses and is accomplished by using the diaphragm instead of the costal muscles.

2. _____ The three 3-month periods into which pregnancy is divided.

3. _____ Hormone responsible for the decreased tone and motility of smooth muscles and decreasing uterine contractility.

4. _____ Hormone responsible for enlargement of uterus and breast, relaxing pelvic ligaments and joints, and a decreased secretion of hydrochloric acid and pepsin.

5. _____ Hormone responsible for preparing breasts for lactation.

6. _____ Hormone responsible for stimulating uterine contractions and milk ejection from breasts after birth.

7. _____ Change in blood pressure that can occur when a pregnant woman lies on her back for an examination of her abdomen. The _____ is compressed by the weight of the abdominal contents, including the uterus.

8. _____ The biologic marker on which pregnancy tests are based. Its presence in urine or serum results in a positive pregnancy test result.

9. _____ Irregular, painless uterine contractions that can be felt through the abdominal wall soon after the fourth month of pregnancy.

10. _____ A rushing or blowing sound of maternal blood flow through the uterine arteries to the placenta that is synchronous with the maternal pulse.

11. _____ Sound of fetal blood coursing through the umbilical cord; it is synchronous with the fetal heart rate.

12. _____ Fetal movements first felt by the pregnant woman as early as 14–16 weeks of gestation.

13. _____ Change in blood pressure as a result of compression of abdominal blood vessels and decrease in cardiac output when a woman lies down on her back.

14. _____ Severe itching of the skin that occurs during pregnancy as a result of retention and accumulation of bile in the liver.

15. _____ Nonfood cravings for substances such as ice, clay, and laundry starch.

MATCHING

Match the assessment finding with the appropriate descriptive term.

16. _____ Excessive salivation.

17. _____ Fundal height decreased, fetal head in pelvic inlet.

18. _____ Cervix and vagina violet-bluish in color.

19. _____ Swelling of ankles and feet at the end of the day.

20. _____ Cervical tip softened.

21. _____ Lower uterine segment is soft and compressible.

22. _____ Fetal head rebounds with gentle upward tapping through the vagina.

23. _____ White or slightly gray mucoid vaginal discharge with faint, musty odor.

24. _____ Enlarged sebaceous glands in areola on both breasts.

25. _____ Plug of mucus fills endocervical canal.

26. _____ Pink stretch marks or depressed streaks on breasts and abdomen.

27. _____ The anterior pituitary stimulates production of this by the end of the first trimester.

28. _____ Blotchy, brownish hyperpigmentation on cheeks, nose, and forehead.

29. _____ Pigmented line extending up abdominal midline to the top of the fundus.

30. _____ A decrease in cardiac output followed by reflex bradycardia caused by compression of the vena cava in the second half of pregnancy.

31. _____ Heartburn.

32. _____ Lumbosacral curve increased.

33. _____ Paresthesia and pain in the hand radiating to elbow.

34. _____ Responsible for slight spotting following cervical palpation or intercourse.

35. _____ State of hemodilution where there is a decrease in normal hemoglobin and hematocrit values.

36. _____ Vascular spiders on neck and thorax.

37. _____ Palms pinkish red, mottled.

38. _____ Abdominal wall muscles separated.

39. _____ Red raised nodule on gums; bleeds after brushing teeth.

a. Colostrum
b. Operculum
c. Ptyalism
d. Angiomata
e. Pyrosis
f. Friability
g. Striae gravidarum
h. Physiologic anemia
i. Linea nigra
j. Ballottement
k. Chadwick sign
l. Diastasis recti abdominis
m. Lordosis
n. Leukorrhea
o. Chloasma (melasma)
p. Lightening
q. Vena caval syndrome
r. Palmar erythema
s. Goodell sign
t. Physiologic/dependent edema
u. Hegar sign
v. Montgomery tubercles
w. Carpal tunnel syndrome
x. Epulis (gingival granuloma gravidarum)

II. REVIEWING KEY CONCEPTS

1. During an examination of a pregnant woman the nurse notes that her cervix is soft on its tip. The nurse would document this finding as:

   a. Friability.

   b. Goodell sign.

   c. Chadwick sign.

   d. Hegar sign.

2. When assessing the pregnant woman, the nurse should keep in mind that baseline vital sign values will change as she progresses through her pregnancy. Describe how each of the following would change:

   a. Blood pressure (BP)

   b. Heart rate and patterns

   c. Respiratory rate and patterns

3. Identify criteria that must be taken into consideration prior to counseling a woman regarding a positive home pregnancy test.

4. Specify the expected changes that occur in the following laboratory tests as a result of physiologic adaptations to pregnancy:

   a. Hematocrit, hemoglobin, white blood cell count

   b. Clotting activity

   c. Acid/base balance

5. Explain the expected adaptations in elimination that occur during pregnancy. Include in your answer the basis for the changes that occur.

   a. Renal

   b. Bowel

6. An essential component of prenatal health assessment of pregnant women is the determination of vital signs. Which of the following would be an expected change in vital sign findings as a result of pregnancy?
   a. Increase in systolic blood pressure by 30 mm Hg or more after assuming a supine position
   b. Increase in diastolic BP by 5–10 mm Hg beginning in the first trimester
   c. Chest breathing replaces abdominal breathing with upward displacement of the diaphragm
   d. Gradual decrease in baseline pulse rate of approximately 20 beats per minute

1. Describe how the nurse should respond to each of the following patient concerns and questions.

   a. Tina is 14 weeks pregnant. She calls the prenatal clinic to report that she noticed slight, painless spotting this morning. She reveals that she did have intercourse with her partner the night before.

   b. Lisa suspects she is pregnant because her menstrual period is already 3 weeks late. She asks her friend, who is a nurse, how to use the pregnancy test that she just bought so that she obtains the most accurate results.

   c. Joan is 3 months pregnant. She tells the nurse that she is worried because a friend told her that vaginal and bladder infections are more common during pregnancy. She wants to know if this could be true and if so, why.

   d. Tammy, who is 20 weeks pregnant, tells the nurse that she has noted some "problems" with her breasts: there are "little pimples" near her nipples and her breasts feel "lumpy and bumpy" and "leak a little" when she performs a breast self-examination (BSE).

   e. Tamara is concerned because she read in a book about pregnancy that a pregnant woman's position could affect her circulation, especially to the baby. She asks what positions are good for her circulation now that she is pregnant.

   f. Carla, a pregnant woman, calls to tell the nurse that she had a nosebleed this morning and has noticed occasional feelings of fullness in her ears. She asks if these occurrences are anything to worry about.

   g. Karen is 7 months pregnant and works as a secretary full time. She asks the nurse if she should take a "water pill" that a friend gave her because she has noticed that her ankles "swell up" at the end of the day.

   h. Fatema is in her third trimester of pregnancy. She tells the nurse that her posture seems to have changed and that she occasionally experiences low back pain.

   i. Monica, who is 36 weeks pregnant with her first baby, calls the clinic stating that she knows the baby is coming because she felt some uterine contractions before getting out of bed in the morning. Monica confirms that they seem to have decreased in intensity and frequency since she has gotten out of bed and walked around.

47

2. Accurate blood pressure readings are critical if significant changes in the cardiovascular system are to be detected as a woman adapts to pregnancy during the prenatal period. Write a protocol for blood pressure assessment that can be used by nurses working in a prenatal clinic to ensure accuracy of the results obtained during blood pressure assessment.

3. The nurse is caring for Nadia, a 32-year-old G4P4 who is admitted to the hospital to rule out preterm labor. She is currently 32 weeks gestation. She has had elevated blood pressures per her report, but she does not know her baseline blood pressure. She states she has had some increased flatulence throughout her pregnancy. She has had irregular and painless contractions, but state they have become more frequent. Admission labs are drawn, and the nurse obtains vital signs and an admission assessment.

- Oral temperature 37.4°C

- Heart rate 88 beats per minute

- Blood pressure 143/94

- Respiratory rate 19

- 2-hour postprandial blood glucose of 134

- WBCs 8,000 mm³

- Hemoglobin 12 g/dL

- Hematocrit 34%

- Platelets 124,000 per mm³

Highlight or place a check mark next to the assessment or history findings that require further follow-up by the nurse.

8 Nursing Care of the Family During Pregnancy

I. LEARNING KEY TERMS

FILL IN THE BLANKS: Insert the term that corresponds to each of the following descriptions.

1. _____ Pregnancy.

2. _____ The number of pregnancies in which the fetus or fetuses have reached 20 weeks of gestation, not the number of fetuses (e.g., twins) born. The numeric designation is not affected by whether the fetus is born alive or is stillborn (i.e., showing no signs of life at birth).

3. _____ A woman who is pregnant.

4. _____ A woman who has never been pregnant.

5. _____ A woman who has not completed a pregnancy with a fetus or fetuses beyond 20 weeks of gestation.

6. _____ A woman who is pregnant for the first time.

7. _____ A woman who has completed one pregnancy with a fetus or fetuses who have reached 20 weeks of gestation or more.

8. _____ A woman who has had two or more pregnancies.

9. _____ A woman who has completed two or more pregnancies to 20 weeks of gestation or more.

10. _____ Capacity to live outside the uterus; there are no clear limits of gestational age or weight.

11. _____ Designation given to a pregnancy that has reached 20 weeks of gestation but ends before completion of 37 weeks of gestation.

12. _____ Designation given to a pregnancy from 39 weeks 0 days to 40 weeks 6 days of gestation.

13. _____ Designation given to a pregnancy that goes beyond 42 weeks 0 days of gestation.

14. _____ Pregnancy-related changes felt by the woman which can include breast changes, nausea, and amenorrhea.

15. _____ Pregnancy-related changes that can be observed by an examiner which can include Goodell sign, a positive pregnancy test, and Hegar sign.

16. _____ Objective signs that can be attributed only to the presence of the fetus which include visualization of fetus by ultrasound.

17. _____ Rule used to determine the estimated day of birth by subtracting _____ months from, adding _____ days to, and one year to the first day of the _____.

18. _____ Measurement performed beginning in the second trimester as one indicator of the progress of fetal growth.

19. _____ Tasks accomplished by women and men as they adapt to the changes of pregnancy; these tasks include _____, _____, _____, _____, and _____.

20. _____ Rapid unpredictable changes in mood.

21. _____ Having conflicting feelings about the pregnancy at the same time.

22. _____ As a pregnant woman establishes a relationship with her fetus,

49

she progresses through three phases. In phase one, she accepts the _____ and needs to be able to state "I am pregnant". In phase two, the woman accepts the growing fetus as distinct from herself. She can now say _____. Finally, in phase three, the woman prepares realistically for the _____ and parenting of the child. She expresses the thought, _____.

23. _____ Change in blood pressure that can occur if a pregnant woman changes her position rapidly from supine to upright.

24. _____ and increases in _____ Techniques used to assess fetal health growth.

25. _____ Professionally trained woman who provides physical, emotional, and informational support to women and their partners during labor and birth and in the postpartum period.

26. _____ Tool that can be used by expectant couples to explore their childbirth options and choose those that are most important to them; it serves as a tentative guide because the reality of what is feasible may change as the actual labor and birth progress.

II. REVIEWING KEY CONCEPTS

1. Describe the obstetric history for each of the following women, using the 5 digit system.

   a. Nancy is currently pregnant. Her first pregnancy resulted in a stillbirth at 36 weeks of gestation and her second pregnancy resulted in the birth of her daughter at 42 weeks of gestation.

   b. Alma is 6 weeks pregnant. Her previous pregnancies resulted in the live birth of a daughter at 40 weeks of gestation, the live birth of a son at 38 weeks of gestation, and a spontaneous abortion at 10 weeks of gestation.

   c. Malak is experiencing her fourth pregnancy. Her first pregnancy ended in a spontaneous abortion at 12 weeks, the second resulted in the live birth of

twin boys at 32 weeks, and the third resulted in the live birth of a daughter at 39 weeks.

2. Calculate the expected date of birth (EDB) for each of the following pregnant women using Naegele's rule.

   a. Delfina's last menses began on May 5, 2022, and its last day occurred on May 10, 2022.
   b. Sara had intercourse on February 4, 2022. She has not had a menstrual period since the one that began on January 19, 2022, and ended 5 days later.

   c. Luiza's last period began on July 4, 2021, and ended on July 10, 2021. She noted that her basal body temperature (BBT) began to rise on July 28, 2021.

3. Cultural beliefs and practices are important influencing factors during the prenatal period.

   a. Describe how cultural beliefs can affect a woman's participation in prenatal care.

4. Outline the assessment measures that should be used and the data that should be collected during each component of the initial prenatal visit and the follow-up prenatal visits.

   INITIAL PRENATAL VISIT

   Health History Interview

   Physical Examination

   Laboratory and Diagnostic Testing

FOLLOW-UP PRENATAL VISITS

Updating History Interview

Physical Examination

Fetal Assessment

Laboratory and Diagnostic Testing

5. Nurses responsible for the care management of pregnant women must be alert for warning signs of potential complications that women could develop as pregnancy progresses from trimester to trimester.

   a. List the clinical manifestations (warning signs) for each of the following potential complications of pregnancy.

      Hyperemesis gravidarum

      Infection

      Miscarriage

      Hypertension conditions including preeclampsia

      Premature rupture of the membranes (PROM)

      Placental disorders (placenta previa; abruptio placentae)

      Fetal jeopardy

   b. Describe the approach a nurse should take when discussing potential complications with a pregnant woman and her family.

6. Create a protocol for fundal measurement that will facilitate accuracy.

7. During the third trimester, parents often make a decision concerning the method they will use to feed their newborn. How would you address questions and concerns related to breastfeeding during a prenatal breastfeeding class?

8. Fathers and nonpregnant partners experience pregnancy in many different ways. Three phases have been identified as characterizing the developmental tasks experienced by expectant partners. Briefly, discuss each phase and how the nurse can help the partner to progress through each phase.

   Announcement Phase

   Moratorium Phase

   Focusing Phase

9. A nurse is assessing a pregnant woman during a prenatal visit. Several presumptive indicators of pregnancy are documented. Which of the following are presumptive indicators? Select all that apply.

   a. Nausea and vomiting
   b. Quickening
   c. Ballottement
   d. Palpation of fetal movement by the nurse
   e. Hegar's sign
   f. Amenorrhea

51

10. A woman's last menstrual period (LMP) began on September 10, 2021, and it ended on September 15, 2021. Using Naegele's rule, the estimated date of birth would be:
    a. June 17, 2022.
    b. June 22, 2022.
    c. August 17, 2022.
    d. December 3, 2022.

11. A woman at 30 weeks of gestation assumes a supine position for a fundal measurement and Leopold's maneuvers. She begins to complain about feeling dizzy and nauseated. Her skin feels damp and cool. The nurse's first action would be to:
    a. assess the woman's respiratory rate and effort.
    b. provide the woman with an emesis basin.
    c. elevate the woman's legs 20 degrees from her hips.
    d. turn the woman on her side.

12. The nurse evaluates a pregnant woman's knowledge about prevention of urinary tract infections at the prenatal visit following a class on infection prevention that the woman attended. The nurse would recognize that the woman needs further instruction when she tells the nurse about which one of the following measures that she now uses to prevent urinary tract infections? Select all that apply.
    a. "I drink about 1 quart of fluid a day."
    b. "I have stopped using bubble baths and bath oils."
    c. "I have started wearing panty hose and underpants with a cotton crotch."
    d. "I have yogurt for lunch or as an evening snack."
    e. "I should stop having intercourse with my partner."

13. Doulas are becoming important members of a laboring woman's health care team. Which of the following activities should be expected as part of the doula's role responsibilities?
    a. Monitoring hydration of the laboring woman, including adjusting IV flow rates
    b. Interpreting electronic fetal monitoring tracings to determine the well-being of the maternal-fetal unit
    c. Eliminating the need for the husband/partner to be present during labor and birth
    d. Providing continuous support throughout labor and birth, including explanations of labor progress

14. A pregnant woman at 10 weeks of gestation exhibits the following signs of pregnancy during a routine prenatal checkup. Which ones would be categorized as probable signs of pregnancy? Select all that apply.
    a. hCG in the urine
    b. Breast tenderness
    c. Ballottement
    d. Fetal heart sounds
    e. Hegar sign
    f. Amenorrhea

15. A pregnant woman who currently has four living children reports the following obstetric history: a stillbirth at 32 weeks of gestation, triplets (two sons and one daughter) born via cesarean section at 30 weeks of gestation, a spontaneous abortion at 8 weeks of gestation, and a daughter born vaginally at 39 weeks of gestation. Which of the following accurately expresses this woman's current obstetric history using the 5 digit system?
    a. 5-1-4-1-4
    b. 4-1-3-1-4
    c. 5-2-2-0-3
    d. 5-1-2-1-4

III. CLINICAL JUDGMENT AND NEXT-GENERATION NCLEX® EXAMINATION-STYLE QUESTIONS

1. A health history interview of the pregnant woman by the nurse is included as part of the initial prenatal visit.

   a. State the purpose of the health history interview.

   b. Write two questions for each component that is included in the initial health history interview. Questions should be clear, concise, and understandable. Most of the questions should be open ended to elicit the most complete response from the patient.

c. Write four questions that should be included in the interview when updating the health history during follow-up visits.

2. Imagine that you are a nurse working in a prenatal clinic. You have been assigned to be the primary nurse for Isidora, an 18-year-old who has come to the clinic for confirmation of pregnancy. She tells you that she knows she is pregnant because she has already missed three periods and a home pregnancy test that she did last week was positive. Isidora states that she has had very little contact with the health care system, and the only reason she came today is because her boyfriend insisted that she "make sure" she is really pregnant. Describe the approach that you would take regarding data collection and nursing interventions appropriate for this woman.

3. Terry is a primigravida in her first trimester of pregnancy. She is accompanied by her husband, Tim, to her second prenatal visit. Answer each of the following questions asked by Terry and Tim:

   a. "At the last visit I was told that my estimated date of birth is December 25, 2022. Can I really count on my baby being born on Christmas Day?"

   b. "Before I became pregnant my friend told me I should be doing Kegel exercises. I was too embarrassed to ask her about them. What are they and is it safe for me to do them while I am pregnant?"

   c. "What effect will pregnancy have on our sex life? We are willing to abstain during pregnancy if we have to keep our baby safe."

   d. "This morning sickness I am experiencing is driving me crazy. I become nauseated in the morning and again late in the afternoon. Occasionally I vomit or have the dry heaves. Will this last for my entire pregnancy? Is there anything I can do to feel better?"

4. Mila is 2 months pregnant. She tells the nurse, at the prenatal clinic, that she is used to being active and exercises every day. Now that she is pregnant she wonders if she should reduce or stop her exercise routine. Discuss what information the nurse's response to Tara should include.

53

5. Write one nursing diagnosis for each of the following situations. State one expected outcome, and list appropriate nursing measures for the nursing diagnosis you identified.

a. Beth is 6 weeks pregnant. During the health history interview, she tells you that she has limited her intake of fluids and tries to hold her urine as long as she can because, "I just hate having to go to the bathroom so frequently."

Nursing diagnosis   Expected outcome   Nursing measures

b. Ananya, who is 23 weeks pregnant, tells you that she is beginning to experience more frequent lower back pain. You note that when she walked into the examining room her posture exhibited a moderate degree of lordosis and neck flexion. She was wearing shoes with 2-inch narrow heels.

Nursing diagnosis   Expected outcome   Nursing measures

c. Maryam, a primigravida at 32 weeks of gestation, comes for a prenatal visit accompanied by her partner, the father of the baby. They both express anxiety about the impending birth of the baby and how they will handle the experience of labor. Maryam is especially concerned about how she will survive the pain, and her partner is primarily concerned about how he will help Maryam cope with labor and make sure she and the baby are safe.

Nursing diagnosis   Expected outcome   Nursing measures

6. Renata is a primigravida in her second trimester of pregnancy. Answer each of the following questions asked by Renata during a prenatal visit.

a. "Why do you measure my abdomen every time I come in for a checkup?"

b. "I am going to start changing the way that I dress now that I am beginning to show. Do you have any suggestions I could follow, especially since I have a limited amount of money to spend?"

c. "What can I do about gas and constipation? I never had much of a problem before I was pregnant."

d. "Since yesterday I have started to feel itchy all over. Do you think I am coming down with some sort of infection?"

e. "I will be flying out to Chicago to visit my father in 1 month. Is airline travel safe for me when I am 5 months pregnant?"

7. While a nurse is measuring a pregnant woman's fundus, the woman becomes pale and diaphoretic. The woman, who is at 23 weeks of gestation, states that she feels dizzy and lightheaded.

   a. State the most likely explanation for the assessment findings exhibited by this woman.

   b. Describe what the nurse's immediate action should be.

8. Kelly is a primigravida in her third trimester of pregnancy. Answer each of the following questions asked by Kelly during a prenatal visit.

   a. "My husband and I have decided to breastfeed our baby, but friends told me it is very difficult if my nipples do not come out. Is there any way I can tell now if my nipples are okay for breastfeeding?"

   b. "My ankles are swollen by the time I get home from work late in the afternoon [Kelly teaches second grade]. I have been trying to drink about 3 liters of fluid every day. Should I reduce the amount of liquid I am drinking or ask my doctor for a water pill?"

   c. "I woke up last night with a terrible cramp in my leg. It finally went away but my husband and I just did not know what to do. What if this happens again tonight?"

9. Marge, a pregnant woman (2-0-0–1-0) beginning her third trimester, expresses concern about preterm birth. "I already had one miscarriage, and my sister's baby died after being born too early. I am so worried that this will happen to me."

   a. Identify one nursing diagnosis with an expected outcome that reflects Marge's concern.

   b. Indicate what the nurse can teach Marge about the signs of preterm labor.

10. Camila is 4 months pregnant and is beginning to "show." She asks the nurse what she should expect as a reaction from her 13-year-old daughter and 3-year-old son. Describe the response the nurse would make.

11. Your neighbor, Renata, is in her second month of pregnancy. Knowing that you are a nurse, her husband, Tom, confides to you, "I just can't figure out Renata. One minute she is happy and the next minute she is crying for no reason at all! I do not know how I will be able to cope with this for 7 more months."

    a. Write a nursing diagnosis and expected outcome that reflects Tom's concern.

    b. Discuss how you would respond to his concern.

12. Jennifer (2-1-0-0-1) and her husband, Santiago, are beginning their third trimester of a low risk pregnancy. As you work with them on their birth plan, they tell you that they are having trouble making a decision about their choice of a birth setting. They experienced a delivery room birth with their first child. Jennifer states, "My first pregnancy was perfectly normal, just like this one, but the birth was disappointing, so medically focused with monitors, IVs, and staying in bed." They ask you for your advice about the different birth settings they have heard and read about, namely labor, delivery, recovery, and postpartum (LDRP) rooms at their local hospital, the birthing center a few miles from their home, and even their own home. Describe the approach that you would take to guide Jennifer and Santiago in their decision regarding a birth setting.

13. Nancy, a pregnant woman (3-2-0-0-2) at 26 weeks of gestation, asks the nurse about doulas. "My friend had a doula and she said that she was amazing. My first two birth experiences were difficult—my husband and I really needed someone to help us. Do you think a doula could be that person?"

    a. Explain the role of the doula so that Nancy will have the information she will need to make an informed decision.

    b. Nancy decides to try a doula for her upcoming labor. Identify what you would tell Nancy about finding a doula.

    c. Specify questions that Nancy should ask when she is making a choice about the doula she will hire for her labor.

14. Tony and Polina are considering the possibility of giving birth to their second baby at home. They have been receiving prenatal care from a certified nurse-midwife who has experience with home birth. Their 5-year-old son and both sets of grandparents want to be present for the birth.

    a. Discuss the decision-making process that Tony and Polina should follow to ensure that they make an informed decision that is right for them and their family.

    b. Tony and Polina decide that home birth is an ideal choice for them. Outline the preparation measures you would recommend to Tony and Polina to ensure a safe and positive experience for everyone.

15. *NGN Item Type: Extended multiple response exercise*

During an early bird prenatal class, a nurse teaches a group of newly diagnosed pregnant women about their emotional reactions during pregnancy. Which of the following should the nurse discuss with the women? Select all that apply.

    a. Sexual desire (libido) is usually increased during the second trimester of pregnancy.
    b. A referral for counseling should be sought if a woman experiences ambivalence in the first trimester.
    c. Rapid, unpredictable mood swings reflect gestational bipolar disorder.
    d. Anxiety can occur as the mother becomes concerned about the birth process.
    e. A woman's own mother will be her greatest source of emotional support during pregnancy.
    f. Attachment to the infant begins late in the third trimester when she begins preparing for birth by attending childbirth preparation classes.
    g. Any fatigue during pregnancy should be associated with depression and immediately reported.
    h. If she does not accept the pregnancy, she will reject the child once it is born.

9 Maternal and Fetal Nutrition

I. LEARNING KEY TERMS

FILL IN THE BLANKS: Insert the term that corresponds to each of the following descriptions.

1. _____ Birth weight of 2500 g or less.

2. _____ Nutrient, particularly important during the periconceptional period. Adequate intake is important for decreasing

   risk for _____ or failures

   in the closure of the neural tube. An intake of ___

   _____ daily is recommended for all women capable of becoming pregnant.

3. _____ Recommendations for nutritional intake that meets the needs of almost all healthy members of the population.

4. _____ Method used to evaluate the appropriateness of weight for height. If the calculated value is less than 18.5, the

   person is considered to be _____. If the calculated value is between 18.5 and 24.9, the person

   is considered to be a _____ weight. If the calculated value is between 25 and 29.9, the person

   is considered to be _____ and if greater

   than 30 the person is considered to be _____.

5. _____ Vegetarian diet that includes milk products.

6. _____ Normal adaptation that occurs during pregnancy when the plasma volume increases more rapidly than RBC mass.

7. _____ Inability to digest milk sugar because of the absence of the lactase enzyme in the small intestine.

8. _____ Practice of consuming nonfood substances or excessive amounts of food stuffs low in nutritional value.

9. _____ Urge to consume specific types of foods such as ice cream, pickles, and pizza during pregnancy.

10. _____ USDA provided guide that can be used to make daily food choices during pregnancy and lactation, just as during other stages of the life cycle.

11. _____ A discomfort most commonly experienced in the first trimester of pregnancy; it usually causes only mild-to-moderate nutritional problems but may be a source of substantial discomfort.

12. _____ Severe and persistent vomiting during pregnancy causing weight loss, dehydration, and electrolyte abnormalities.

13. _____ Discomfort of pregnancy that is often related to iron supplement intake and may be relieved with increased water and fiber intake.

14. _____ Discomfort of pregnancy that is usually caused by reflux of gastric contents into the esophagus.

II. REVIEWING KEY CONCEPTS

1. Indicate the importance of each of the following nutrients for healthy maternal adaptation to pregnancy and optimum fetal growth and development. Indicate three food/fluid sources for each of the nutrients.

Nutrient	Importance for Pregnancy	Major Food Sources
Protein		
Iron		
Calcium		
Sodium		
Zinc		
Fat-soluble vitamins		
Water-soluble vitamins		

2. When assessing pregnant women, it is critical that nurses are alert for factors that could place women at nutritional risk so that early intervention can be implemented. Name five such indicators or risk factors of which the nurse should be aware.

3. Cite the pregnancy-related risks associated with the following nutritional problems.

   a. Underweight women

   b. Inappropriate weight gain during pregnancy (inadequate; excessive)

   c. Obese women

59

4. At her first prenatal visit, Marie, a 20-year-old primigravida, reports that she has been a strict vegetarian for the past 3 years. Identify two major guidelines that the nurse should follow when planning menus with Marie.

5. Evaluation of nutritional status is an essential part of a thorough physical assessment of pregnant women. Cite four signs of good nutrition and four signs of inadequate nutrition that the nurse should observe for during the assessment of a pregnant woman.

6. Calculate the BMI for each of the following women, and then determine the recommended weight gain and pattern for each woman based on her BMI.

Woman	BMI Meaning	Weight Gain (total; pattern)
a. June: 5 feet 3 inches, 120 pounds		
b. Alisa: 5 feet 6 inches, 180 pounds		
c. Siobhan 5 feet 5 inches, 95 pounds		

7. A nurse teaching a pregnant woman about the importance of iron in her diet would tell her to avoid consuming which of the following foods at the same time as her iron supplement because they will decrease iron absorption? Select all that apply.
   a. Tomatoes
   b. Spinach
   c. Meat
   d. Eggs
   e. Milk
   f. Bran

8. A 25-year-old pregnant woman is at 10 weeks of gestation. Her BMI is calculated to be 24. Which one of the following is recommended in terms of weight gain during pregnancy?
   a. Total weight gain of 18 kg
   b. First trimester weight gain of 1–2 kg
   c. Weight gain of 0.45 kg each week for 40 weeks
   d. Weight gain of 3 kg per month during the second and third trimesters

9. A pregnant woman at 6 weeks of gestation tells her nurse-midwife that she has been experiencing nausea with occasional vomiting every day. The nurse could recommend which of the following as an effective relief measure?
   a. Drink a large glass of water in the morning before getting out of bed.
   b. Avoid eating before going to bed at night.
   c. Alter eating patterns to a schedule of small meals every 2–3 hours.
   d. Skip a meal if nausea is experienced.

10. A woman demonstrates an understanding of the importance of increasing her intake of foods high in folic acid (100 mcg or more) when she includes which of the following foods in her diet? Select all that apply.
    a. Seafood
    b. Legumes
    c. Eggs
    d. Liver (beef)
    e. Asparagus
    f. Oranges

III. CLINICAL JUDGMENT AND NEXT-GENERATION NCLEX® EXAMINATION-STYLE QUESTIONS

1. Nutrition and weight gain are important areas of consideration for nurses who care for pregnant women. In addition, weight gain is often a source of stress and body image alteration for the pregnant woman. Discuss the approach you would use in each of the following situations.

   a. Zehra (5' 8" and 120 pounds) complains to you that her physician recommended a weight gain of approximately 30 pounds during her pregnancy. She states, "Babies only weigh about 7 pounds when they are born. Why do I have to gain much more than that?"

   b. Kate (5' 4" and 125 pounds) has just found out that she is pregnant. She states, "I am so glad to be pregnant. I love to eat, and now I can start eating for two. It will be great not to have to watch the scale or what I eat."

   c. June tells you that she does not have to worry about her nutrient intake during her pregnancy. "I take plenty of vitamins—everything from A to Z."

   d. Sylvie, a primigravida beginning her second month of pregnancy, asks you why she needs to increase her intake of so many nutrients during pregnancy and states, "I work every weekday and rely on fast foods to get through the week, though I try to eat better over the weekends."

   e. Sara (BMI = 28.7) is 1 month pregnant. She asks you for dietary guidance, including a weight reduction diet because she does not want to gain too much weight with this pregnancy.

   f. Alma is 2 months pregnant. She states, "I have cut down on my water intake. I do get a little thirsty, but it's worth it since I don't have to urinate so often."

   g. Hedy is 2 months pregnant and has come for her second prenatal visit. During a discussion about nutritional needs during pregnancy she states, "I know I will never get enough calcium because I get sick when I drink milk."

2. Yvonne's hemoglobin is 13 g/dL and her hematocrit is 37% at the onset of her pregnancy. She asks the nurse if she will have to take iron during her pregnancy if she tries to follow a good diet. "My friend took iron when she was pregnant and it made her sick to her stomach." Discuss the appropriate response by the nurse.

3. Identify three nursing measures appropriate for each of the following nursing diagnoses:

a. Imbalanced nutrition: less than body requirements related to inadequate intake associated with moderate nausea and vomiting (morning sickness) associated with pregnancy

b. Constipation related to decreased intestinal motility associated with increased progesterone levels during pregnancy

c. Pain related to reflux of gastric contents into esophagus following dinner

4. The nurse is caring for a 30-year-old pregnant woman with a BMI of 33. She tells the nurse that she is concerned about her weight, but also wants to make sure she is healthy for her baby. She asks the nurse about recommendations for diet and weight gain during pregnancy.

Use an X to indicate whether the health teaching below is Indicated (appropriate or necessary) or Not-Indicated (not necessary or contraindicated) at this time.

Health Teaching	Indicated	Not Indicated
Counsel her to begin a lifestyle change for weight reduction		
Recommend a total weight gain goal of 4 kg during pregnancy		
Set a weight gain goal of 0.2 kg per week during the second and third trimesters		
Limit her third trimester calorie increase to no more than 600 kcal more than prepregnant needs		
Her recommended total weight gain is 11–20 pounds during pregnancy		
Recommend a low calorie, low-carbohydrate, high-protein diet during the second and trimesters		

10 Assessment of High-Risk Pregnancy

I. LEARNING KEY TERMS

FILL IN THE BLANKS: Insert the term that corresponds to each of the following descriptions.

1. _____ A pregnancy in which the life or health of the mother or her fetus is jeopardized by a disorder coincidental with or unique to pregnancy.

2. _____ Assessment of fetal activity by the mother is a simple yet valuable method for monitoring the condition of the fetus.

   _____ Term used to refer to the cessation of fetal movements entirely for 12 hours.

3. _____ Diagnostic test that involves the use of sound having a frequency higher than that detectable by humans to examine structures inside the body. During pregnancy, it can be done by using either the _____ or _____ approach.

4. _____ Noninvasive study of blood flow in the fetus and placenta with ultrasound.

5. _____ Noninvasive dynamic assessment of the fetus and its environment that is based on acute and chronic markers of fetal disease.

   It uses real-time _____ to permit a detailed assessment. This test includes assessment of variables by ultrasound, namely _____, _____, _____, _____, and fetal heart rate reactivity by a _____.

6. _____ Noninvasive radiologic technique used for obstetric and gynecologic diagnosis by providing excellent pictures of soft tissue without the use of ionizing radiation.

7. _____ Prenatal diagnostic test that is performed to obtain amniotic fluid to examine the fetal cells it contains.

8. _____ Prenatal diagnostic test that provides direct access to the fetal circulation during the second and third trimesters.

9. _____ Procedure that involves the removal of a small tissue specimen from the fetal portion of the placenta. Because this tissue originates from the zygote, it reflects the genetic makeup of the fetus and is performed between 10 and 13 weeks of gestation.

10. _____ Test used as a screening tool for neural tube defects in pregnancy. The test is ideally performed between 16 and 18 weeks of gestation.

11. _____ Test used to screen for Down syndrome, which are available beginning in the first trimester at 11–14 weeks gestation.

12. _____ Screening test for Rh incompatibility by examining the serum of Rh-negative women for Rh antibodies.

13. _____ Noninvasive test based on the fact that the heart rate of a healthy fetus with an intact central nervous system will usually accelerate in response to its own movement.

14. _____ Test that determines fetal response to the stimulation of vibration and sound; the expected response is acceleration of the fetal heart rate.

15. _____ Test used to identify the jeopardized fetus that is stable at rest but shows evidence of compromise when exposed to the stress of uterine contractions. If the resultant hypoxia of the fetus is sufficient, a deceleration of the FHR will result. Two methods used for this test are the _____ test and the _____ test.

II. REVIEWING KEY CONCEPTS

1. Identify factors that would place the pregnant woman and fetus/neonate at risk, for each of the following categories:

   a. Biophysical factors

   b. Psychosocial factors

   c. Sociodemographic factors

   d. Environmental factors

2. Discuss the role of the nurse when caring for high-risk pregnant women who are required to undergo antepartum assessment testing to determine fetal well-being.

3. State two risk factors for each of the following pregnancy-related problems:

   a. Polyhydramnios

   b. Intrauterine growth restriction

   c. Oligohydramnios

   d. Chromosomal abnormalities

4. A 34-year-old woman at 36 weeks of gestation has been scheduled for a biophysical profile. She asks the nurse why the test needs to be performed. The nurse would tell her that the test:
   a. determines how well her baby will breathe after it is born.
   b. evaluates the response of her baby's heart to uterine contractions.
   c. measures her baby's head size and length.
   d. observes her baby's activities in utero to predict fetal well-being.

5. As part of preparing a 24-year-old woman at 42 weeks of gestation for a nonstress test, the nurse would:
   a. tell the woman to fast for 8 hours before the test.
   b. explain that the test will evaluate how well her baby is moving inside her uterus.
   c. have her sit in a semi-Fowler's position for at least 10 minutes during the test.
   d. attach a spiral electrode to the presenting part to determine FHR patterns.

6. A 40-year-old woman at 18 weeks of gestation is having a multiple marker test performed. She is obese, and her health history reveals that she is Rh negative. The primary purpose of this test is to screen for:
   a. spina bifida.
   b. Down syndrome.
   c. gestational diabetes.
   d. Rh antibodies.

7. During a contraction stress test, four contractions lasting 45–55 seconds were recorded in a 10-minute period. A late deceleration was noted during the third contraction. The nurse conducting the test would document that the result is:
   a. negative.
   b. positive.
   c. suspicious.
   d. unsatisfactory.

8. A pregnant woman is scheduled for a transvaginal ultrasound test to establish gestational age. In preparing this woman for the test, the nurse would:
   a. place the woman in a supine position with her hips elevated on a folded pillow.
   b. instruct her to come for the test with a full bladder.
   c. administer an analgesic 30 minutes before the test.
   d. lubricate the vaginal probe with transmission gel.

III. CLINICAL JUDGMENT AND NEXT-GENERATION NCLEX® EXAMINATION-STYLE QUESTIONS

1. Annie is a primigravida who is at 10 weeks of gestation. Her prenatal history reveals that she was treated for pelvic inflammatory disease 2 years ago. She describes irregular menstrual cycles and is therefore unsure about the first day of her last menstrual period. Annie is scheduled for a transvaginal ultrasound.

    a. Cite the likely reasons for the performance of this test.

    b. Describe how the nurse should prepare Annie for this test.

2. Latisha, a pregnant woman at 20 weeks of gestation, is scheduled for a series of transabdominal ultrasounds to monitor the growth of her fetus. Describe the nursing role as it applies to Latisha and transabdominal ultrasound examinations.

3. Aanya is a G1P0 at 42 weeks of gestation. She is pregnant with a female. Her physician has ordered a biophysical profile (BPP). She is very upset and tells the nurse, "All my doctor told me is that this test will see if my baby is okay. I do not know what is going to happen and if it will be painful to me or harmful for my baby." **Choose the most likely options for the information missing from the nurse's statements below by selecting from the lists of options provided**.

    A biophysical profile is a <u>1</u> used to see how your baby is developing. It shows us how the baby is moving, how her tone is, and we can see her heart rate activity and generally tell how she is doing. If your baby is in <u>2</u> state, we may need to watch her longer to get the information we need. The test will not be painful to you or harm your baby. The BPP will get scored based on her breathing movements, fetal movements, fetal tone, amniotic fluid, and the results of the nonstress test. A score of <u>3</u> is considered a normal result.

Options for 1	Options for 2	Options for 3
small intrauterine probe	an active	4–6
type of amniocentesis	a disturbed sleep	6–8
noninvasive ultrasound	an irritable	8–10
MRI	a quiet sleep	10–12

4. Jan, age 42, is 18 weeks pregnant. Because of her age, Jan's fetus is at risk for genetic anomalies. Jan's blood type is A negative and her partner's, the father of her baby, is B positive. Her primary health care provider has suggested an amniocentesis. Describe the nurse's role in terms of each of the following:

    a. Preparing Jan for the amniocentesis

    b. Supporting Jan during the procedure

c. Providing Jan with postprocedure care and instructions

5. Marisol, who has diabetes and is in week 36 of pregnancy, has been scheduled for a nonstress test.

   a. Discuss what you would tell Marisol about the purpose of this test and what will be learned about her baby's well-being.

   b. Describe how you would prepare Marisol for this test.

   c. Discuss how you would conduct the test.

   d. Indicate the criteria you would use to determine whether the result of the test was:

      i. Reactive

      ii. Nonreactive

6. Chi is scheduled for a contraction stress test following a nonreactive result on a nonstress test. Nipple stimulation will be used to stimulate the required contractions.

   a. Discuss what you would tell Beth about the purpose of this test and what will be learned about the well-being of her fetus.

   b. Describe how you would prepare Chi for the test.

   c. Indicate how you would conduct the test.

   d. State how you would conduct the test differently if exogenous oxytocin (Pitocin) is used instead of nipple stimulation.

e. Indicate the criteria you would use to determine whether the result of the test was:

   i. Negative

   ii. Positive

   iii. Equivocal-Suspicious

   iv. Equivocal

   v. Unsatisfactory

11 High-Risk Perinatal Care: Preexisting Conditions

I. LEARNING KEY TERMS

FILL IN THE BLANKS: Insert the term that corresponds to each of the following descriptions related to diabetes mellitus.

1. _____ A group of metabolic diseases characterized by hyperglycemia resulting from defects in insulin secretion, insulin action, or both.

2. _____ Accumulation of excessive glucose in the blood.

3. _____ A normal blood glucose level.

4. _____ Blood glucose level that is too low.

5. _____ Excretion of large volumes of urine.

6. _____ Excessive thirst.

7. _____ Excessive eating.

8. _____ Excretion of unusable glucose into the urine.

9. _____ Accumulation of ketones in the blood resulting from hyperglycemia and leading to metabolic acidosis.

10. _____ Classification of diabetes mellitus primarily caused by pancreatic islet beta cell destruction and prone to ketoacidosis; persons with this form of diabetes usually have an absolute insulin deficiency.

11. _____ Most prevalent classification of diabetes mellitus; persons with this form of diabetes have insulin resistance and usually relative (rather than absolute) insulin deficiency.

12. _____ Label given to diabetes mellitus that existed before pregnancy.

13. _____ Diabetes mellitus diagnosed during the second or the third trimester that was clearly not present prior to pregnancy.

14. _____ Blood test that provides a measurement of glycemic control over time, specifically over the previous 2–6 weeks.

15. _____ Excessive fetal growth; birth weight greater than 4000–4500 g or greater than the 90th percentile.

16. _____ Excessive amniotic fluid.

17. _____ Secreting large amounts of insulin.

FILL IN THE BLANKS: Insert the term that corresponds to each of the following descriptions related to selected preexisting medical disorders during pregnancy.

18. _____ Inability of the heart to maintain a sufficient cardiac output. Physiologic stress on the heart is greatest between week _____ and _____ of gestation because the cardiac output is at its peak.

19. _____ Classification system for cardiovascular disorders developed by the New York Heart Association. Class I implies _____. Class II implies _____. Class III implies _____ Class IV implies _____.

20. _____ Cardiac disorder characterized by the development of congestive heart failure in the last month of pregnancy or within 5 postpartum months, lack of another cause for heart failure, and the absence of heart disease before the last month of pregnancy; etiology for the disorder may be related to genetic predisposition, autoimmunity, and viral infections.

21. _____ Damage of the heart valves and the chordae tendineae cordis as a result of an infection originating from an inadequately treated group A beta-hemolytic streptococcal infection of the throat.

22. _____ Narrowing of the valve between the left atrium and the left ventricle of the heart by stiffening of the valve leaflets, which obstructs blood flow from the atrium to the ventricles. _____ Narrowing of the opening of the aortic valve.

23. _____ Acute ischemic event involving cardiac muscle.

24. _____ Inflammation of the innermost lining of the heart caused by invasion of bacteria.

25. _____ Common, usually benign, cardiac condition that involves the protrusion of the leaflets of the mitral valve back into the left atrium during ventricular systole, allowing some backflow of blood.

26. _____ A hemoglobin level of less than 11 g/dL in the first and third trimester and less than 10.5 gm/dL in the second trimester; it is mainly a result of an _____ deficiency.

27. _____ Disease caused by the presence of abnormal hemoglobin in the blood. It is a recessive, hereditary, familial hemolytic anemia that affects those of African or Mediterranean ancestry.

28. _____ Relatively common anemia in which an insufficient amount of hemoglobin is produced to fill red blood cells.

29. _____ Chronic respiratory inflammatory disorder caused by allergens, irritants, marked changes in ambient temperature, certain medications, or exercise. In response to stimuli, there is widespread but reversible narrowing of the hyperactive airways making it difficult to breathe.

30. _____ Common autosomal recessive genetic disorder in which the exocrine glands produce excessive viscous secretions, causing problems with both respiratory and digestive functions.

31. _____ Generalized itching during pregnancy without the presence of a rash.

32. _____ Integumentary condition during pregnancy characterized by itching and urticarial papules and plaques most often appearing during the mid to late third trimester.

33. _____ Liver disorder unique to pregnancy that is characterized by generalized pruritus, usually beginning during the third trimester, most severely affecting the palms and soles, and is worse at night.

34. _____ Disorder of the brain causing recurrent seizures; it is the most common neurologic disorder accompanying pregnancy.

35. _____ Patchy demyelinization of the spinal cord and CNS may be viral in origin.

36. _____ Acute idiopathic facial paralysis that can occur during pregnancy.

37. _____ Chronic, multisystem, inflammatory disease characterized by autoimmune antibody production that affects the skin, joints, kidneys, lungs, central nervous system (CNS), liver, and other body organs.

II. REVIEWING KEY CONCEPTS

1. Identify the major maternal and fetal/neonatal risks and complications associated with pregnancies complicated by diabetes mellitus. Indicate the underlying pathophysiologic basis for each of the complications you identify.

2. Explain the current recommendations for screening for and diagnosing of gestational diabetes mellitus.

3. State how hyperthyroidism and hypothyroidism can affect reproductive well-being and pregnancy.

4. Identify the maternal and fetal complications that are more common among pregnant women who have cardiac problems.

5. State how the 4*P*s Plus Screening Tool could be used during pregnancy and the information it is designed to gather.

6. A pregestational diabetic woman at 20 weeks of gestation exhibits the following: thirst, nausea and vomiting, abdominal pain, drowsiness, and increased urination. Her skin is flushed and dry and her breathing is rapid with a fruity odor. A priority nursing action when caring for this woman would be to:
   a. provide the woman with a simple carbohydrate immediately.
   b. request an order for an antiemetic.
   c. assist the woman into a lateral position to rest.
   d. administer insulin according to the woman's blood glucose level.

7. During her pregnancy, a woman with pregestational diabetes has been monitoring her blood glucose level several times a day. Which of the following levels would require further assessment?
   a. 85 mg/dL—before breakfast
   b. 90 mg/dL—before lunch
   c. 135 mg/dL—2 hours after supper
   d. 126 mg/dL—1 hour after breakfast

8. A nurse is working with a woman with pregestational diabetes mellitus to plan the diet she will follow during pregnancy. Which of the following nutritional guidelines should be used to ensure a euglycemic state and appropriate weight gain? Select all that apply.
   a. Substantial bedtime snack composed of complex carbohydrates with some protein and fat

   b. Average calories per day of 2200 during the first trimester and 2500 during the second and third trimesters
   c. Caloric distribution among three meals and one or two snacks
   d. Minimum of 45% carbohydrate daily
   e. Protein intake of at least 30% of the total kilo-calories in a day
   f. Fat intake of 50%–55% of the daily caloric intake

9. An obese pregnant woman with gestational diabetes is learning self-injection of insulin. While evaluating the woman's technique for self-injection of a mixture of NPH and Rapid-Acting Insulin, the nurse would recognize that the woman understood the instructions when she:
   a. washed her hands and put on a pair of clean gloves.
   b. shook the NPH insulin vial vigorously to fully mix the insulin.
   c. drew the NPH insulin into her syringe first.
   d. spread her skin taut and punctured the skin at a 90-degree angle.

10. When assessing a pregnant woman at 28 weeks of gestation who is diagnosed with mitral valve stenosis, the nurse must be alert for signs indicating cardiac decompensation. Signs of cardiac decompensation would include which of the following? Select all that apply.
    a. Dry, hacking cough
    b. Increasing fatigue
    c. Wheezing with inspiration and expiration
    d. Bradycardia
    e. Progressive generalized edema
    f. Orthopnea with increasing dyspnea

11. A woman at 30 weeks of gestation with a class II cardiac disorder calls her primary health care provider's office and speaks to the nurse practitioner. She tells the nurse that she has been experiencing a frequent, moist cough for the past few days. In addition, she has been feeling more tired and is having difficulty completing her routine activities because of some difficulty with breathing. The nurse's best response would be:
    a. "Have someone bring you to the office so we can assess your cardiac status."
    b. "Try to get more rest during the day because this is a difficult time for your heart."
    c. "Take an extra diuretic tonight before you go to bed, since you may be developing some fluid in your lungs."
    d. "Ask your family to come over and do your housework for the next few days so you can rest."

12. A pregnant woman with a cardiac disorder will begin anticoagulant therapy to prevent clot formation. In preparing this woman for this treatment measure, the nurse would expect to teach the woman about self-administration of which of the following medications?
    a. Furosemide
    b. Propranolol
    c. Heparin
    d. Ibuprofen

13. At a previous antepartum visit, the nurse taught a pregnant woman diagnosed with a class II cardiac disorder about measures to use to lower her risk for cardiac decompensation. This woman will demonstrate need for further instruction if she tells the nurse she will use which of the following measures?
    a. Increase roughage in her diet
    b. Remain on bed rest, getting out of bed only to go to the bathroom
    c. Sleep 10 hours every night and take a short nap after meals
    d. Will call the nurse immediately if she experiences any pain or swelling in her legs

III. CLINICAL JUDGMENT AND NEXT-GENERATION NCLEX® EXAMINATION-STYLE QUESTIONS

1. Mary is a 24-year-old woman with diabetes. When Mary informed her gynecologist that she and her husband are trying to get pregnant, she was referred to her endocrinologist for preconception counseling. Mary tells the nurse that she just cannot understand why this is necessary. "I have had diabetes since I was 12 years old, and I have not had many problems. All I want to do is get pregnant!" Discuss how the nurse should respond to Mary's comments.

2. Luann is a 25-year-old nulliparous woman in her first trimester of pregnancy (6th week of gestation). She has had type 1 diabetes since she was 15 years old. Recently, she has been experiencing some nausea and is eating less as a result. She took her usual dose of regular and NPH insulin before eating a very light breakfast of tea and a piece of toast. Just before her midmorning snack at work, she began to experience nervousness and weakness. She felt dizzy and became diaphoretic and pale. The nurse obtains vital signs and a blood glucose, and the findings are outlined below:

   ■ Oral temperature 37.5 °C

   ■ Respiration rate 20

   ■ Heart rate 108

   ■ Blood pressure 112/65

   ■ Blood glucose 67

   Highlight or place a check mark next to the history and assessment findings that require further follow-up by the nurse.

3. Judy's first pregnancy has just been confirmed. She also has type 1 diabetes.

   a. As a result of her high-risk status, a variety of additional assessment measures are emphasized during her prenatal period to evaluate her status and that of her fetus. Identify these additional assessment measures and their relevance in a diabetic pregnancy.

   b. Discuss the stressors that might confront Judy and her family as a result of her status as a diabetic woman who is pregnant.

   c. Indicate the activity and exercise recommendations that Judy should be given.

   d. Outline the nursing interventions and health teaching for self-management in terms of nutrition, blood glucose monitoring, and insulin requirements at each stage of Judy's pregnancy.

      i. Antepartum

      ii. Intrapartum

      iii. Postpartum

   e. Judy expresses a desire to breastfeed her baby and wonders if this is a good idea for her and her baby. What should the nurse tell Judy about breastfeeding?

   f. Discuss the birth control options that would be best for Judy and her partner.

4. Elena (2-1-0-0-1) is a 32-year-old woman in week 28 of her pregnancy. She is obese. Her mother, who is 59, was recently diagnosed with type 2 diabetes. Elena's first pregnancy resulted in the birth of a 10-pound 6-ounce daughter who is now 2 years old. A 1-hour, 50-g glucose tolerance test last week revealed a glucose level of 152 mg/dL. A 3-hour glucose tolerance test was done yesterday with the following results: Fasting—108 mg/dL, 1 hr—195 mg/dL, 2 hr—170 mg/dL, 3 hr—140 mg/dL.

   a. Identify the complication of pregnancy Elena is exhibiting. State the rationale for your answer.

b. List the risk factors for this health problem that are present in Elena's assessment data.

c. Describe the pathophysiology involved in creating Elena's problem.

d. Identify the maternal and fetal/neonatal risks and complications that are possible in this situation.

e. Outline the ongoing assessment measures necessitated by Elena's health problem.

f. State two nursing diagnoses for Elena and her fetus.

g. Describe how Elena should be advised to maintain euglycemia for the remainder of her pregnancy. Explain to her why euglycemia is so important.

h. Before discharge after the birth of her second daughter, Elena asks the nurse whether the health problem she experienced during this pregnancy will continue now that she has had her baby. She also wonders if it will happen with her next pregnancy because she wants to get pregnant again soon so she can "try for a son." Discuss the response the nurse should give to Elena's concerns.

5. Linda, age 26, had rheumatic fever as a child and subsequently developed mitral valve stenosis. She is presently 6 weeks pregnant. She is classified as class II according to the New York Heart Association functional classification of heart disease. This is the first pregnancy for Linda and her husband, Sam.

a. Discuss a recommended therapeutic plan for Linda that will reduce her risk for cardiac decompensation in terms of each of the following:

i. Rest/sleep/activity patterns

ii. Prevention of infection

iii. Nutrition

iv. Bowel elimination

Chapter **11** **High-Risk Perinatal Care: Preexisting Conditions**

b. Identify physiological and psychosocial factors that could increase the stress placed on Linda's heart during her pregnancy.

Physiologic factors   Psychosocial factors

c. List the subjective symptoms that the nurse should teach Linda and her family to look for as indicators of possible cardiac decompensation.

d. List the objective signs that could indicate that Linda is experiencing signs of cardiac decompensation and heart failure.

e. Linda is admitted to the labor unit. Her cardiac condition is still classified as class II. Outline the nursing measures designed to assess Linda and promote optimum cardiac function during labor and birth.

f. Linda should be observed carefully during the postpartum period because cardiac risk continues. Indicate the physiologic events after birth that place Linda at risk for cardiac decompensation.

g. Discuss the measures the nurse can use to reduce the stress placed on Linda's heart during the postpartum period.

h. Linda indicates that she wishes to breastfeed her infant. Describe the nurse's response.

i. Identify the important factors to be considered when preparing Linda's discharge plan.

6. Allison is a pregnant woman at risk for thromboembolism. As part of her medical regimen, her primary health care provider has prescribed subcutaneous heparin.

a. Allison states, "I cannot give myself a shot! Why can't I just take the medication orally?" Discuss how you would respond as to the purpose of heparin and the indications for use during pregnancy.

b. Indicate the information that the nurse should give Allison to ensure safe use of the heparin.

7. Jean is a primigravida at 4 weeks of gestation. She has been an epileptic for several years and her seizures have been controlled with levetiracetam (Keppra). Jean expresses concern regarding how her medication use will affect her pregnancy and her baby. She wants to stop taking the levetiracetam. Describe the approach you would take in addressing Jean's concern and the course of action she is contemplating.

8. Imagine that you are an advanced practice nurse who specializes in the treatment of men and women who are alcohol and drug dependent. You have been asked to establish a treatment program specifically designed for pregnant women. Outline the approach you would take to ensure that the program you establish takes into consideration the unique characteristics and needs of women in general and pregnant women who abuse alcohol and drugs.

Chapter **11** **High-Risk Perinatal Care: Preexisting Conditions**

12 High-Risk Perinatal Care: Gestational Conditions

I. LEARNING KEY TERMS

FILL IN THE BLANKS: Insert the term that corresponds to each of the following descriptions related to fetal assessment.

1. _____ A systolic BP greater than 140 mm Hg or a diastolic BP greater than 90 mm Hg recorded on two separate occasions at least 4–6 hours apart.

2. _____ Development of hypertension after week 20 of pregnancy in a previously normotensive woman without proteinuria.

3. _____ Pregnancy-specific syndrome in which hypertension and proteinuria develop after 20 weeks of gestation in a woman who previously had neither condition.

4. _____ Presence of a BP of 160/110 mm Hg or greater on 2 or more occasions at least 4 hours apart. Other signs and symptoms reflective of multisystem organ involvement are also present.

5. _____ Onset of seizure activity in the woman with preeclampsia.

6. _____ Hypertension present before pregnancy or diagnosed during pregnancy but persists postpartum.

7. _____ Process which results in poor tissue perfusion in organ systems, increased peripheral resistance and blood pressure, and increased cellular permeability. Protein and fluid loss occurs and plasma volume is reduced.

8. _____ Laboratory diagnosis for a variant of severe preeclampsia that involves hepatic dysfunction; it is characterized by _____, _____, and _____.

9. _____ Protein concentration of ≥300 mg/24 hours or a protein/creatinine ratio greater than 0.3.

10. _____ Preeclampsia usually resolves within this timeframe after birth.

11. _____ Excessive vomiting during pregnancy that leads to significant weight loss along with dehydration, electrolyte imbalance, nutritional deficiency, and ketonuria.

12. _____ Pregnancy that ends as a result of natural causes before 20 weeks of gestation or less than 500 g birthweight.

13. _____ Pregnancy in which the fetus has died but the products of conception are retained in utero for up to several weeks.

14. _____ Three or more consecutive pregnancy losses before 20 weeks of gestation. Some authorities now recommend the definition to be two or more pregnancy losses before 20 weeks.

15. _____ Passive and painless dilation of the cervix during the second trimester leading to recurrent preterm births during the second trimester in the absence of other causes.

16. _____ Procedure that involves placement of a suture around the cervix beneath the mucosa to constrict the internal os of the cervix.

17. _____ Pregnancy in which the fertilized ovum is implanted outside the uterine cavity, most often in the uterine tube.

18. _____ A benign proliferative growth of the placental trophoblast in which the chorionic villi develop into edematous, cystic, avascular transparent vesicles that hang in a grapelike cluster.

19. _____ Disorder that results when an egg without an active nucleus has been fertilized.

20. _____ Disorder that results when two sperms fertilize an apparently normal ovum.

21. _____ Implantation of the placenta in the lower uterine segment totally covering the internal cervical os.

22. _____ Implantation of the placenta in the lower uterine segment without reaching the os.

23. _____ Detachment of part or all of the placenta from its implantation site.

24. _____ Condition in which the fetal vessels are implanted into the fetal membranes rather than the placenta. They often lie over the cervical os. _____ Variation of vasa previa in which the cord vessels begin to branch at the membranes and then course into the placenta. _____ A second variation of vasa previa in which the placenta is divided into two or more lobes rather than remaining as a single mass. Fetal vessels run between the lobes and collect at the periphery, eventually uniting to form the vessels of the umbilical cord.

25. _____ Marginal insertion of the cord into the placenta, which also increases the risk for fetal hemorrhage.

26. _____ Pathologic form of clotting that is diffuse and consumes large amounts of clotting factors, causing widespread external or internal bleeding or both.

27. _____ Persistent presence of bacteria within the urinary tract of women who have no symptoms.

28. _____ Bladder infection characterized by dysuria, urgency, and frequency, along with lower abdominal or suprapubic pain.

29. _____ Renal infection that is a common serious medical complication of pregnancy and the leading cause of septic shock during pregnancy.

30. _____ The most common nonobstetric surgical emergency during pregnancy.

31. _____ Presence of gallstones in the gallbladder.

32. _____ Inflammation of the gallbladder.

II. REVIEWING KEY CONCEPTS

1. Describe the differences between preeclampsia and preeclampsia with severe features.

2. Describe the assessment technique used to determine whether the following findings are present in women with preeclampsia. (Note: You may wish to review this information in a physical assessment textbook for a complete explanation of each technique.)

   a. Hyperreflexia and ankle clonus

   b. Proteinuria

   c. Pitting edema

MATCHING: Match the client description with the appropriate diagnosis.

3. _____ At 30 weeks of gestation, a woman's BP is consistently above 140/90; her latest urinalysis indicated a protein level of 2+ on dipstick; biceps and patellar reflexes are 2+.

4. _____ At 24 weeks of gestation, a normotensive woman's BP rose from a prepregnant baseline of 118/70 to 148/92 and 151/93 on separate occasions. No other problematic signs and symptoms including proteinuria were noted.

5. _____ A 34-year-old pregnant woman has had a consistently high BP ranging from 148/92 to 160/98 since she was 28 years old. Her weight gain has followed normal patterns, and urinalysis remains normal as well.

6. _____ At 32 weeks of gestation, a woman, with hypertension since 28 weeks, hyperactive DTRs with clonus, and proteinuria of 4+, has a convulsion.

7. _____ A pregnant woman has been hypertensive since her 24th week of pregnancy. Urinalysis indicates a protein content of 3+. Further testing reveals a platelet count of 95,000 and elevated AST and ALT levels; she has begun to experience nausea with some vomiting and epigastric pain.

a. Eclampsia

b. Chronic hypertension

c. Gestational hypertension

d. HELLP syndrome

e. Preeclampsia

MATCHING: Match the medication description with the appropriate medication.

8. _____ Drug of choice in the prevention and treatment of seizure activity (eclampsia) caused by severe preeclampsia.

9. _____ Intravenous antihypertensive agent that works primarily by dilating peripheral arterioles; use cautiously in the presence of maternal tachycardia.

10. _____ Antihypertensive agent of choice for the treatment of chronic hypertension during pregnancy.

11. _____ Antiemetic medication that is recommended to treat hyperemesis gravidarum.

12. _____ Synthetic prostaglandin E_1 analog administered orally or vaginally as part of the medical management of a miscarriage.

13. _____ Antimetabolite and folic acid antagonist that is used to destroy rapidly dividing cells; it is used for the medical management of an unruptured ectopic pregnancy.

14. _____ Prostaglandin derivative that can be administered intramuscularly to contract the uterus and treat excessive bleeding following evacuating the products of conception when a miscarriage has occurred.

15. _____ Antihypertensive medication that reduces systemic vascular resistance and can be used if blood pressure not adequately controlled with labetalol.

a. Pyridoxine

b. Methotrexate

c. Magnesium sulfate

d. Labetalol

e. Nifedipine

f. Methylcarboprost tromethamine

g. Hydralazine

h. Misoprostol

16. When measuring the BP to ensure consistency and to facilitate early detection of BP changes consistent with gestational hypertension, the nurse should:
    a. place the woman in a supine position.
    b. allow the woman to rest for at least 15 minutes before measuring her BP.
    c. use the same arm for each BP measurement.
    d. use a proper sized cuff that covers at least 50% of her upper arm.

17. When caring for a woman with mild preeclampsia, it is critical that during assessment the nurse is alert for

signs of progress to severe preeclampsia. Progress to severe preeclampsia would be indicated by which one of the following assessment findings?
   a. Severe persistent epigastric or right upper quadrant pain
   b. Platelet level of 200,000/mm^3
   c. Deep tendon reflexes 2+, ankle clonus is absent
   d. BP of 154/94 and 156/100, 6 hours apart

18. A woman's preeclampsia has advanced to the severe stage. She is admitted to the hospital and her primary health care provider has ordered an infusion of magnesium sulfate be started. In fulfilling this order the nurse would implement which of the following? Select all that apply.
   a. Prepare a loading dose of 2 g of magnesium sulfate in 200 mL of 5% glucose in water to be given over 15 minutes.
   b. Prepare the maintenance solution by mixing 40 g of magnesium sulfate in 1000 mL of lactated Ringer solution.
   c. Monitor maternal vital signs, fetal heart rate (FHR) patterns, and uterine contractions every 2 hours.
   d. Expect the maintenance dose to be approximately 2 g/hour.
   e. Report a respiratory rate of 14 breaths or less per minute to the primary health care provider immediately.
   f. Recognize that urinary output should be at least 25–30 mL per hour.

19. The primary expected outcome for care associated with the administration of magnesium sulfate would be met if the woman exhibits which of the following?
   a. Exhibits a decrease in both systolic and diastolic BP
   b. Experiences no seizures
   c. States that she feels more relaxed and calm
   d. Urinates more frequently, resulting in a decrease in pathologic edema

20. A woman has just been admitted with a diagnosis of hyperemesis gravidarum. She has been unable to retain any oral intake and as a result has lost weight and is exhibiting signs of dehydration with electrolyte imbalance and acetonuria. The care management of this woman would include which of the following?
   a. Administering labetalol to control nausea and vomiting
   b. Assessing the woman's urine for ketones
   c. Avoiding oral hygiene until the woman is able to tolerate oral fluids
   d. Providing small frequent meals consisting of bland foods and warm fluids together once the woman begins to respond to treatment

21. A primigravida at 10 weeks of gestation reports slight vaginal spotting without passage of tissue and mild uterine cramping. When examined, no cervical dilation is noted. The nurse caring for this woman would:
   a. anticipate that the woman will be sent home and placed on bed rest with instructions to avoid stress and orgasm.
   b. prepare the woman for a dilation and curettage.
   c. inform the woman that frequent blood tests will be required to check the level of estrogen.
   d. tell the woman that the doctor will most likely perform a cerclage to help her maintain her pregnancy.

22. A woman is admitted through the emergency room with a medical diagnosis of ruptured ectopic pregnancy. The primary nursing diagnosis at this time would be:
   a. acute pain related to irritation of the peritoneum with blood.
   b. risk for infection related to tissue trauma.
   c. deficient fluid volume related to blood loss associated with rupture of the uterine tube.
   d. anticipatory grieving related to unexpected pregnancy outcome.

23. A woman diagnosed with an ectopic pregnancy is given an intramuscular injection of methotrexate. The nurse would tell the woman which of the following?
   a. Methotrexate is an analgesic that will relieve the dull abdominal pain she is experiencing.
   b. Gastric distress, nausea and vomiting, stomatitis, and dizziness are common. Rare side effects include severe neutropenia, reversible hair loss, and pneumonitis.
   c. Follow-up blood tests will be required every other month for 6 months after the injection of the methotrexate.
   d. She should continue to take her prenatal vitamin and folic acid to enhance healing.

24. A pregnant woman at 32 weeks of gestation comes to the emergency room because she has begun to experience bright red vaginal bleeding. She reports that she is experiencing no pain. The admission nurse suspects:
   a. abruptio placentae.
   b. disseminated intravascular coagulation.
   c. placenta previa.
   d. preterm labor.

25. A pregnant woman, at 38 weeks of gestation diagnosed with marginal placenta previa, has just given birth to a healthy newborn male. The nurse recognizes that the immediate focus for the care of this woman would be:
   a. preventing hemorrhage.
   b. relieving pain.
   c. preventing infection.
   d. fostering attachment of the woman with her new son.

1. Jean (1-0-0-0-0) is at 30 weeks of gestation and has been diagnosed with mild preeclampsia. The treatment plan includes home care with limited activity consisting of bed rest with bathroom privileges and out of bed twice a day for meals, appropriate nutrition, and stress reduction. She and her husband are very anxious about the diagnosis and are also concerned about how they will manage the care of their active 3-year-old adopted daughter, Anne.

    a. What factors could be present in Jean's history that would increase her risk for developing preeclampsia?

    b. Indicate the clinical manifestations that would be present to indicate this diagnosis.

    c. Describe how you would help this couple organize their home care routine.

    d. Specify what you would teach them about the assessment of Jean's status in terms of each of the following:

        i. BP

        ii. Protein in urine

        iii. Fetal well-being

        iv. Signs of a worsening condition

    e. Describe the instructions you would give Jean regarding her nutrient and fluid intake.

    f. Discuss the measures Jean can use to cope with the boredom and alteration in circulation and muscle tone that accompany bed rest.

    g. Limited activity can lead to a nursing diagnosis of constipation related to changes in bowel function associated with pregnancy and limited activity. Cite two measures that Jean can use to enhance bowel elimination and prevent constipation.

2. Aaliyah, a pregnant woman at 37 weeks of gestation, is admitted to the hospital with a diagnosis of severe preeclampsia.

   a. Indicate the signs and symptoms that would be present to indicate this diagnosis.

   b. Specify the precautionary measures that should be taken to protect Aaliyah and her fetus from injury.

   c. Aaliyah's physician orders magnesium sulfate to be infused at 4 g in 20 minutes as a loading dose, and then a maintenance intravenous infusion of 2 g/hr.

   - Identify the guidelines that must be followed when preparing and administering the magnesium sulfate infusion.

   - Explain the expected therapeutic effect of magnesium sulfate to Aaliyah and her family.

   d. List the maternal–fetal assessments that should be accomplished on a regular basis during the infusion of magnesium sulfate.

   - Identify the progressive signs of magnesium sulfate toxicity.

   - State the interventions that must be instituted immediately if magnesium sulfate toxicity occurs.

   e. Despite all prevention efforts, Aaliyah has a convulsion.

   - Specify the nursing measures that should be implemented at the onset of the convulsion and immediately afterward.

   - List the problems that can occur as a result of the convulsion that Aaliyah experienced.

   f. Aaliyah successfully gave birth vaginally despite her high-risk status. Describe Aaliyah's care management during the first 48 hours of her postpartum recovery period.

Chapter **12** **High-Risk Perinatal Care: Gestational Conditions**

3. Marie, an 18-year-old obese primigravida at 9 weeks of gestation, is diagnosed with hyperemesis gravidarum. She is unmarried and lives at home with her parents. Marie is admitted to the high risk antepartal unit. During the admission interview, Marie confides to the nurse that her parents have been very unhappy about her pregnancy. She now is worried that she may have made the wrong decision to continue with her pregnancy and raise her baby as a single parent.

   a. Identify the etiologic factors that may have contributed to Marie's current health problem.

   b. List the physiologic and psychologic factors that the nurse should be alert for when assessing Marie upon her admission.

   c. State one nursing diagnosis related to Marie's current health status.

   d. Outline the nursing care measures appropriate for Marie while hospitalized.

   e. Once stabilized, Marie is discharged to home care. She is able to tolerate oral food and fluid intake. Explain the important care measures that the nurse should discuss with Marie and her family before she goes home.

4. Andrea is admitted to the hospital, where a diagnosis of acute unruptured ectopic pregnancy in her fallopian tube is made.

   a. State the risk factors associated with ectopic pregnancy.

   b. Describe the findings that were most likely experienced and exhibited by Andrea as her ectopic pregnancy progressed and then ruptured.

   c. Identify the other health care problems that share the same or similar clinical manifestations as ectopic pregnancy.

   d. State the major care management problem at this time. Support your answer.

   e. Outline the nursing measures Andrea will require during the preoperative and postoperative period.

5. Janet is 10 weeks pregnant. She comes to the clinic and states that she has been experiencing slight bleeding with mild cramping for about 4 hours. No tissue has been passed and pelvic examination reveals that the cervical os is closed.

   a. Indicate the most likely basis for Janet's signs and symptoms.

   b. Outline the expected care management of Janet's problem.

6. Denise, a primigravida, calls the clinic. She is crying while she tells the nurse that she has noted "a lot of bleeding" and that she is sure she is losing her baby.

   a. Write several questions the nurse should ask Denise to obtain a more definitive picture of the bleeding she is experiencing.

   b. Based on the data collected, Denise is admitted to the hospital for further evaluation. A medical diagnosis of incomplete abortion is made. Describe the assessment findings that would indicate the diagnosis of incomplete abortion.

   c. State the nursing diagnosis that would take priority at this time.

   d. Outline the nursing measures that would be appropriate for the priority nursing diagnosis you identified and for the expected medical management of Denise's health problem.

   e. Specify the instructions that Denise should receive before her discharge from the hospital.

   f. List the nursing measures appropriate for the following nursing diagnosis: Anticipatory grieving related to unexpected outcome of pregnancy.

7. Saira has been diagnosed with hydatidiform mole (complete).

   a. Identify the typical signs and symptoms Saira would most likely exhibit to establish this diagnosis.

b. Specify the posttreatment instructions that the nurse must stress when discussing follow-up management with Saira.

c. Name the major concern associated with complete hydatidiform mole and indicate the signs that would indicate that it is occurring.

8. Two pregnant women are admitted to the labor unit with vaginal bleeding. Sara is at 29 weeks of gestation and is diagnosed with marginal placenta previa. Jane is at 34 weeks of gestation and is diagnosed with a moderate (grade II) premature separation of the placenta (abruptio placentae).

a. Compare the clinical picture each of these women is likely to exhibit during assessment.

Sara	Jane

b. Identify one priority nursing diagnosis for both Sara and Jane.

c. Contrast the care management approach required by each of the women as it relates to their diagnosis and the typical medical management.

Sara	Jane

d. Indicate the considerations that must be given top priority following birth for each of these women.

Sara	Jane

9. Trauma continues to be a common complication during pregnancy that may require obstetric critical care.

a. Discuss the significance of this complication using statistical data to describe the scope of the problem in terms of incidence, timing during pregnancy, and forms of trauma.

b. Indicate the effects trauma can have on pregnancy.

c. Describe the potential impact of trauma on the fetus.

d. Identify the priorities of care for the pregnant woman following trauma.

e. Outline the major components of the assessment and care of a pregnant woman who has experienced trauma.

Primary survey

Secondary survey

f. Explain how cardiopulmonary resuscitation (CPR) should be adapted for a pregnant woman.

10. *NGN Item Type: Extended multiple response exercise*

A woman has been diagnosed with mild preeclampsia and will be treated at home. The nurse, in teaching this woman about her treatment regimen for mild preeclampsia, would tell her to do which of the following? Select all that apply.

a. Check her respirations before and after taking her oral dose of magnesium sulfate.

b. Monitor blood pressure and report any increases to health care provider.

c. Reduce her fluid intake to four to five 8-ounce glasses each day.

d. Do gentle exercises such as hand and feet circles and gently tensing and relaxing arm and leg muscles.

e. Avoid excessively salty foods.

f. Maintain strict bed rest in a quiet dimly lighted room with minimal stimuli.

g. Monitor for headaches, right upper quadrant pain, or epigastric pain

h. Take 325 mg aspirin every 6 hours as needed for headache

13 Labor and Birth Processes

I. LEARNING KEY TERMS

FILL IN THE BLANKS: Insert the term that corresponds to each of the following descriptions

1. _____, _____, _____, _____, and _____ The five factors or "Ps" of labor and birth.

2. _____ Membrane-filled spaces that are located where more than two bones meet on the fetal skull.

3. _____ Slight overlapping of the bones of the fetal skull that occurs during childbirth; it permits the skull to adapt to the various pelvic diameters.

4. _____ Part of the fetus that enters the pelvic inlet first. The three main types are _____ (head first), _____ (buttocks first), and _____.

5. _____ Part of the fetal body first felt by the examining finger during a vaginal examination. The three parts are _____, _____, and _____.

6. _____ Relationship of the long axis (spine) of the fetus to the long axis (spine) of the mother. There are two types: _____, when the spines are parallel to each other, and _____, when the spines are at right angles or diagonal to each other.

7. _____ Relationship of the fetal body parts to one another. The most common type is one of general _____.

8. _____ Largest transverse diameter of the fetal skull. _____ Smallest anteroposterior diameter of the fetal skull

to enter the maternal pelvis when the fetal head is in complete flexion.

9. _____ Relationship of a reference point on the fetal presenting part to the four quadrants of the maternal pelvis.

10. _____ Term that indicates that the largest transverse diameter of the presenting part has passed through the maternal pelvic brim or inlet into the true pelvis, reaching the level of the ischial spines.

11. _____ Relationship of the presenting part of the fetus to an imaginary line drawn between the maternal ischial spines; this is a measure of the degree of fetal descent through the birth canal.

12. _____ and _____ The two components of the maternal passageway or birth canal.

13. _____ Shortening and thinning of the cervix during the first stage of labor; it is expressed as a percentage.

14. _____ Enlargement or widening of the cervical opening (os) and the cervical canal, which occurs once labor has begun; degree of progress is expressed in centimeters (cm) from less than 1 cm to 10 cm.

15. _____ Descent of the fetal presenting part into the true pelvis approximately 2 weeks before term for the primigravida and after uterine contractions are established and true labor is in progress for the multipara.

16. _____ Primary powers of labor.

17. _____ Secondary powers of labor.

18. _____ Brownish or blood-tinged cervical mucus representing the passage of the mucus plug as the cervix ripens in preparation for labor.

19. _____ The seven turns and adjustments of the fetal head, to facilitate passage through the birth canal. In a vertex presentation, these turns and adjustments include _____, _____, _____, _____, _____, _____, and finally birth by _____.

20. _____ Pushing method discouraged during the second stage of labor characterized by a closed glottis with prolonged bearing down.

21. _____ The second stage of labor is composed of two phases: _____ and _____.

22. _____ Process of moving the fetus, placenta, and membranes out of the uterus and through the birth canal.

23. _____ Maternal urge to bear down that occurs when the fetal presenting part reaches the perineal floor and stretching of the cervix and vagina occur; oxytocin is released.

24. _____ The stage of labor which is considered to last from the onset of _____ to full dilation of the cervix. It is traditionally divided into two phases, namely _____ and _____.

25. _____ The stage of labor which lasts from the time the cervix is fully _____ to the _____.

26. _____ The stage of labor which lasts from the birth of the infant until the _____ is delivered.

27. _____ The stage of labor which is the period of time immediately after the _____ and lasts until the woman's condition is considered stable.

28. _____, _____, _____, and _____ The four factors that affect fetal circulation during labor.

29. _____ Morphine-like chemicals produced naturally in the body, which raise the pain threshold and produce sedation.

II. REVIEWING KEY CONCEPTS

1. Describe how the five factors (the five Ps) affect the process of labor and birth.

2. A vaginal examination during labor reveals the following information: LOA, −1, 75%, 3 cm. An accurate interpretation of this data would include which of the following? Select all that apply.
   a. Attitude: flexed
   b. Station: 3 cm below the ischial spines
   c. Presentation: cephalic
   d. Lie: longitudinal
   e. Effacement: 75% complete
   f. Dilation: 9 cm more to reach full dilation

3. Changes occur as a woman progresses through labor. Which of the following maternal adaptations would be expected during labor? Select all that apply.
   a. Increase in both systolic and diastolic blood pressure during uterine contractions in the first stage of labor
   b. Decrease in white blood cell count
   c. Slight increase in heart rate during the first and second stages of labor
   d. Decrease in gastric motility leading to nausea and vomiting during the first stage of labor
   e. Hypoglycemia
   f. Proteinuria up to 1+

4. A nurse is instructing a group of primigravid women about the onset of labor. Which of the following signs could the women observe preceding the onset of their labors? Select all that apply.
   a. Urinary frequency
   b. Weight gain of 2 kg
   c. Quickening
   d. Energy surge
   e. Bloody show
   f. Shortness of breath

1. As part of their care of the laboring woman, nurses perform vaginal examinations and interpret the results. State the meaning of each of the following vaginal examination findings.

Exam I	Exam II	Exam III	Exam IV
ROP	RMA	LST	OA
−1	0	+1	+3
50%	25%	75%	100%
3 cm	2 cm	6 cm	10 cm

2. Brooke is a primigravida at 36 weeks of gestation. She is pregnant with a male and desires an unmedicated birth. During a prenatal visit at 34 weeks of gestation, she asks you the following questions regarding her approaching labor. **Indicate which nursing response listed in the far-left column is most appropriate for each of Brooke's questions. Note that not all responses will be used.**

Nurse's Responses	Mother's Statements	Appropriate Nurse's Response for each Question
"Labor starts when your progesterone levels increase to a high enough level to start uterine contractions."	"What gets labor to start?"	
"Yes, this is an excellent way to push while having your baby."	"Are there things I should watch for that would tell me my labor is getting closer to starting?"	
"There is no one single cause, there will be changes to your hormones, uterus, and cervix as true labor begins."	"My friend just had a baby and she told me the nurses kept helping her change her position and even encouraged her to walk! Isn't that dangerous for the baby and painful for the mom?"	
"Unfortunately, there is no way to tell."	"I have heard that the best way to push is to bear down and hold my breath, is this true?"	
"Frequent position changes can actually increase your comfort and reduce fatigue. You should work to find positions that are comfortable for you with the help of your nurse."		
"You may notice a surge of energy, bloody show, a backache, or feeling less pressure below your ribcage."		
"You should try and stay as calm and still as possible during your labor to save your energy for when you need to push."		
"You are actually encouraged to not hold your breath and bear down; this is called the Valsalva maneuver."		

Chapter **13** **Labor and Birth Processes**

14 Maximizing Comfort for the Laboring Woman

I. LEARNING KEY TERMS

FILL IN THE BLANKS: Insert the term that corresponds to each of the following descriptions related to childbirth discomfort and its management.

1. _____ Decreased blood flow to the uterus during a contraction leading to an oxygen deficit.

2. _____ Pain that predominates during the first stage of labor; it results from cervical changes, distention of the lower uterine segment, and uterine ischemia.

3. _____ Pain that predominates during the second stage of labor; it results from stretching and distention of perineal tissues and the pelvic floor to allow passage of the fetus, from distention and traction on the peritoneum and uterocervical supports during contractions, and from lacerations of soft tissues.

4. _____ Pain in labor and birth that originates in the uterus and radiates to the abdominal wall, lumbosacral area of the back, iliac crests, gluteal area, and down the thighs.

5. _____ Level of pain a person is willing to endure.

6. _____ Theory of pain based on the premise that pain sensations travel along sensory nerve pathways to the brain, but only a limited number of sensations or messages can travel through these nerve pathways at one time; by using distraction techniques (e.g., massage, music, focal points, imagery) the capacity of nerve pathways are diminished.

7. _____ Endogenous opioids secreted by the pituitary gland that act on the central and peripheral nervous systems to reduce pain; their level increases during pregnancy and birth, thereby enhancing a woman's ability to tolerate acute pain and reducing anxiety.

8. _____ Relaxed deep breath in through the nose and out through the mouth that begins each breathing pattern and ends each contraction.

9. _____ Paced breathing technique during which a woman breathes at approximately 6–8 breaths per minute (half the normal breathing rate).

10. _____ Paced breathing technique during which a woman breathes at approximately 32–40 breaths per minute (twice the normal breathing rate).

11. _____ Paced breathing technique during which a woman breathes at approximately 32–40 breaths per minute interspersed with blowing out of air in a ratio of 3:1 or 4:1; this technique enhances concentration.

12. _____ Undesirable reaction to a rapid-paced breathing pattern characterized by rapid deep respirations that lead to signs of respiratory alkalosis such as lightheadedness, dizziness, tingling of the fingers, or circumoral numbness. Breathing into a paper bag held tightly around the mouth will help to reestablish normal breathing.

13. _____ Light massage (stroking) of the abdomen or other body part in rhythm with breathing during contractions.

14. _____ Steady pressure against the sacrum using the fist or heel of the hand or a firm object to help the woman cope with the sensations of internal pressure and pain in the lower back.

15. _____ Bathing, showering, or whirlpool baths using warm water to promote comfort and relaxation during labor, stimulate the release of endorphin, close the gate on pain, promote circulation and oxygenation, and help to soften the perineum.

16. _____ Method that involves placement of two pairs of electrodes on either side of the woman's thoracic and sacral spine to provide continuous low-intensity electrical impulses that can be increased during a contraction, thereby stimulating the release of endorphins that make the pain less disturbing

17. _____ Application of pressure over the skin of specific points on the body to promote pain relief.

18. _____ Insertion of fine needles into specific areas of the body to restore the flow of qi (energy) and decrease pain, which is thought to be obstructing the flow of energy.

19. _____ Use of oils distilled from plants, flowers, herbs, and trees to promote health and to treat and balance the mind, body, and spirit.

20. _____ Injection of small amounts of sterile water by using a fine-gauge needle into four locations on the lower back to relieve back pain; effectiveness of this method may be related to the mechanism of counterirritation, gate control, or an increase in the level of endorphins.

II. REVIEWING KEY CONCEPTS

1. Describe the factors that could influence the following nursing diagnosis identified for a woman in labor: Acute pain related to the processes involved in labor and birth.

2. Explain the theoretic basis for using techniques such as massage, stroking, music, and imagery to reduce the sensation of pain during childbirth.

MATCHING: Match the description with the appropriate pharmacologic method for discomfort management during childbirth.

3. _____ Abolition of pain perception by interrupting nerve impulses going to the brain. Loss of sensation (partial or complete) and sometimes loss of consciousness occurs.

4. _____ Method used to repair a tear or hole in the dura mater around the spinal cord as a result of spinal anesthesia; the goal is to prevent or treat postdural puncture headaches (PDPH).

5. _____ Single-injection, subarachnoid anesthesia useful for pain control during birth but not for labor; it is often used for cesarean birth.

6. _____ Systemic analgesic such as nalbuphine and butorphanol that relieves pain without causing significant maternal or neonatal respiratory depression and is less likely to cause nausea and vomiting.

7. _____ Provides rapid perineal anesthesia for performing and repairing an episiotomy or lacerations.

8. _____ Gas mixed with oxygen to provide analgesia during all stages of labor.

9. _____ Medication such as phenothiazines and benzodiazepines that can be used to relieve anxiety, to induce sleep, to augment the effectiveness of analgesics, and to reduce nausea and vomiting.

10. _____ Technique that can be used to block pain transmission without compromising motor ability because an opioid with or without a local anesthetic is injected intrathecally prior to epidural catheter placement; with this technique women are able to walk if they choose to do so.

11. _____ Drug that promptly reverses the effects of opioids, including maternal and neonatal CNS depression, especially respiratory depression.

12. _____ Use of a medication such as an opioid analgesic that is administered IM or IV for pain relief during labor.

13. _____ Alleviation of pain sensation or raising of the pain threshold without loss of consciousness.

14. _____ Relief from pain of uterine contractions and birth by injecting a local anesthetic agent, an opioid, or both into the epidural space.

15. _____ Anesthetic that relieves pain in the lower vagina, vulva, and perineum, making it useful if an episiotomy is to be performed or forceps or vacuum assistance is required to facilitate birth.

16. _____ Systemic analgesic such as morphine or fentanyl that relieves pain and creates a feeling of well-being but can also result in respiratory depression (maternal and neonate), nausea, and vomiting.

a. Opioid agonist-antagonist analgesic

b. Anesthesia

c. Analgesia

d. Combined spinal-epidural analgesic

e. Epidural analgesia/anesthesia (block)

f. Autologous epidural blood patch

g. Local perineal infiltration anesthesia

h. Spinal anesthesia (block)

i. Opioid antagonist

j. Nitrous oxide

k. Pudendal nerve block

l. Systemic analgesic

m. Sedative

n. Opioid agonist analgesic

17. Compare each of the following commonly used methods for nerve block analgesia and anesthesia. Indicate the effects, timing of administration, advantages and disadvantages, and nursing care management for each method in your comparison.

Local perineal infiltration anesthesia

Spinal anesthesia (block)

Epidural anesthesia/analgesia (block)

Combined spinal–epidural analgesia

Epidural and intrathecal opioids

18. Systemic analgesics cross the placenta and affect the fetus.

a. List three factors that influence the effect systemic analgesics have on the fetus.

b. Identify the fetal effects of systemic analgesics.

19. Explain why the intravenous route is preferred to the intramuscular route for the administration of systemic analgesics during labor.

20. In her birth plan, a woman requests that she be allowed to use the new whirlpool bath during labor. When implementing this woman's request the nurse would do which of the following?

a. Assist the woman to maintain a reclining position when in the tub.
b. Tell the woman she will need to leave the tub as soon as her membranes rupture.
c. Limit her to no longer than 1 hour in the tub.
d. Maintain the water temperature between 36° C/96.8° F and 37.5° C/99.5° F.

21. The use of benzodiazepines can potentiate the action of analgesics and reduce nausea. When preparing to administer a benzodiazepine to a laboring woman, the nurse could expect to give which one of the following medications?
a. Diazepam (Valium)
b. Promethazine (Phenergan)
c. Butorphanol tartrate (Stadol)
d. Fentanyl (Sublimaze)

22. The nurse has just administered metoclopramide (Reglan) to a woman in labor. Which of the following would be an expected effect of this medication?
a. Analgesia
b. Nausea and vomiting
c. Potentiation of opioid analgesics
d. Respiratory depression

23. The doctor has ordered meperidine (Demerol) 25 mg IV q2–3 hr prn for pain associated with labor. In fulfilling this order, the nurse should consider which of the following?
a. Abstinence syndrome will occur if the woman is opioid dependent.
b. Prepare naloxone for use in case of respiratory depression due to normeperidine metabolite.
c. Maternal respiratory depression is more likely to occur when compared with morphine.
d. The newborn should be observed for respiratory depression if birth occurs within 4 hours of the dose.

24. Following administration of fentanyl (Sublimaze) IV for labor pain, a woman's labor progresses more rapidly than expected. The physician orders that a stat dose of naloxone (Narcan) 1 mg be administered intravenously to the woman to reverse respiratory depression in the newborn after its birth. In fulfilling this order the nurse would:
a. question the route because this medication should be administered orally.
b. recognize that the dose is too low.
c. monitor maternal condition for possible side effects.
d. observe the woman for bradycardia and lethargy.

25. Administering an opioid antagonist to a woman who is opioid dependent will result in the opioid abstinence syndrome. The nurse would recognize which of the following clinical manifestations as evidence that this syndrome is occurring? Select all that apply.
    a. Yawning
    b. Piloerection
    c. Anorexia
    d. Coughing
    e. Dry skin, eyes, and nose
    f. Tachypnea

26. After induction of a spinal block in preparation for an elective cesarean birth, a woman's blood pressure decreases from 124/76 to 96/60. The nurse's initial action would be to do which of the following?
    a. Administer a vasopressor intravenously to raise the blood pressure.
    b. Change the woman's position from supine to lateral.
    c. Begin to administer oxygen by mask at 10–12L/min.
    d. Notify the woman's health care provider.

III. CLINICAL JUDGMENT AND NEXT-GENERATION NCLEX® EXAMINATION-STYLE QUESTIONS

1. A nurse working with a group of expectant fathers is asked if there really is "a physical reason for all the pain women say they feel when they are in labor." Describe the response that this nurse should give.

2. On admission to the labor unit in the latent phase of labor, a pregnant woman (2-0-0–1-0) and her partner tell you that they are so glad they took Lamaze classes and did so much reading about childbirth. "We will not need any medication now that we know what to do. But most importantly our baby will be safe." Describe how you would respond if you were their primary nurse for childbirth.

3. Imagine you are the nurse manager of a labor and birth unit. Major renovations are being planned for your unit and your input is required. You and your staff nurses believe that water therapy, including the use of showers and whirlpool baths, is a beneficial nonpharmacologic method to relieve pain and discomfort and to enhance the progress of labor. Discuss the rationale you would use to convince planners that installation of a shower and a whirlpool bath into each birthing room is cost effective.

4. Tara has been in labor for 4 hours. Her blood pressure had been stable, averaging 130/80 when assessed between contractions, and the FHR pattern consistently exhibited criteria of a reassuring pattern. A lumbar epidural block was initiated. Shortly afterward, during assessment of maternal vital signs and FHR, Tara's blood pressure decreased to 102/60 and the FHR pattern began to exhibit a decrease in rate and variability.

    a. State what Tara is experiencing. Support your answer and explain the physiologic basis for what is happening to Tara.

    b. List the immediate nursing actions.

5. Moira, a primigravida, has elected for epidural anesthesia as her pharmacologic method of choice during childbirth.

    a. Identify the assessment procedures that should be used to determine Moira's readiness for the initiation of the epidural anesthesia.

    b. Describe the preparation methods that should be implemented.

    c. Describe two positions you could help Moira to assume for the induction of the epidural.

    d. Outline the nursing care management interventions recommended while Moira is receiving the anesthesia to ensure her well-being and that of her fetus.

6. You are caring for Raquel, a first-time mother who has been in labor for 14 hours. She has requested an epidural for pain relief. The Certified Nurse Anesthetist prepares to begin a continuous epidural block using a combination local anesthetic and opioid analgesic for Raquel.

Use an X to indicate whether the nursing actions below are Indicated (appropriate or necessary) or Not-Indicated (not necessary or contraindicated) at this time.

Nursing Actions	Indicated	Not Indicated
Assist the woman into a modified left lateral recumbent position or upright position with back curved for administration of the block.		
Alternate her position from side to side every hour.		
Assess the woman for headaches because they commonly occur in the postpartum period if an epidural is used for labor.		
Assist the woman to urinate every 2 hours during labor to prevent bladder distention.		
Prepare the woman for use of forceps- or vacuum-assisted birth because she will be unable to bear down.		
Assess blood pressure frequently because severe hypotension can occur.		

Chapter **14** **Maximizing Comfort for the Laboring Woman**

15 Fetal Assessment During Labor

I. LEARNING KEY TERMS

FILL IN THE BLANKS: Insert the term that corresponds to each of the following descriptions related to fetal assessment

1. _____ Listening to fetal heart sounds at periodic intervals to assess fetal heart rate.

2. _____ Instrument used to assess the fetal heart rate through the transmission of ultrahigh-frequency sound waves reflecting movement of the fetal heart and the conversion of these sounds into an electronic signal that can be counted.

3. _____ Method used to continuously assess the FHR pattern. _____ and _____ are the two modes used to accomplish this method of assessment.

4. _____ Device used in external monitoring to assess fetal heart rate and pattern.

5. _____ Device used in external monitoring to measure uterine activity transabdominally; it can determine the frequency, regularity, and approximate duration of uterine contractions but not their intensity.

6. _____ Device used in internal monitoring to obtain a continuous assessment of the fetal heart rate and pattern.

7. _____ Device used in internal monitoring to measure the frequency, duration, and intensity of uterine contractions as well as uterine resting tone.

8. _____ _____ Deficiency of oxygen in the blood that results in abnormal FHR patterns.

9. _____ The interventions initiated when an abnormal FHR pattern is detected; these interventions involve providing supplemental oxygen, instituting maternal position changes, and increasing intravenous fluid administration.

10. _____ Assessment method that uses digital pressure or vibroacoustic stimulation to elicit an acceleration of the FHR of 15 beats/min for at least 15 seconds and/or to improve FHR variability.

11. _____ Abnormally small amount of amniotic fluid.

12. _____ Absence of amniotic fluid.

13. _____ Instillation of room temperature isotonic fluid into the uterine cavity when the volume of amniotic fluid is low for the purpose of adding fluid around the umbilical cord and thus preventing its compression during uterine contractions or fetal movement.

14. _____ Relaxation of the uterus achieved through the administration of drugs that inhibit uterine contractions.

II. REVIEWING KEY CONCEPTS

MATCHING: Match the definition with the appropriate term related to FHR pattern.

1. _____ Average of FHR during a 10-minute segment that excludes periodic or episodic changes, periods of marked variability, and segments of the baseline that differ by more than 25 beats per minute; it is assessed during the absence of uterine activity or between contractions.

2. _____ Amplitude range of the FHR fluctuations not detectable to the unaided eye.

3. _____ Amplitude range detectable by the unaided eye, but is <5 beats/min.

4. _____ Persistent (≥10 minutes) baseline FHR <110 beats/min.

5. _____ Visually apparent decrease in the FHR of 15 beats/min or more below the baseline, which lasts between 2 and 10 minutes.

6. _____ Changes from baseline patterns in FHR that occur with uterine contractions.

7. _____ Persistent (≥10 minutes) baseline FHR >160 beats/min.

8. _____ Irregular fluctuations or waves in the baseline FHR of ≥2 cycles/min.

9. _____ Visually apparent gradual decrease in and return to baseline FHR in response to transient fetal head compression during a uterine contraction; it is considered a normal and benign finding.

10. _____ Visually apparent gradual decrease in and return to baseline FHR in response to uteroplacental insufficiency resulting in a transient disruption of oxygen transfer to the fetus; lowest point occurs after the peak of the contraction and baseline rate is not usually regained until the uterine contraction is over.

11. _____ Visually abrupt decrease in FHR below baseline of 15 beats or more, lasting 15 seconds and returning to baseline in less than 2 minutes from the time of onset, which can occur at any time during a contraction as a result of umbilical cord compression.

12. _____ Visually apparent abrupt increase in the FHR of 15 beats/min or greater above the baseline, which lasts 15 seconds or more with return to baseline less than 2 minutes from the beginning of the increase.

13. _____ Changes from baseline patterns in FHR that are not associated with uterine contraction.

a. Acceleration

b. Early deceleration

c. Variability

d. Late deceleration

e. Variable deceleration

f. Tachycardia

g. Prolonged deceleration

h. Bradycardia

i. Baseline FHR

j. Absent variability

k. Periodic changes

l. Episodic changes

m. Minimal variability

14. Describe the factors associated with a reduction in fetal oxygen supply.

    b. Internal fetal monitoring

    c. Portable telemetry

15. It is critical that a nurse working on a labor unit be knowledgeable concerning the characteristics of normal (reassuring) and abnormal (nonreassuring) FHR patterns, and characteristics of normal and abnormal uterine activity. List the required information for each of the following:

    a. Characteristics of a normal (reassuring) FHR pattern

    b. Characteristics of abnormal (nonreassuring) FHR patterns

    c. Characteristics of normal uterine activity

16. Nurses caring for women in labor must review FHR tracings on a regular basis. Name several essential components that the nurse must evaluate each time the monitor tracing is observed.

17. Nurses caring for laboring women use a variety of methods to assess fetal health and well-being during labor. State the advantages and disadvantages of each of the following methods to assess FHR and pattern as well as uterine activity. Outline the nursing care measures required for each of the monitoring methods.

    a. External fetal monitoring

18. State the legal responsibilities related to fetal monitoring for nurses who care for women during childbirth.

19. A laboring woman's uterine contractions are being internally monitored. When evaluating the monitor tracing, which of the following findings would be a source of concern and require further assessment?
    a. Frequency every 2.5–3 minutes
    b. Duration of 80–85 seconds
    c. Intensity during a uterine contraction of 55–80 mm Hg
    d. Average resting pressure of 25–30 mm Hg

20. External electronic fetal monitoring will be used for a woman just admitted to the labor unit in active labor. Guidelines the nurse should follow when implementing this form of monitoring would be which of the following? Select all that apply.
    a. Use Leopold maneuvers to determine correct placement of the ultrasound transducer.
    b. Assist woman to maintain a dorsal recumbent position to ensure accurate monitor tracings for evaluation.
    c. Reposition the tocotransducer, cleanse abdomen, and reapply gel when the fetus changes position.
    d. Tell the woman she can perform effleurage along the sides of her abdomen.
    e. Palpate the fundus to estimate the intensity of uterine contractions.

21. When evaluating the external fetal monitor tracing of a woman whose labor is being induced, the nurse identifies signs of persistent late deceleration patterns and begins intrauterine resuscitation interventions. Which of the following reflects that the appropriate interventions were implemented in the recommended order of priority?
    1. Increase rate of maintenance intravenous solution.
    2. Palpate uterus for tachysystole.
    3. Discontinue Pitocin infusion.
    4. Change maternal position to a lateral position; then elevate her legs if woman is hypotensive.

5. Administer oxygen at 8–10 L/min with a tight face mask.
   a. 2, 1, 5, 4, 3
   b. 4, 1, 2, 3, 5
   c. 5, 3, 4, 1, 2
   d. 4, 5, 1, 2, 3

c. Acceleration with fetal movement
d. Late deceleration patterns approximately every 3 contractions
e. FHR of 155 beats/min between contractions
f. Early deceleration patterns

22. The nurse caring for women in labor should be aware of signs characterizing normal (reassuring) and abnormal (nonreassuring) FHR patterns. Which of the following would be nonreassuring signs? Select all that apply.
   a. Moderate baseline variability
   b. Average baseline FHR of 100 beats/min

23. A laboring woman's temperature is elevated as a result of an upper respiratory infection. The FHR pattern that reflects maternal fever would be:
   a. diminished variability.
   b. variable decelerations.
   c. tachycardia.
   d. early decelerations.

III. CLINICAL JUDGMENT AND NEXT-GENERATION NCLEX® EXAMINATION-STYLE QUESTIONS

1. Darlene, a primigravida in active labor, has just been admitted to the labor unit. She becomes very anxious when external electronic monitoring equipment is set up. She tells the nurse that her father had a heart attack 2 months ago. "He was so sick they had to put him on a monitor, too. Does this mean that my baby has a heart problem just like my father?" Describe the nurse's expected response.

2. Terry is a primigravida at 43 weeks of gestation. Her labor is being stimulated with oxytocin administered IV. Her contractions have been increasing in intensity with a frequency of every 2–2.5 minutes and a duration of 80–85 seconds. She is currently in a supine position with a 30-degree elevation of her head. On observation of the monitor tracing, you note that during the last two contractions the FHR decreased after the contraction peaked and did not return to baseline until about 10 seconds into the rest period. A slight decrease in variability and baseline rate was observed.

   a. Identify the pattern described and the possible factors responsible for it.

   b. Describe the actions you would take. State the rationale for each action.

3. Taisha is a multiparous woman in active labor. Her membranes rupture and the nurse caring for her immediately evaluates the EFM tracing.

   a. What type of periodic FHR pattern would the nurse be alert for when evaluating the tracing? Explain the rationale for your answer.

   b. State the actions the nurse should take in order of priority if the pattern is noted.

4. Marianna is a primigravida in labor. On the labor and birth unit where she is a patient, intermittent auscultation (IA) with a Doppler device is used for low risk pregnant women during the latent phase and early active phases if the admission FHR monitor tracing reflects a reassuring FHR pattern. State the guidelines the nurse caring for Marianna should follow when using IA.

5. A nulliparous woman is in the active phase of labor and her cervix has progressed to 6 cm dilation. The nurse caring for this woman evaluates the external monitor tracing and notes the following: decrease in FHR shortly after onset of several uterine contractions returning to baseline rate by the end of the contraction; shape is uniform. Based on these findings the nurse should do which of the following?

Use an X to indicate whether the nursing actions below are Indicated (appropriate or necessary) or Not-Indicated (not necessary or contraindicated) at this time.

Nursing Actions	Indicated	Not Indicated
Change the woman's position to her left side.		
Document the finding on the woman's chart.		
Notify the physician.		
Perform a vaginal examination to check for cord prolapse.		
Reassure her that this finding is not a cause for concern.		
Administer oxygen via nonrebreather.		

16 Nursing Care of the Family During Labor and Birth

I. LEARNING KEY TERMS

FILL IN THE BLANKS: Insert the term that corresponds to each of the following descriptions associated with stages of labor.

1. The first stage of labor begins with the onset of

   _____ and ends with complete cervi-

   cal _____ and _____.

2. During the latent phase of the first stage of labor the

   cervix dilates up to _____ cm. Cervical dilation pro-

   gresses from _____ to _____ cm during the active phase
   of the first stage of labor.

3. The second stage of labor is divided into two phases. It
   begins with full cervical dilation and complete efface-

   ment, and it ends with the _____.

4. The third stage of labor lasts from the _____

   until the _____. Detachment of the placenta from the
   wall of the uterus or separation is indicated by a firmly

   contracted _____; change in the shape of the

   uterus from _____ to _____; a sudden

   _____ from the introitus; apparent _____; and

   the finding of apparent lengthening of the _____

   and appearance of _____ at the introitus.

5. The fourth stage of labor is considered to be the first

   _____ hours after birth. During this
   stage, the mother and newborn recover from the physical process of childbirth and get to know each other.

MATCHING: Match the description with the appropriate term.

6. _____ Prolonged breath holding while bearing down (closed glottis pushing).

7. _____ Burning sensation of acute pain as vagina stretches and crowning occurs.

8. _____ Artificial rupture of membranes (AROM).

9. _____ Occurs when widest part of the head (parietal diameter) distends the vulva just before birth.

10. _____ Incision into perineum to enlarge the vaginal outlet.

11. _____ Test to determine whether membranes have ruptured by assessing pH of the fluid.

12. _____ Pink, sticky, mucoid vaginal discharge.

13. _____ Also referred to as delayed pushing, laboring down, or passive descent.

14. _____ Cord encircles the fetal neck.

a. Bloody show

b. Episiotomy

c. Oxytocic

d. Ferguson reflex

e. Valsalva maneuver

f. Ring of fire

g. Crowning

h. Amniotomy

i. Nuchal cord

j. Prolapse of umbilical cord

k. Nitrazine test

l. Leopold maneuvers

m. Ferning

n. Latent phase

o. Open glottis pushing

15. _____ Method used to palpate fetus through abdomen.

16. _____ Occurs when pressure of presenting part against pelvic floor stretch receptors results in a woman's perception of an urge to bear down.

17. _____ Frondlike crystalline pattern created by amniotic fluid when it is placed on a glass slide.

18. _____ Classification of medication that stimulates the uterus to contract (a uterotonic).

19. _____ Protrusion of umbilical cord in advance of the presenting part.

FILL IN THE BLANKS: Insert the term that corresponds to each of the following descriptions related to the characteristics of the powers of labor.

20. _____ The primary powers of labor that act involuntarily to expel the fetus and the placenta from the uterus.

21. _____ "Building up" of a contraction from its onset.

22. _____ The peak of a contraction.

23. _____ "Letting down" of a contraction.

24. _____ How often uterine contractions occur; the time that elapses from the beginning of one contraction to the beginning of the next contraction.

25. _____ The strength of a contraction at its peak.

26. _____ The time that elapses between the onset and the end of a contraction.

27. _____ The tension of the uterine muscle between contractions.

28. _____ Period of rest between contractions.

29. _____ An involuntary urge to push in response to the Ferguson reflex.

II. REVIEWING KEY CONCEPTS

1. Laura (3-1-1-0-2) has just been admitted in the latent phase of the first stage of labor. As part of the admission procedure, you review her prenatal record and interview her regarding what she has observed regarding her labor and discuss her current health status.

   a. List the essential data you would need to obtain from her prenatal record to plan appropriate care for Laura.

   b. Identify the information required regarding the status of Laura's labor.

   c. State the information required regarding Laura's current health status.

2. Identify two advantages for each of the following labor positions:

   Semirecumbent

   Lateral

Upright

Hands-and-knees

3. Outline the critical factors to be included in the physical assessment of the maternal–fetal unit during labor.

4. Indicate the laboratory and diagnostic tests that are recommended during labor. State the purpose for each.

5. Identify the factors that can influence the duration of the second stage of labor.

6. Describe the maternal positions recommended to enhance the effectiveness of a woman's bearing-down efforts during the second stage of labor. State the basis for each position's effectiveness in facilitating the descent and birth of the fetus.

7. Explain why the nurse should encourage a woman planning to breastfeed to begin breastfeeding during the fourth stage of labor.

8. Identify signs of the second stage of labor that the nurse would see in the patient.

   a. Describe what physical assessment would be appropriate.

9. A primigravida calls the hospital and tells a nurse on the labor unit that she knows that she is in labor. The nurse's initial response would be which of the following?

   a. "Tell me what is happening to indicate to you that you are in labor."
   b. "How far do you live from the hospital?"
   c. "When is your expected date of birth?"
   d. "Have your membranes ruptured?"

10. A woman's amniotic membranes have apparently ruptured. The nurse assesses the fluid to determine its characteristics and confirm membrane rupture. Which of the following would be an expected assessment finding?
    a. pH 5.5
    b. Absence of ferning
    c. Pale straw-colored fluid with white flecks
    d. Strong odor

11. When admitting a primigravida to the labor unit, the nurse observes for signs that indicate the woman is in true labor and should be admitted. The nurse would recognize which of the following as signs indicative of true labor? Select all that apply.
    a. Woman reports that her contractions seem stronger since she walked from the car to her room on the labor unit.
    b. Progressive change in the cervix that feels soft and is 50% effaced.
    c. Woman perceives pain to be in her back or abdomen above the level of the navel.
    d. Progressive descent of the fetus that is engaged in the pelvis at zero station.
    e. Cervix is in the posterior position.
    f. Woman continues to feel her contractions intensify following a backrub and with use of effleurage.

12. A vaginal examination is performed on a multiparous woman who is in labor. The results of the examination were documented as 6 cm, 75%, +2, LOT. Which of the following would be an accurate interpretation of this data?
    a. Woman is in the latent phase of the first stage of labor.
    b. Station is 2 cm above the ischial spines.
    c. Presentation is cephalic.
    d. Lie is transverse.

13. A physical care measure for a laboring woman that has been identified as unlikely to be beneficial and may even be harmful would be:
    a. allowing the laboring woman to drink fluids and eat light solids as tolerated.
    b. administering a Fleet enema at admission.
    c. ambulating periodically throughout labor as tolerated.
    d. using a whirlpool bath once active labor is established.

1. Alice, a primigravida, calls the labor unit. She tells the nurse that she thinks she is in labor. "I have had some pains for about 2 hours. Should my husband bring me to the hospital now?"

   a. Describe how the nurse should approach this situation.

   b. Write several questions the nurse could use to elicit the appropriate information required to determine the course of action required.

   c. Based on the data collected during the telephone interview, the nurse determines that Alice is in very early labor. Because she lives fairly close to the hospital, she is instructed to stay home until her labor progresses. Outline the instructions and recommendations for care Alice and her husband should be given.

2. Analyze the assessment findings documented for each of the following women.

	Denise (2-0-0-1-0)	**Teresa (4-3-0-0-3)**	**Danielle (2-1-0-0-1)**
Dilation	6 cm	9 cm	2 cm
Contraction strength	Moderate	Very strong	Mild
Contraction frequency	q4min	q2-3min	q6-8min
Contraction length	40–55 sec	65–75 sec	30–35 sec
Pelvic station	0	+2	−1

   a. Identify the phase of labor being experienced by each woman.

   b. Describe the behavior and appearance you would expect to be exhibited by each woman.

   c. Specify the physical care and emotional support measures you would implement if you were caring for each of these women.

   d. Denise's husband, Sam, is her major support person during labor. The nurse observes that he is beginning to appear fatigued and "stressed" after being with Denise since her admission 5 hours ago. Describe the actions this nurse can take to support Sam and his efforts to care for Denise.

3. Describe the procedure that should be followed before auscultating the FHR or applying an ultrasound transducer to the abdomen of a laboring woman. Explain the rationale for utilizing this procedure.

4. Tonya, a woman in active labor, begins to cry during a vaginal examination to assess her status. "Why not watch the monitor to see how I am progressing instead of doing these vaginal exams? They really hurt and they are embarrassing!"

   a. Describe the response the nurse should make in regard to Tonya's concern.

   b. Discuss the measures the nurse could use to meet Tonya's safety and comfort needs during a vaginal examination.

5. Tasha is dilated 6 cm. Her coach comes to tell you that her "water just broke with a gush!" Identify each action you would take in this situation, in order of priority. State the rationale for the actions you have identified.

6. Sara, a 17-year-old primigravida, is admitted in the latent phase of stage 1 labor. Her boyfriend, Dan, is with her as her only support. They appear committed to each other. During the admission interview, Sara tells you that they did not go to any classes because she was embarrassed about not being married. Both Sara and Dan appear very nervous and assessment indicates they know little about what is happening, what to expect, and how to work together with the process of labor. Identify the labor support Sara and Dan should expect. State one expected outcome and list nursing measures appropriate for their care.

7. Identifying a laboring couple's cultural and religious beliefs and practices regarding childbirth is a critical factor in providing culturally sensitive care that enhances the couple's sense of control and eventual satisfaction with their childbirth experience.

   a. List the questions you would ask when assessing a couple's cultural and religious preferences for childbirth.

   b. Discuss the problems that can occur if the nurse does not consider the couple's cultural and religious preferences when planning and implementing care.

Chapter **16** **Nursing Care of the Family During Labor and Birth**

8. Cori (4-3-0-0-3) is in the latent phase of stage 1 labor. She and her husband are being oriented to the birthing room. Their last birth occurred in a delivery room 10 years ago. Both Cori and her husband are amazed by the birthing room and the birthing bed that will allow her to give birth in an upright position. They are also informed that changes in bearing-down efforts in the active phase of stage 2 labor now allow a woman to follow her own body feelings and even to vocalize with pushing. Both Cori and her husband state that with every other birth they put her legs in stirrups; she held her breath for as long as she could, and pushed quietly. "Everything turned out okay, so why should we change?" **Choose the most likely options for the information missing from the nurse's statements below by selecting from the lists of options provided.**

"You can deliver however you are most comfortable; however, upright positions may be more pleasant than lying in bed. Upright positions have shown more efficient uterine contractions, shorter labors, a decreased need for pain medications, increased feelings of maternal control, a greater satisfaction with the birth experience, and a reduced risk of <u>1</u>. There are several positions you may want to try, including squatting or standing and leaning forward which are considered <u>2</u> positions; a <u>3</u> position, where you can alternate between left and right side-lying positions; or the <u>4</u> position where you assume "all fours" or you can lean over an object like a birth ball."

Options for 1	Options for 2	Options for 3	Options for 4
cesarean birth	semirecumbent	semirecumbent	semirecumbent
spinal headaches	lateral	lateral	lateral
orthostatic hypotension	hands-and-knees	hands-and-knees	hands-and-knees
breech delivery	upright	upright	upright

9. A nurse living in a rural area is called to her neighbor's home to assist his wife who is in labor. "Everything is happening so fast. She says she is ready to deliver!"

a. Identify the measures the nurse can use to reassure and comfort the woman.

b. Shortly after the nurse arrives, crowning begins. State what the nurse should do.

c. Describe the action the nurse should take after the birth of the head.

d. List the measures the nurse should use to prevent excessive neonatal heat loss after the birth.

e. Identify the infection control measures that should be implemented during a home birth.

f. Specify the measures the nurse should use to prevent excessive maternal blood loss or hemorrhage until the ambulance arrives.

g. Outline the information the nurse should document regarding the childbirth.

10. Jada is in the active phase of the second stage of labor. She is actively pushing/bearing down to facilitate birth. Indicate the criteria a nurse would use to evaluate the correctness of Jada's technique.

11. Imagine that you are participating in a panel discussion on childbirth practices. Your topic is "Episiotomy—is it needed to ensure the safety and well-being of the laboring woman and her fetus?" Outline the information you would include in your presentation.

12. Imagine that you are a staff nurse on a childbirth unit. Your hospital is instituting a change in policy that would allow the participation of children in the labor and birth process of their mother. You are asked to be a part of the committee that will formulate the guidelines regarding sibling participation during childbirth. Discuss the suggestions you would make to help ensure a positive outcome for parents, children, and health care providers.

13. Annie is a primipara in the fourth stage of labor following a long and difficult childbirth process.

a. Identify the essential nursing assessment and care measures required to ensure Annie's safety and recovery during this stage of her labor.

b. As she performs the first assessment, the nurse notes that Annie seems disinterested in her baby. She looks him over quickly and then asks the nurse to take him back to the nursery. Identify the factors that could be accounting for Annie's behavior.

c. Discuss the nursing measures you would use to encourage future maternal-newborn interactions and facilitate the attachment process.

17 Labor and Birth Complications

I. LEARNING KEY TERMS

FILL IN THE BLANKS: Insert the term that corresponds to each of the following descriptions.

1. _____ Regular uterine contractions and cervical change occurring between 20 and 36 6/7 weeks of pregnancy.

2. _____ Any birth that occurs after 20 weeks and before the completion of 37 weeks of pregnancy regardless of birth weight.

3. _____ Weight at the time of birth of 2500 g or less.

4. _____ Glycoproteins found in plasma and produced during fetal life; their reappearance in the cervical canal between 24 and 34 weeks of gestation could predict preterm labor.

5. _____ Characteristic of the cervix that could be a predictor for preterm labor.

6. _____ Spontaneous rupture of the amniotic sac and leakage of amniotic fluid beginning before the onset of labor at any gestational age.

7. _____ Spontaneous rupture of the amniotic sac and leakage of fluid before the completion of 37 weeks of gestation often associated with weakening of the membranes caused by inflammation, stress from uterine contractions, or other factors that cause increased intrauterine pressure.

8. _____ A bacterial infection of the amniotic cavity that is potentially life threatening for the fetus and the woman.

9. _____ Long, difficult, or abnormal labor caused by various conditions associated with the lack of labor progress.

10. _____ or _____

_____ Abnormal uterine activity often experienced by an anxious first-time mother who is having painful and frequent contractions that are ineffective in causing cervical dilation and effacement to progress. It usually occurs in the latent phase of the first stage of labor.

11. _____ Abnormal uterine activity that usually occurs when a woman initially makes normal progress into the active phase of the first stage of labor and then uterine contractions become weak and inefficient or stop altogether.

12. _____ Abnormal labor caused by contractures of the pelvic diameters that reduce the capacity of the bony pelvis, including the inlet, midpelvis, outlet, or any combination of these planes.

13. _____ Abnormal labor caused by obstruction of the birth passage by an anatomic abnormality other than that involving the bony pelvis; the obstruction may result from placenta previa, leiomyomas (uterine fibroid tumors), ovarian tumors, or a full bladder or rectum.

14. _____ Abnormal labor caused by fetal anomalies, excessive fetal size, malpresentation, malposition, or multifetal pregnancy.

15. _____ Abnormal labor caused by excessive fetal size and the size of maternal pelvis.

16. _____ The most common fetal malposition.

17. _____ The most common form of malpresentation.

18. _____ Gestation of twins, triplets, quadruplets, or more infants.

19. _____, _____, _____,

_____, _____,

and _____ Six abnormal labor patterns identified according to the nature of the cervical dilation and fetal descent.

20. _____ Labor pattern that lasts 3 hours from the onset of contractions to the time of birth, often resulting from hypertonic uterine contractions that are tetanic in intensity.

21. _____ Attempt to turn the fetus from a breech or shoulder presentation to a vertex presentation for birth by exerting gentle, constant pressure on the abdomen.

108

22. _____ Observance of a woman and her fetus for a reasonable period of spontaneous active labor to assess the safety of a vaginal birth for both.

23. _____ Chemical or mechanical initiation of uterine contractions before their spontaneous onset for the purpose of bringing about the birth.

24. _____ Rating system used to evaluate the inducibility of the cervix.

25. _____ Artificial rupture of the membranes often used to induce labor when the cervix is ripe or to augment labor if the progress begins to slow.

26. _____ Stimulation of uterine contractions after labor has started spontaneously but progress is unsatisfactory. Common methods include infusion of oxytocin and rupture of membranes.

27. _____ Chemical, mechanical, and physical methods used to prepare the cervix for stimulation of labor by making it more inducible by making it softer and thinner.

28. _____ Term applied to the occurrence of more than five contractions in 10 minutes averaged over a 30-minute window; it can occur in both spontaneous and stimulated labors.

29. _____ Birth method in which an instrument with two curved blades is used to assist the birth of the fetal head.

30. _____ Birth method involving the attachment of a vacuum cup to the fetal head, using negative pressure.

31. _____ Birth of the fetus through a transabdominal incision of the uterus.

32. _____ Pregnancy that extends beyond the end of week 42 of gestation.
_____ Syndrome that can occur in a neonate born after pregnancy that extends beyond 42 weeks; the neonate exhibits dry, cracked, peeling skin, long nails, meconium staining of skin, nails, and umbilical cord, and loss of subcutaneous fat and muscle mass.

33. _____ Uncommon obstetric emergency in which the head of the fetus is born but the anterior shoulder cannot pass under the pubic arch.

34. _____ Obstetric emergency in which the umbilical cord lies below the presenting part of the fetus; it may be occult (hidden) or more commonly frank (visible).

35. _____ Obstetric emergency in which a foreign substance present in the amniotic fluid enters the maternal circulation triggering a rapid, complex series of pathophysiologic events that lead to life threatening maternal symptoms including acute hypoxia, hypotension, cardiovascular collapse, and coagulopathies.

II. REVIEWING KEY CONCEPTS

1. Compare and contrast spontaneous and indicated preterm birth.

2. Explain why bed rest may be more harmful than helpful as a component of preterm labor care management.

MATCHING: Match the description of medications used as part of the management of preterm labor with the appropriate medication.

3. _____ An antenatal glucocorticoid used to accelerate fetal lung maturity when there is risk for preterm birth.

4. _____ Beta2-adrenergic receptor agonist often administered subcutaneously; it inhibits uterine activity and causes bronchodilation.

5. _____ A calcium channel blocker that relaxes smooth muscles including those of the contracting uterus; maternal hypotension is a major concern.

a. Tocolytic

b. Betamethasone

c. Terbutaline (Brethine)

d. Magnesium sulfate

6. _____ Classification of drugs used to arrest labor after uterine contractions and cervical changes have occurred.

7. _____ A central nervous system (CNS) depressant used during preterm labor for its ability to relax smooth muscles including the uterus; it is administered intravenously.

8. _____ A prostaglandin synthesis inhibitor that relaxes uterine smooth muscle; it is administered orally.

e. Nifedipine (Procardia)

f. Indomethacin (Indocin)

Match the description of medications used during the process of stimulating uterine contractions and cervical ripening with the medication listed.

9. _____ Tocolytic medication administered subcutaneously to suppress uterine tachysystole.

10. _____ Classification of medications that can be used to ripen the cervix, stimulate uterine contractions, or both.

11. _____ Cervical ripening agent in the form of a vaginal insert that is placed in the posterior fornix of the vagina.

12. _____ Cervical ripening agent in the form of a gel that is inserted into the cervical canal just below the internal os or into the posterior fornix.

13. _____ Pituitary hormone used to stimulate uterine contractions in the augmentation or induction of labor.

14. _____ Natural cervical dilator made from seaweed.

15. _____ Synthetic cervical dilator containing magnesium sulfate.

16. _____ Cervical ripening agent, used in the form of a tablet that is most commonly inserted intravaginally into the posterior fornix.

a. Oxytocin (Pitocin)

b. Misoprostol (Cytotec)

c. Dinoprostone (Cervidil)

d. Dinoprostone (Prepidil)

e. Terbutaline (Brethine)

f. Prostaglandin

g. Laminaria tent

h. Lamicel

17. Describe factors that cause labor to be long, difficult, or abnormal. Explain how they interrelate.

18. Explain the treatment approach of therapeutic rest.

19. Angela (1-0-0-0-0) is experiencing hypertonic uterine dysfunction and Helena (3-1-0-1-1) is experiencing hypotonic uterine dysfunction. Compare and contrast each woman's labor in terms of causes/precipitating factors, maternal–fetal effects, change in pattern of progress, and care management.

a. Angela—hypertonic uterine dysfunction

b. Helena—hypotonic uterine dysfunction

20. Identify four indications for oxytocin induction and four contraindications to the use of oxytocin to stimulate the onset of labor.

    Indications

    Contraindications

21. Bed rest for the prevention of preterm birth can result in which of the following effects? Select all that apply.
    a. Bone loss
    b. Weight gain
    c. Muscle atrophy
    d. Increase in cardiac output
    e. Emotional lability

22. A woman's labor is being suppressed using intravenous magnesium sulfate. Which of the following measures should be implemented during the infusion?
    a. Limit fluid intake to 2500–3000 mL per day.
    b. Discontinue infusion if maternal respirations are 12 breaths per minute.
    c. Ensure that calcium gluconate is available should toxicity occur.
    d. Assist woman to maintain a comfortable semirecumbent position when in bed.

23. The physician has ordered that dinoprostone (Cervidil) be administered to ripen a pregnant woman's cervix in preparation for an induction of her labor. In fulfilling this order, the nurse would do which of the following?
    a. Insert the Cervidil into the posterior fornix of the cervical canal just below the internal os.
    b. Tell the woman to remain in bed for at least 2 hours.
    c. Observe the woman for signs of tachysystole.
    d. Begin induction using oxytocin (Pitocin) 30–60 minutes after removal of the insert.

24. A nulliparous woman experiencing a postterm pregnancy is admitted for labor induction. Assessment reveals a Bishop score of 9. The nurse would:
    a. call the woman's primary health care provider to order a cervical ripening agent.
    b. mix 20 units of oxytocin (Pitocin) in 500 mL of 5% glucose in water.
    c. piggyback the Pitocin solution into the port nearest the drip chamber of the primary IV tubing.
    d. begin the Pitocin infusion at a rate between 0.5 and 2 milliunits/min as determined by the induction protocol.

25. A woman's labor is being induced. The nurse assesses the woman's status and that of her fetus and the labor process just before a Pitocin infusion increment of 2 milliunits/min. The nurse would discontinue the infusion and notify the woman's primary health care provider if which of the following had been noted during the assessment?
    a. Frequency of uterine contractions: every 1.5 minutes
    b. Variability of FHR: present
    c. Deceleration patterns: early decelerations noted with several contractions
    d. Strong uterine contractions lasting 80–90 seconds each.

26. A laboring woman's vaginal examination reveals the following: 3 cm, 50%, LSA, 0. The nurse caring for this woman would:
    a. place the ultrasound transducer in the left lower quadrant of the woman's abdomen.
    b. recognize that passage of meconium would be a definitive sign of fetal distress.
    c. expect the progress of fetal descent to be slower than usual.
    d. assist the woman into a knee-chest position for each contraction.

27. A nurse is caring for a pregnant woman at 30 weeks of gestation in preterm labor. The woman's physician orders Betamethasone 12 mg for two doses with the first dose to be given at 11 A.M. In implementing this order, the nurse would do which of the following?
    a. Consult with the physician because the dose is too high.
    b. Administer the medication orally.
    c. Schedule the second dose for 11 P.M.
    d. Assess the woman for signs of hyperglycemia.

28. A nurse caring for a pregnant woman suspected of being in preterm labor would recognize which of the following as diagnostic of preterm labor?
    a. Cervical dilation of at least 2 cm
    b. Uterine contractions occurring every 15 minutes
    c. Spontaneous rupture of the membranes
    d. Presence of fetal fibronectin in cervical secretions

1. Imagine that you are a nurse-midwife working at an inner-city women's health clinic. You are concerned about the rate of preterm labor and birth among the pregnant women who come to your clinic for care. Outline a preterm labor and birth prevention program that you would implement at your clinic to reduce the rate of preterm labors and birth.

2. Sara, a multiparous woman (2-0-1-0-1) at 22 weeks of gestation, comes to the clinic for her scheduled prenatal visit. She is anxious because her last labor began at 26 weeks and she is worried that this will happen again. "I had no warning the last time. Is there anything I can do this time to have my baby later or at least know that labor is starting so I can let you know?"

    a. Identify the signs of preterm labor that the nurse-midwife should teach Sara.

    b. Explain how the nurse-midwife could help Sara implement a plan to reduce her risk for preterm labor.

    c. Sara calls the clinic 3 weeks later and tells her nurse-midwife that she has been having uterine contractions about every 8 minutes or so for the last hour. She is admitted for possible tocolytic therapy. Specify the criteria that Sara must meet before tocolysis can be safely initiated.

    d. Sara is started on a tocolysis regimen that involves the intravenous administration of magnesium sulfate. Outline the nursing care measures that must be implemented during the infusion to ensure the safety of Sara and her fetus.

    e. The nurse is preparing to give Sara a dose of betamethasone as ordered by the physician.

        1. State the purpose of this medication.

        2. Explain the protocol that the nurse should follow in fulfilling this order.

3. Debra has been experiencing signs of preterm labor. After a period of hospitalization, her labor was successfully suppressed and she was discharged to be cared for at home. Debra is receiving nifedipine (Procardia) 30 mg every 12 hours orally. She will palpate her uterine activity twice a day. Debra must also remain on bed rest with only bathroom privileges.

    a. State what the nurse should tell Debra about how the nifedipine works.

b. Identify the side effects of nifedipine that the nurse should teach Debra before discharge.

c. Describe the instructions that Debra should be given regarding palpating her uterus for contractions.

d. Debra has two children who are 5 years old and 8 years old. Specify the suggestions you would give to help Debra and her children cope with the bed rest requirement ordered by Debra's primary health care provider.

4. Denise, a primigravida, has reached the second stage of her labor with her fetus at zero station and positioned LOP. She is experiencing intense low back pain. Denise did not attend any childbirth classes and is having difficulty pushing effectively. No anesthesia has been used.

a. Identify the factors that can have a negative effect on the secondary powers of labor (bearing-down efforts).

b. Describe how you would help Denise use her expulsive forces to facilitate the descent and birth of her baby.

c. Specify the positions that would be recommended based on the position of the presenting part of Denise's fetus.

5. Anne, a primigravida, attended childbirth classes with her husband, Mark. They were looking forward to working together during the labor and birth of their baby. Because of fetal distress with meconium staining, an emergency low-segment cesarean section with a transverse incision was performed after 18 hours of labor. Even though Anne and her son are in stable condition and she is glad that "everything turned out okay" for her son, she expresses a sense of failure, stating, "I could not manage to give birth to my son in the normal way and now I never will!"

a. List the preoperative nursing measures that should have been implemented to prepare Anne physically and emotionally for the unexpected cesarean birth.

b. Describe the major focus of care for Anne's care immediately after unplanned cesarean section.

c. Specify the assessment measures that are critical when Anne is in the recovery room following the birth of her son.

d. Identify the nursing diagnosis reflected in Anne's statement, "I could not manage to give birth to my son in the normal way and now I never will!" Specify the support measures the nurse could use to put her cesarean birth into perspective.

6. A vaginal examination reveals that Marie's fetus is RSA. Specify the considerations that the nurse should keep in mind when providing care for Marie.

7. Angela (2-0-0-1-0) is at 42 weeks of gestation and has been admitted for induction of her labor.

   a. Assessment of Angela at admission included determination of her Bishop score. State the purpose of the Bishop score and identify the factors that are evaluated.

   b. Angela's score was 5. Interpret this result in terms of the planned induction of her labor.

   c. Angela's primary health care provider ordered that dinoprostone (Cervidil) be inserted. State the purpose of the Cervidil, method of application, and potential side effects that can occur.

   d. Before induction of her labor, Angela's primary health provider performs an amniotomy. State the rationale for performing an amniotomy at this time. Specify the nursing responsibilities before, during, and after this procedure.

   e. Indicate which of the following actions reflect appropriate care (A) for Angela during the induction of her labor with intravenous oxytocin. If the action is not appropriate (NA), state what the correct action would be.

      1. _____ Assist Angela into a lateral or upright position.

      2. _____ Apply an external electronic fetal monitor and evaluate the tracing every 30 minutes throughout labor.

      3. _____ Explain to Angela what to expect and techniques used.

      4. _____ Add 10 units of oxytocin (Pitocin) into 1000 mL of an isotonic electrolyte solution.

      5. _____ Piggyback the oxytocin (Pitocin) solution to the proximal port (port nearest the venous insertion site) of the primary IV.

6. _____ Begin infusion at 4 milliunits/min.

7. _____ Increase oxytocin by 1–2 milliunits/min at 5- to 10-minute intervals after the initial dose until the desired pattern of contractions is achieved.

8. _____ Stop increasing the dosage and maintain level of oxytocin when strong contractions occur every 2–3 minutes, and last 80–90 seconds each.

9. _____ Monitor maternal blood pressure and pulse every 15 minutes and after every increment.

10. _____ Limit IV intake to 1500 mL/8 hours.

f. State the reportable conditions associated with oxytocin (Pitocin) induction for which the nurse must be alert when managing Angela's labor.

g. The nurse notes a uterine hyperstimulation pattern when evaluating Angela's monitor tracing. List the actions the nurse should take in order of priority.

8. Lora is a 37-year-old nulliparous woman beginning her 42nd week of pregnancy. She and her primary health care provider have decided on a conservative "watchful waiting" approach because both she and her fetus are not experiencing distress.

a. In helping Lora make this decision, the risks she and her fetus face as a result of a postterm pregnancy were explained. Identify the risks that Lora should have considered in making her decision.

b. State the clinical manifestations that Lora is likely to experience as her pregnancy continues.

c. Outline the typical care management measures that should be implemented to ensure the safety of Lora and her fetus.

d. Specify the instructions that the nurse should give to Lora regarding her self-care as she awaits the onset of labor.

9. Julia is in latent labor. Her BMI prior to pregnancy was 35 and she gained 80 pounds during her pregnancy. If you were the nurse caring for Julia, what considerations related to her BMI would you keep in mind as you manage her care?

10. The nurse is caring for Erin, a 24-year-old G1P0 pregnant with twins. She is currently 25 weeks gestation. Erin is currently a smoker, but she states she has decreased her cigarette use by half since she found out she was pregnant. Her BMI is 18.9. She has states that she does not feel like eating most of the time because she has been nauseous her whole pregnancy. She states "I am so scared to deliver this baby early. My sister delivered both of her kids early and it was terrifying. My mom said both me and my sister were also born early. It feels like a curse." **Highlight or place a check mark next to the assessment findings and statements that the nurse identifies as placing Erin at a higher risk for spontaneous preterm labor**.

18 Postpartum Physiologic Changes

I. LEARNING KEY TERMS

FILL IN THE BLANKS: Insert the term that corresponds to each of the following descriptions.

1. _____ Increased sweating that occurs after birth, especially at night for the first 2–3 days, to rid the body of fluid retained during pregnancy.

2. _____ Uncomfortable uterine cramping that occurs during the early postpartum period as a result of periodic relaxation and vigorous contractions.

3. _____ Lactogenic hormone secreted by the pituitary gland of lactating women. _____ Pituitary hormone that is responsible for uterine contraction and suppression of ovulation.

4. _____ Surgical incision of the perineum at birth.

5. _____ Chloasma or "mask of pregnancy."

6. _____ Anal varicosity.

7. _____ Return of the uterus to a nonpregnant state.

8. _____ Self-destruction of excess hypertrophied uterine tissue as a result of the decrease in estrogen and progesterone level following birth.

9. _____ Terms used interchangeably with postpartum to refer to the period of recovery after childbirth when reproductive organs return to their nonpregnant state; it lasts approximately 6 weeks though the time can vary from woman to woman.

10. _____ Separation of the abdominal wall muscles related to the effect of the enlargement of the uterus on the abdominal musculature.

11. _____ Postbirth uterine discharge or flow.

12. _____ Dark red, bloody uterine discharge that occurs for the first few days following birth; it consists primarily of blood, decidual tissue, trophoblastic debris, and sometimes small clots.

13. _____ Pink to brownish uterine discharge that begins about 3–4 days after birth; it consists of old blood, serum, leukocytes, and tissue debris.

14. _____ Yellowish white flow that begins about 10 days after birth and continues for 4–8 weeks; it consists of leukocytes, decidua, epithelial cells, mucus, serum, and bacteria.

15. _____ Term that describes distended, firm, tender, and warm breasts during the postpartum period.

16. _____ Failure of the uterus to return to a nonpregnant state. The most common causes for this failure are _____ and _____.

17. _____ Medication most commonly administered intravenously immediately after expulsion of the placenta to ensure that the uterus remains firm and well contracted.

18. _____ Coital discomfort or pain with intercourse.

19. _____ Exercises that help to strengthen perineal muscles and encourage healing.

20. _____ Yellowish fluid produced in the breasts before transitioning to mature milk.

21. _____ Increased production of urine that occurs in the postpartum period to rid the body of fluid retained during pregnancy.

22. _____ Stretch marks that appear during pregnancy on the breasts, abdomen, and thighs.

II. REVIEWING KEY CONCEPTS

1. When caring for a woman following vaginal birth, it is of critical importance for the nurse to assess the woman's bladder for distention.

   a. Explain why bladder distention is more likely to occur during the immediate postpartum period.

   b. Identify the problems that can occur if the bladder is allowed to become distended.

2. Cite the factors that can interfere with bowel elimination in the postpartum period.

3. Explain why hypovolemic shock is less likely to occur in the postpartum woman experiencing a normal or average blood loss.

4. Indicate the factors that place a postpartum woman at increased risk for the development of thrombophlebitis.

5. Compare and contrast the characteristics of lochial bleeding and nonlochial bleeding.

6. A nurse has assessed a woman who gave birth vaginally 12 hours ago. Which of the following findings would require further assessment?
   a. Bright to dark red uterine discharge
   b. Midline episiotomy—approximated, moderate edema, slight erythema, absence of ecchymosis
   c. Protrusion of abdomen with sight separation of abdominal wall muscles
   d. Fundus firm at 1 cm above the umbilicus and to the right of midline

7. A woman, 24 hours after giving birth, complains to the nurse that her sleep was interrupted the night before because of sweating and the need to have her gown and bed linen changed. The nurse's first action would be to:
   a. assess this woman for additional clinical manifestations of infection.
   b. explain to the woman that the sweating represents her body's attempt to eliminate the fluid that was accumulated during pregnancy.
   c. notify her physician of the finding.
   d. document the finding as postpartum diaphoresis.

8. Which of the following women at 24 hours after giving birth is least likely to experience afterpains?
   a. Primipara who is breastfeeding her twins that were born at 38 weeks of gestation
   b. Multipara who is breastfeeding her 10-pound full-term baby girl
   c. Multipara who is bottle-feeding her 8-pound baby boy
   d. Primipara who is bottle-feeding her 7-pound baby girl

1. Describe how you would respond to each of the following typical questions/concerns of postpartum women.

    a. Esi is a primipara who is breastfeeding. "Why am I experiencing so many painful cramps in my uterus? I thought this happens only in women who have had babies before."

    b. Asia is being discharged after giving birth 20 hours ago. "For how many days should I be able to palpate my uterus to make sure it is firm?"

    c. Jazmine is a primipara. "My friend, who had a baby last year, said she had a flow for 6 weeks. Isn't that a long time to bleed after having a baby?"

    d. Jean is at 24 hours postpartum. "I cannot believe it—I look as if I am still pregnant! How can this be?"

    e. Marion is 1 day postpartum. "It seems like I am urinating all the time; do you think that I have a bladder infection?"

    f. Joan is a primipara who is breastfeeding her baby. "My friend told me that I cannot get pregnant as long as I continue to breastfeed. This is great because I do not like to use birth control."

    g. Alice, a primiparous, bottle-feeding woman, is concerned. She states, "My mother told me that I should be getting a drug to dry up my breasts like she got after she gave birth. How will my breasts ever stop making milk and get back to normal?"

2. Andrea, a primipara, is 1 day postpartum. She has a 2nd degree perineal laceration, which was repaired after delivery. While breastfeeding her baby she confides to the nurse that she does not know how long she will continue to breast-feed. "My husband and I have always had a satisfying sex life, but my friend told me that as long as I breastfeed, intercourse is painful. I am also worried about this tear. Will I be ok to have sex again?" **Choose the most likely options from the information missing from the nurse's statements below by selecting from the lists of options provided**.

"Initial healing of your laceration will begin in 1 week, but it can take 2 months for it to heal completely. You may notice 3 in vaginal dryness caused by decreased estrogen. This dryness is 4 among breastfeeding mothers, but a water-soluble lubricant can help during sexual intercourse. You will want to follow-up with your provider at your follow-up appointment before resuming sexual intercourse with your husband."

Options for 1	Options for 2	Options for 3	Options for 4
1–2	1–3	a decrease	less common
2–3	2–4	an increase	more common
3–4	4–6	no difference	chronic

19 Nursing Care of the Family During the Postpartum Period

I. LEARNING KEY TERMS

FILL IN THE BLANKS: Insert the term that corresponds to each of the following descriptions regarding the postpartum period.

1. _____ Nursing care management approach in which one nurse cares for both the mother and her infant. It is also called _____ or _____.

2. _____ Major intervention to alleviate uterine atony and restore uterine muscle tone.

3. _____ Classification of medications that stimulate contraction of the uterine smooth muscle.

4. _____ Failure of the uterine muscle to contract firmly. It is the most frequent cause for excessive bleeding following childbirth.

5. _____ Perineal treatment that involves sitting in warm water for approximately 20 minutes to soothe and cleanse the site and to increase blood flow, thereby enhancing healing.

6. _____ Menstrual-like cramps experienced by many women as the uterus contracts after childbirth.

7. _____ Dilation of the blood vessels supplying the intestines as a result of the rapid decrease in intraabdominal pressure after birth. It causes blood to pool in the viscera and thereby contributes to the development of _____ when the woman who has recently given birth sits or stands, first ambulates, or takes a warm shower.

8. _____ Exercises that can assist women to regain muscle tone that is often lost when pelvic tissues are stretched and torn during pregnancy and birth.

9. _____ Swelling of breast tissue caused by increased blood and lymph supply to the breasts as the body begins the process of lactation.

10. _____ Vaccine that can be given to postpartum women whose antibody titer is less than 1:8 or whose EIA level is less than 0.8. It is used to prevent nonimmune women from contracting this TORCH infection during a subsequent pregnancy.

11. _____ Blood product that is administered to Rh-negative, antibody (Coombs)-negative women who give birth to Rh-positive newborns. It is administered at 28 weeks of gestation and again within 72 hours after birth.

12. _____ Telephone-based postpartum consultation service that can provide information and support; it is not a crisis intervention line to be used for emergencies.

II. REVIEWING KEY CONCEPTS

1. Explain to a woman who has just given birth why breastfeeding her newborn during the fourth stage of labor is beneficial to her and to her baby.

2. A postpartum woman at 6 hours after a vaginal birth is having difficulty voiding. List the measures that you would try to help this woman void spontaneously.

3. Identify the measures the nurse should teach a postpartum woman in an effort to prevent the development of thrombophlebitis.

4. Identify the measures you would teach a mother who is formula feeding to suppress lactation naturally and to relieve discomfort during breast engorgement.

5. State the two most important interventions that can be used to prevent excessive postpartum bleeding in the early postpartum period. Indicate the rationale for the effectiveness of each intervention you identified.

6. Identify the signs of potential psychosocial complications that may occur during the postpartum period.

7. The nurse is prepared to assess a postpartum woman's fundus. The nurse would tell the woman to:
   a. elevate the head of the bed.
   b. place her hands under her head.
   c. flex her knees.
   d. lie flat with legs extended and toes pointed.

8. A nurse is preparing to administer RhoGAM to a postpartum woman. Before implementing this care measure the nurse should:
   a. ensure that medication is given at least 24 hours after the birth.
   b. verify that the Coombs test results are negative.
   c. make sure that the newborn is Rh negative.
   d. cancel the administration of the RhoGAM if it was given to the woman during her pregnancy at 28 weeks of gestation.

9. When teaching a postpartum woman with an episiotomy about using a sitz bath, the nurse should emphasize:
   a. using sterile equipment.
   b. filling the sitz bath basin with hot water (at least 42°C).
   c. taking a sitz bath once a day for 10 minutes.
   d. squeezing her buttocks together before sitting down, then relaxing them.

10. Prior to discharge at 2 days postpartum, the nurse evaluates a woman's level of knowledge regarding the care of her second-degree perineal laceration. Which of the following statements if made by the woman would indicate the need for further instruction before she goes home? Select all that apply.
    a. "I will wash my stitches at least once a day with mild soap and warm water."
    b. "I will change my pad every time I go to the bathroom—at least 4 times each day."
    c. "I will use my squeeze bottle filled with warm water to cleanse my stitches after I urinate."
    d. "I will take a sitz bath once a day before bed for about 10 minutes."
    e. "I will apply the anesthetic cream to my stitches at least 6 times per day."

III. CLINICAL JUDGMENT AND NEXT-GENERATION NCLEX® EXAMINATION-STYLE QUESTIONS

1. Tara is a breastfeeding woman at 12 hours postpartum. She requests medication for pain. Describe the approach that you would take when fulfilling Tara's request.

2. When caring for a woman who gave birth 4 hours earlier, the nurse notes an excessive rubra flow and early signs of hypovolemic shock.

   a. State the criteria that the nurse should have used to determine that the flow is rubra and excessive and that the early signs of hypovolemic shock are being exhibited.

   b. Identify the nurse's priority action in response to these assessment findings.

   c. Identify additional interventions that a nurse may need to implement to ensure this woman's safety and to prevent the development of further complications.

3. Carrie is a postpartum woman awaiting discharge. Because her rubella titer indicates that she is not immune, a rubella vaccination has been ordered before discharge. State what you would tell Carrie with regard to this vaccination.

4. The physician has written the following order for a postpartum woman: "Administer RhoGAM (Rh immunoglobulin) if indicated." Describe the actions the nurse should take in fulfilling this order.

5. Susan, a postpartum breastfeeding woman, confides to the nurse, "My partner and I have always had a very satisfying sex life, even when I was pregnant. My sister told me that this will definitely change now that I have had a baby." Describe what the nurse should tell Susan regarding sexual changes and activity after birth.

6. Identify the priority nursing diagnosis as well as one expected outcome and appropriate nursing management for each of the following situations.

   a. Tina is 2 days postpartum. During a home visit the nurse notes that Tina's episiotomy is edematous and slightly reddened, with approximated wound edges and no drainage. A distinct odor is noted and there is a buildup of secretions and Hurricaine gel Tina uses for discomfort. During the interview, Tina reveals that she is afraid to wash the area. "I rinse with a little water in my peri bottle in the morning and again at night. I also apply plenty of my gel."

   Nursing Diagnosis   Expected Outcome   Nursing Management

   b. Erin, who gave birth 3 days ago, has not had a bowel movement since a day or two before labor. She tells the visiting nurse during the interview that she has been avoiding "fiber" foods for fear that the baby will get diarrhea. Her activity level is low. "My family is taking good care of me. I do not have to lift a finger! Besides I would prefer to wait until my 'bottom' is less sore before trying to have a bowel movement."

   Nursing Diagnosis   Expected Outcome   Nursing Management

   c. Mary gave birth 24 hours ago. She complains of perineal discomfort. "My hemorrhoids and stitches are killing me, but I do not want to take any medication because it will get into my breast milk and hurt my baby."

   Nursing Diagnosis   Expected Outcome   Nursing Management

7. Dawn gave birth 8 hours ago. Upon palpation, her fundus was found to be 2 fingerbreadths above the umbilicus and deviated to the right of midline. It was also assessed to be less firm than previously noted.

   a. State the most likely basis for these findings.

   b. Describe the action that the nurse should take based on these assessment findings.

8. Jill gave birth 3 hours ago. During labor, epidural anesthesia was used for pain relief. Jill's primary health care provider has written the following order: "Out of bed and ambulating when able." Discuss the approach the nurse should take in safely fulfilling this order.

9. Taisha and her husband, Raushaun, are expecting their first baby. They have been given the option by their nurse-midwife of early postpartum discharge but are unsure of what to do.

   a. Describe the approach the nurse-midwife could take to help this couple make a decision that is right for them.

   b. Taisha and Raushaun decide to take the option of early discharge within 12 hours of birth. Identify the criteria for discharge that Taisha and her newborn must meet before discharge from the hospital to home.

   c. Outline the essential content that must be taught before discharge. A home visit by a nurse is planned for Taisha's third postpartum day.

10. Cultural beliefs and practices must be considered when planning and implementing care in the postpartum period. Discuss the importance of using a culturally competent approach when providing care to postpartum women and their families.

11. Tamara delivered vaginally 2 hours ago. She has a midline episiotomy.

   a. Describe the position that Tamara should assume in order to facilitate palpation of her fundus.

   b. Identify the characteristics of Tamara's fundus that should be assessed.

   c. Describe the position Tamara should assume in order to facilitate the examination of her episiotomy.

   d. Identify the characteristics that should be assessed to determine progress of healing and adequacy of Tamara's perineal self-care measures.

   e. State the characteristics of Tamara's uterine blood flow that should be assessed.

12. Imagine that you are the nurse who cared for a woman during her labor and birth and her recovery during the fourth stage of labor. Outline the information that you would report to the mother-baby nurse when you transfer the new mother and her baby to her room on the postpartum unit.

Chapter **19** **Nursing Care of the Family During the Postpartum Period**

13. Infection control measures should guide the practice of nurses working on a postpartum unit.

    a. Discuss the measures designed to prevent transmission of infection from person to person.

    b. Discuss measures a postpartum woman should be taught to reduce her risk of infection.

14. *NGN Item Type: Extended multiple response exercise*
    When assessing postpartum women during the first 24 hours after birth, the nurse must be alert for signs that could indicate the development of postpartum physiologic complications. Which of the following signs would be of concern to the nurse? Select all that apply.

    a. Temperature—38°C

    b. Fundus—midline, boggy

    c. Heart rate of 88 beats per minute

    d. Anorexia

    e. Voids approximately 150–200 mL of urine for each of the first three voidings after birth.

    f. Saturated perineal pad in 10 minutes

    g. Sore nipples after 3 breastfeeding sessions

    h. Fatigue

20 Transition to Parenthood

I. LEARNING KEY TERMS

FILL IN THE BLANKS: Insert the appropriate term for each of the following descriptions regarding parent-infant interaction and parenting.

1. _____ Process by which a parent comes to love and accept a child and a child comes to love and accept a parent. The term _____ is often used to refer to this process.

2. _____ Process that occurs as parents interact with their newborn and maintain close proximity as they identify the infant as an individual and claim him or her as a member of the family; parents will touch, talk to, make eye contact with, and explore their newborn.

3. _____ Infant behaviors and characteristics call forth a corresponding set of maternal behaviors and characteristics.

4. _____ Infant behaviors such as crying, smiling, and cooing that initiate the contact and bring the caregiver to the child.

5. _____ Infant behaviors such as rooting, grasping, and postural adjustments that maintain the contact.

6. _____ Process in which parents identify the new baby, first in terms of likeness to other family members, second in terms of differences, and third in terms of uniqueness.

7. _____ Position used for mutual gazing in which the parent's face and the infant's face are approximately 8 inches apart and are on the same plane.

8. _____ Newborns move in time with the structure of adult speech by waving their arms, lifting their heads, and kicking their legs, seemingly "dancing in tune" to a parent's voice.

9. _____ Personal biorhythm developed by the infant; parents facilitate this process by giving consistent loving care and using their infant's alert state to develop responsive behavior and thereby increase social interaction and opportunities for learning.

10. _____ Type of body movement or behavior that provides the observer with cues. The observer or receiver interprets those cues and responds to them.

11. _____ The "fit" between the infant's cues and the parents' response.

12. _____ Developmental transition period from the decision to conceive through the first months of having a child.

13. _____ Parents action of looking at their baby demonstrating interest in them, which often makes them feel closer to them.

14. _____ Involves a stabilization of tasks and coming to terms with commitments to the parental role.

15. _____ Classes that allow time for questions to be answered and for mothers to lend support to one another.

16. _____ Process of transformation and growth of the mother identity during which the woman learns new skills and increases her confidence in herself as she meets new challenges in caring for her child(ren).

17. _____ Period surrounding the first day or two after giving birth, characterized by heightened joy and feelings of well-being.

_____ Period following birth that is characterized by emotional lability, depression, a let-down feeling, restlessness, fatigue, insomnia, anxiety, sadness, and anger. Lability peaks around the 5th day postpartum and subsides by the 10th day.

18. _____ Father's absorption, preoccupation, and interest in his infant.

19. _____ Contingent responses that occur within a specific time and are similar in form to a stimulus behavior.

II. REVIEWING KEY CONCEPTS

1. Attachment of the newborn to parents and family is critical for optimum growth and development.

   a. List conditions that must be present for the parent-newborn attachment process to begin favorably.

   b. Discuss how you would assess the progress of attachment between parents and their new baby.

   c. Identify what nurses can do to facilitate the process of attachment in the immediate postbirth period.

2. Describe three parental tasks and responsibilities that are part of parental adjustment to a new baby.

3. Discuss how each of the following forms of parent–infant contact can facilitate attachment and promote the family as a focus of care.

   a. Early contact

   b. Extended contact

4. Describe how a mother's touching of her newborn progresses during the immediate postbirth period.

5. Describe how each of the following factors influences the manner in which parents respond to the birth of their child. State two nursing implications/actions related to each factor.

   Adolescent parents

   Parental age older than 35

   Lesbian couple

   Social support

   Culture

   Socioeconomic conditions

   Personal aspirations

   Sensory impairment

6. During maternal attachment and bonding with the newborn, which of the following might a mother say?
   a. "She has her grandfather's nose."
   b. "His ears lay nice and flat against his head, not like mine and his sister's, which stick out."
   c. "She gave me nothing but trouble during pregnancy, and now she is so stubborn she won't wake up to breastfeed."
   d. "He has such a sweet disposition and pleasant expression. I have never seen a baby quite like him before."

128

7. Which of the following nursing actions would be least effective in facilitating parent attachment to their new infant?
   a. Referring the couple to a lactation consultant to ensure continuing success with breastfeeding
   b. Keeping the baby in the nursery as much as possible for the first 24 hours after birth so the mother can rest
   c. Extending visiting hours for the woman's partner or significant other as desired
   d. Providing guidance and support as the parents care for their baby's nutrition and hygiene needs

8. Which of the following behaviors illustrates engrossment?
   a. A father is sitting in a rocking chair, holding his new baby boy, touching his toes, and making eye contact.
   b. A mother tells her friends that her baby's eyes and nose are just like hers.
   c. A mother picks up and cuddles her baby girl when she begins to cry.
   d. A grandmother gazes into her new grandson's face, which she holds about 8 inches away from her own; she and the baby make eye-to-eye contact.

9. Which of the following infant behaviors affect parental attachment? Select all that apply.
   a. Grasp reflex
   b. Unpredictable feeding and sleeping schedule
   c. Seeks attention from any adult in room
   d. Differential crying, smiling and vocalizing
   e. Approaches through locomotion

III. CLINICAL JUDGMENT AND NEXT-GENERATION NCLEX® EXAMINATION-STYLE QUESTIONS

1. Tiara and Andrew are parents of a newborn girl. Describe what you would teach them regarding the communication process as it relates to their newborn.

   a. Techniques they can use to communicate effectively with their newborn.

   b. The manner in which the baby is able to communicate with them.

2. Allison had a difficult labor that resulted in an emergency cesarean birth under general anesthesia. She did not see her baby until 12 hours after her birth. Allison tells the nurse who brings the baby to her room, "I am so disappointed. I had planned to breastfeed my baby and hold her close, skin to skin, right after her birth just like all the books say. I know that this is so important for our relationship." Describe how the nurse should respond to Allison's concern.

3. Diamond is the mother of a 1-day-old boy and a 3-year-old girl. As you prepare Diamond for discharge, she states, "My little girl just saw her brother. She says she loves him and cannot wait for him to come home. I am so glad that I do not have to worry about any of that sibling rivalry business!" Indicate how you would respond to Diamond's comments.

4. Dania and Ben have just experienced the birth of their first baby. They are very happy with their baby boy but appear very unsure of themselves and are obviously anxious about how to tell what their baby needs. Sara is trying very hard to breastfeed and is having some success but not as much as she had hoped. Both parents express self-doubt about their ability to succeed at the "most important role in our lives."

   a. State the nursing diagnosis that is most appropriate for this couple.

   b. Describe what the nurse caring for this family can do to facilitate the attachment process.

5. Mary and Fynn are the parents of three sons. They very much wanted to have a girl this time, but after a long and difficult birth they had another son who weighed 10 pounds. His appearance reflects the difficult birth process: occipital molding, caput succedaneum, and forceps marks on each cheek. Mary and Jim express their disappointment not only in the appearance of their son but also in the fact that they had another boy. "This was supposed to be our last child—now we just do not know what we will do." Discuss how you would facilitate Mary and Jim's attachment to their son and reconcile their fantasy ("dream") child with the reality of their actual child.

6. Dawn and Hakeem have just given birth to their first baby. This is the first grandchild for both sets of grandparents. The grandmothers approach the nurse to ask how they can help the new family, stating, "We want to help Dawn and Hakeem but at the same time not interfere with what they want to do." Discuss the role of the nurse in helping these grandparents to recognize their importance to the new family and to develop a mutually satisfying relationship with Dawn, Hakeem, and the new baby.

7. Jane is 2 days postpartum. When the nurse makes a home visit, Jane is found crying. Jane states, "I have such a let-down feeling. I cannot understand why I feel this way when I should be so happy about the healthy outcome for myself and my baby." Jane's husband confirms her behavior and expresses confusion as well, stating, "I wish I knew what to do to help her." Identify the priority nursing diagnosis and one expected outcome for this situation. Describe the recommended nursing management for the nursing diagnosis you have identified.

Nursing Diagnosis   Expected Outcome   Nursing Management

8. Ali has just become a father with the birth of his first child, a baby boy.

   a. Describe the process Ali will follow as he adjusts to fatherhood.

   b. Identify several measures the nurse caring for Ali's wife and baby boy can use to facilitate his adjustment to fatherhood and attachment to his baby.

9. The nurse is caring for a first-time mother and her newborn. She is breastfeeding well and had an uncomplicated vaginal delivery 2 days prior to discharge. Before discharge, she asks the nurse about the baby blues. She states that "my friend said she felt so let down after she had her baby, and I have heard that some women actually become very depressed. Is there anything I can do to prevent this from happening to me or at least to cope with the blues if they occur?"

   Use an X to indicate which of the following health teaching by the nurse below is Indicated (appropriate or necessary) or Not-Indicated (not necessary or contraindicated) at this time.

Health Teaching	Indicated	Not Indicated
"Postpartum blues usually happen in pregnancies that are high risk or unplanned, so there is no need for you to worry."		
"Try to become skillful in breastfeeding and caring for your baby as quickly as you can."		
"Get as much rest as you can and sleep when the baby sleeps, because fatigue can precipitate the blues or make them worse."		
"I will call your doctor before you leave to get you a prescription for an antidepressant to prevent the blues from happening."		
"The 'baby blues' can cause you to cry for no apparent reason, and may experience anxiety, anger, or insomnia."		
"As long as you love your baby, you don't need to worry about depression after delivery."		

21 Postpartum Complications

I. LEARNING KEY TERMS

FILL IN THE BLANKS: Insert the term that corresponds to each of the following descriptions of postpartum complications.

1. _____ Loss of 500 mL or more of blood after vaginal birth or 1000 mL or more after cesarean birth. ____ Excessive blood loss that occurs within 24 hours after birth; it is most often caused by marked uterine hypotonia.

   _____ Blood loss that occurs more than 24 hours after birth but less than 6 weeks after birth.

2. _____ Marked hypotonia of the uterus; the uterus fails to contract well or maintain contraction.

3. _____ Collection of blood in the connective tissue as a result of blood vessel damage. _____ are the most common type.

4. _____ Unusual placental adherence in which there is slight penetration of the myometrium by placental trophoblast.

5. _____ Unusual placental adherence in which there is deep penetration of the myometrium by the placenta.

6. _____ Unusual placental adherence in which there is perforation of the uterus by the placenta.

7. _____ Turning of the uterus inside out after birth.

8. _____ Delayed return of the enlarged uterus to normal size and function.

9. _____ Emergency situation in which profuse blood loss (hemorrhage) can result in severely compromised perfusion of body organs. Death may occur.

10. _____ and _____ Coagulopathies which places the woman at risk for postpartum hemorrhage.

11. _____ Pathologic form of clotting that is diffuse and consumes large amounts of clotting factors; can result from severe postpartum hemorrhage when there is a depletion of clotting factors.

12. _____ Results from a formation of a blood clot or clots inside a blood vessel.

13. _____ Inflammation of a vein with clot formation.

14. _____ Clot involves the superficial saphenous venous system.

15. _____ Clot involvement can extend from the foot to the iliofemoral region.

16. _____ Complication occurring when part of a blood clot dislodges and is carried to the pulmonary artery, where it occludes the vessel and obstructs blood flow to the lungs.

17. _____ or _____ Clinical infection of the genital canal that occurs within 28 days after miscarriage, induced abortion, or childbirth. In the United States, it is defined as a temperature of 38° C or more on 2 successive days of the first 10 postpartum days (not counting the first 24 hours after birth).

18. _____ Infection of the lining of the uterus; it is the most common postpartum infection and usually begins as a localized infection at the placental site.

19. _____ Infection of the breast with symptoms such as fever, malaise, flu-like symptoms, and a sore area on the breast.

20. _____ Downward displacement of the uterus, with varying degrees of displacement from into the vagina to complete protrusion outside the introitus.

21. _____ Predominant classification of mental health disorders in the postpartum period.

22. _____ Characterized by mood swings, feelings of sadness and anxiety, crying, difficulty sleeping, and loss of appetite; however, resolves within a few days and does not need treatment.

23. _____ This is considered the most significant risk factor for postpartum depression.

24. _____ An intense and pervasive sadness with severe and labile mood swings; it is serious and persistent. Intense fears, anger, anxiety, and despondency that persist past the baby's first few weeks are not a normal part of postpartum blues.

25. _____ Syndrome most often characterized by depression, delusions, and thoughts by the mother of harming either herself or her infant.

26. _____ Depression of men during the period of time from the first trimester of pregnancy through the first year after birth.

27. _____ Symptoms of postpartum depression that may include not feeling love for the newborn.

28. _____ Treatment of mild postpartum depression without the use of medication.

29. _____ Most common pharmacological treatment for postpartum depression.

30. _____ Mood disorder defined by the presence of one or more episodes of abnormally elevated energy levels, cognition, and mood and one or more depressive episodes.

31. _____ and _____ Most widely used screening tool to assess postpartum depression.

32. _____, _____, _____, and _____ Four criteria used to measure the seriousness of a suicidal plan.

33. _____ Disorder characterized by pervasive feeling of anxiety most of the time and excessive worry about multiple concerns.

34. _____ Disorder characterized by panic symptoms or "panic attacks".

II. REVIEWING KEY CONCEPTS

1. State the twofold focus of medical management of hemorrhagic shock.

2. Identify the priority nursing interventions for postpartum hemorrhage and hypovolemic shock. Include the rationale for each intervention identified.

3. State the standard of care for bleeding emergencies.

4. Identify measures found to be effective in preventing genital tract infections during the postpartum period.

5. Describe nursing interventions that may help families anticipate postpartum mood disorders.

6. Describe how you, as a nurse, would help family members with maternal death.

7. A woman has been diagnosed with severe postpartum depression. The nurse caring for this woman is concerned that she may harm herself, her baby, or both of them.

   a. What questions should the nurse ask to determine whether the woman is considering such a harmful action?

   b. The woman admits that she has been thinking that her family and even her baby might be better off without her. Identify the four criteria the nurse could use to determine how serious the woman might be.

8. Methylergonovine (Methergine) 0.2 mg is ordered to be administered intramuscularly to a woman who gave birth vaginally 1 hour ago for a profuse lochial flow with clots. Her fundus is boggy and does not respond well to massage. She is still being treated for preeclampsia with intravenous magnesium sulfate at 1 g/hr. Her blood pressure, measured 5 minutes ago, was 155/98. In fulfilling this order, the nurse would do which of the following?
   a. Measure the woman's blood pressure again 5 minutes after administering the medication.
   b. Question the order based on the woman's hypertensive status.
   c. Recognize that Methergine will counteract the uterine relaxation effects of the magnesium sulfate infusion the woman is receiving.
   d. Tell the woman that the medication will lead to uterine cramping.

9. A postpartum woman in the fourth stage of labor received prostaglandin F_{2a} (Hemabate) 0.25 mg intramuscularly. The expected outcome of care for the administration of this medication would be which of the following?
   a. Relief from the pain of uterine cramping
   b. Prevention of intrauterine infection
   c. Reduction in the blood's ability to clot
   d. Limitation of excessive blood loss that is occurring after birth

10. The nurse responsible for the care of postpartum women should recognize that the first sign of puerperal infection would most likely be which of the following?

a. Fever with body temperature at 38° C or higher after the first 24 hours following birth
b. Increased white blood cell count
c. Foul-smelling profuse lochia
d. Bradycardia

11. A breastfeeding woman's cesarean birth occurred 2 days ago. Investigation of the pain, tenderness, and swelling in her left leg led to a medical diagnosis of deep vein thrombosis (DVT). Care management for this woman during the acute stage of the DVT would involve which of the following actions? Select all that apply.
   a. Explaining that she will need to stop breastfeeding until anticoagulation therapy is completed
   b. Administering heparin via continuous intravenous drip
   c. Placing the woman on bed rest with her left leg elevated
   d. Encouraging the woman to change her position frequently when on bed rest
   e. Teaching the woman and her family how to administer warfarin (Coumadin) subcutaneously after discharge
   f. Telling the woman to use acetaminophen (Tylenol) for discomfort

12. Which of the following would be a priority question to ask a woman experiencing postpartum depression?
   a. Have you thought about hurting yourself?
   b. Does it seem like your mind is filled with cobwebs?
   c. Have you been feeling insecure, fragile, or vulnerable?
   d. Does the responsibility of motherhood seem overwhelming?

13. Which disorder is prostaglandin F_{2a} (Hemabate) contraindicated
   a. Hypertension
   b. von Willebrand disease
   c. Asthma
   d. Cardiac disease

14. Signs of pulmonary embolus include:
   a. decreased pulse.
   b. elevated blood pressure.
   c. skin warm to touch.
   d. tachypnea.

15. Which of the following are management techniques used in postpartum hemorrhage? Select all that apply.
   a. Bimanual compression
   b. Administration of uterotonic medications
   c. Call the hemorrhage team
   d. Start an IV with lactated Ringer with magnesium sulfate

1. Cameron is a multiparous woman (6-5-1-0-7) who gave birth to full-term twins vaginally 1 hour ago. Pitocin was used to augment her labor when hypotonic uterine contractions protracted the active stage of her labor. Special forceps were used to assist the birth of the second twin. Currently her vital signs are stable, her fundus is at the umbilicus, midline and firm, and her lochial flow is moderate to heavy without clots.

   a. Early postpartum hemorrhage is a major concern at this time. State the factors that have increased Cameron's risk for hemorrhage at this time.

   b. During the second hour after birth, the nurse notes that Cameron's perineal pad became saturated in 15 minutes and a large amount of blood had accumulated on the bed under her buttocks. Describe the nurse's initial response to this finding. State the rationale for the action you described.

   c. The nurse prepares to administer 10 units of Pitocin intravenously as ordered by Cameron's physician. Explain the guidelines the nurse should follow in fulfilling this order.

   d. During the assessment of Cameron, the nurse must be alert for signs of developing hypovolemic shock. Cite the signs the nurse would be watching for.

   e. Describe the measures that the nurse should use to support Cameron and her family in an effort to reduce their anxiety.

2. Nurses working on a postpartum unit must be constantly alert for signs and symptoms of puerperal infection in their patients.

   a. List the factors that can increase a postpartum woman's risk for puerperal infection.

b. State the typical clinical manifestations of endometritis for which the nurse should be alert when assessing postpartum women.

c. Describe the critical nursing measures that are essential in care management related to puerperal infection.

3. Kiara is a 36-year-old obese multiparous woman (5-4-0–1-4) who experienced a cesarean birth 2 days ago. During this pregnancy, she was able to reduce her smoking of 1 pack of cigarettes each day to 1/2 pack per day. Although she has never experienced a deep vein thrombosis (DVT) or thrombophlebitis, she did develop varicose veins in both legs with her third pregnancy. A major complication of the postpartum period is the development of thromboembolic disease.

a. State the risk factors for this complication that Kiara presents.

b. When assessing Kiara on the afternoon of her second postpartum day, the nurse notes signs indicative of DVT. List the signs the nurse most likely observed.

c. A medical diagnosis of DVT is confirmed. State one nursing diagnosis appropriate for this situation.

d. Outline the expected care management for Kiara during the acute phase of the DVT.

e. Upon discharge Kiara will be taking warfarin for at least 3 months. Specify the discharge instructions that Kiara and her family should receive.

4. Denise (1-0-0-0-0), a 25-year-old postpartum woman, has been diagnosed with a pelvic hematoma.

    a. Describe the signs and symptoms Denise most likely exhibited that lead to this diagnosis.

    b. State the risk factors for this complication that Denise presents.

    c. Outline the care management approach recommended for Denise's diagnosis.

5. Mary, a 35-year-old primiparous woman beginning her second week postpartum, is bottle-feeding her baby. She and her husband, Tom, moved from Buffalo, where they lived all their lives, to Los Angeles 2 months ago to take advantage of a career opportunity for Tom. They live in a community with many other young couples who are also starting families. Last month they joined the Catholic church near their home. Tom tries to help Mary with the baby but he has to spend long hours at work to establish his position. Mary's prenatal record reveals that she often exhibited anxiety about her well-being and that of her baby. During a home visit by a nurse, as part of an early discharge program, Mary tells the nurse that she always wants to sleep and just cannot seem to get enough rest. Mary is very concerned that she is not being a good mother and states, "Sometimes I just do not know what to do to care for my baby the right way, and I am not even breastfeeding my baby. It seems that Tom enjoys spending what little time he has at home with the baby and not with me. I even find myself yelling at him for the silliest things." The nurse is concerned about postpartum depression based on her assessment and some of Mary's comments. **Highlight or place a check mark next to the assessment findings that require further assessment by the nurse**.

6. Nitaya gave birth vaginally to a newborn at 41 weeks of gestation. Her infant was 10 pounds. After the birth, Nitaya experienced a postpartum hemorrhage. Explain the care for Nitaya involving an interprofessional health care team.

7. Anita gave birth to a baby boy by cesarean section after a prolonged labor. She was later diagnosed with a urinary tract infection.

    a. Discuss risk factors that place Anita at risk for a urinary tract infection.

    b. Review a possible management plan for Anita after her diagnosis.

22 Physiologic and Behavioral Adaptations of the Newborn

I. LEARNING KEY TERMS

FILL IN THE BLANKS: Insert the term that corresponds to each of the following descriptions related to newborn characteristics and care.

1. _____ Environment that allows the newborn to maintain a stable normal body temperature.

2. _____ Heat production or generation; for the newborn, it occurs as a result of increased muscle activity.

3. _____ Heat production process unique to the newborn accomplished primarily by brown fat and secondarily by increased metabolic activity in the brain, heart, and liver.

4. _____ Flow of heat from the body surface to cooler ambient air. Two measures to reduce heat loss by this method would be to keep the ambient air at 24° C and wrap the infant.

5. _____ Loss of heat from the body surface to a cooler, solid surface not in direct contact but in relative proximity. To prevent this type of heat loss, cribs and examining tables are placed away from outside windows and care is taken to avoid direct air drafts.

6. _____ Loss of heat that occurs when a liquid is converted to vapor; in the newborn heat loss occurs when moisture from the skin is vaporized. This heat loss can be intensified by failure to dry the newborn directly after birth or by drying the newborn too slowly after a bath.

7. _____ Loss of heat from the body surface to cooler surfaces in direct contact. When admitted to the nursery, the newborn is placed in a warmed crib to minimize heat loss. Placing a protective cover on the scale when weighing the newborn will also minimize heat lost by this method.

8. _____ High body temperature that develops more rapidly in the newborn than in the adult. The newborn has a decreased ability to increase evaporative skin water losses because sweat glands do not function sufficiently to allow the newborn to sweat; serious overheating can cause cerebral damage from dehydration or heat stroke and death.

9. _____ Caused by heat loss that exceeds the capacity to produce heat; this condition can lead to metabolic and respiratory complication.

10. _____ Pinkish, easily blanched areas on the upper eyelids, nose, upper lip, back of head, and nape of neck. They are also known as "stork bites" or "angel kisses."

11. _____ Overlapping of cranial bones to facilitate movement of the fetal head through the maternal pelvis during the process of labor and birth.

12. _____ Generalized, easily identifiable edematous area of the scalp usually over the occiput.

13. _____ Collection of blood between a skull bone and its periosteum as a result of pressure during birth.

14. _____ Bluish-black pigmented areas usually found on back and buttocks but can occur anywhere on the exterior surface of the body including the extremities.

15. _____ Bluish discoloration of the hands and feet, especially when chilled as a result of vasomotor instability and capillary stasis; it occurs for the first 7–10 days of life.

16. _____ White, cheesy substance that coats and protects the fetus's skin while in utero.

17. _____ Distended, small, white sebaceous glands on the newborn face.

18. _____ Yellowish skin discoloration caused by increased levels of serum bilirubin.

19. _____ Thick, tarry, dark green-black stool usually passed within 24 hours of birth.

20. _____ Transient newborn rash characterized by erythematous macules, papules, and small vesicles; it may appear suddenly anywhere on the body.

21. _____ Substance present in the urine of newborns that cause a pink-tinged stain or "brick dust" on the diaper; it is a normal finding during the first week and not representative of bleeding.

22. _____ Contraction of the anal sphincter in response to touch; it is a sign of good sphincter tone.

23. _____ Accumulation of fluid in the scrotum, around the testes.

24. _____ Bruising.

25. _____ Heart sound heard when fetal shunts (foramen ovale, ductus arteriosus) remain fully or partially open after birth.

26. _____ Soft, downy hair on face, shoulders, and back.

27. _____ Bleeding into a potential space in the brain that contains loosely arranged connective tissue; it is located beneath the tendinous sheath that connects the frontal and occipital muscles and forms the inner surface of the scalp. The injury occurs as a result of forces that compress and then drag the head through the pelvic outlet.

28. _____ Peeling of the skin that occurs in the term infant a few days after birth; if present at birth, it may be an indication of postmaturity.

29. _____ Flat red to purple birthmark composed of a plexus of newly formed capillaries in the papillary layer of the corium; it varies in size, shape, and location but is usually found on the neck and face. It does not blanch under pressure or disappear.

30. _____ Birthmark consisting of dilated, newly formed capillaries occupying the entire dermal and subdermal layers with associated connective tissue hypertrophy; it is typically a raised, sharply demarcated bright or dark red, rough-surfaced swelling that may proliferate and become more vascular as the infant grows; usually is found as a single lesion on the head.

31. _____ Slightly blood-tinged mucoid vaginal discharge associated with an estrogen decrease after birth.

32. _____ Foreskin.

33. _____ Lipoprotein that lines the alveoli resulting in a lower surface tension and alveolar stability with inspiration and expiration.

34. _____ Small, white, firm cysts that can be found on the gum margins.

35. _____ Extra digits, fingers or toes. _____ Missing digits.

36. _____ Fused fingers or toes.

37. _____ Variations in the state of consciousness of newborn infants.

38. _____ and _____ The two sleep states. The newborn sleeps about 17 hours a day, with periods of wakefulness _____ gradually.

39. _____, _____, _____, and _____ The four wake states.

40. _____ The optimum state of arousal in which the infant can be observed smiling, responding to voices, watching faces, vocalizing, and moving in synchrony.

41. _____ Ability of the newborn to modulate its state of consciousness, develop predictable sleep and wake states, and react appropriately to stress.

42. _____ Protective mechanism that allows the infant to become accustomed to environmental stimuli. It is a psychologic and physiologic phenomenon in which the response to a constant or repetitive stimulus is decreased.

43. _____ Quality of alert states and ability to attend to visual and auditory stimuli while alert.

44. _____ Ability of the new-
born to comfort itself and reduce stress; one behavior
a newborn uses is hand-to-mouth movements with or
without sucking.

45. _____ Individual variations
in a newborn's primary reaction pattern.

46. _____ The language an
infant uses to signal hunger, discomfort, pain, desire
for attention, or fussiness.

MATCHING: Match the description with the appropriate newborn reflex.

2. _____ Place infant supine and then partially flex both legs and apply
light pressure with fingers to the soles of the feet—legs extend
against examiner's pressure.

3. _____ Place infant supine on flat surface and make a loud abrupt noise
(e.g., sharp hand clap)—symmetric abduction and extension of
arms, fingers fan out, thumb and forefinger form a C; arms are
then adducted into an embracing motion and return to relaxed
flexion and movement.

4. _____ Place finger in palm of hand or at base of toes—infant's fingers
curl around examiner's finger; toes curl downward.

5. _____ Place infant prone on flat surface, run finger down side of back
first on one side and then down the other 4–5 cm lateral to
spine—body flexes and pelvis swings toward stimulated side.

6. _____ Tap over forehead, bridge of nose, or maxilla when eyes are
open—blinks for first four to five taps.

7. _____ Use finger to stroke sole of foot beginning at heel, upward
along lateral aspect of sole, and then across ball of foot—all
toes hyperextend, with dorsiflexion of big toe.

8. _____ Touch infant's lip, cheek, or corner of mouth with nipple or
finger—turns head toward stimulus, opens mouth, takes hold,
and sucks.

9. _____ Place infant in a supine neutral position, turn head quickly to
one side—arm and leg extend on side to which head is turned
while opposite arm and leg flex.

10. _____ Hold infant vertically under the arms or around the trunk
allowing one foot to touch a flat surface—alternates flexion
and extension of its feet; term infants will use soles of feet and
preterm infants will use toes.

11. _____ Touch or depress tip of tongue—infant forces tongue outward.

12. _____ Place infant supine and then extend one leg, press knee
downward, and stimulate the bottom of the foot—opposite leg
flexes, adducts, and then extends as if the infant is attempting
to push away the stimulation.

1. The most critical adjustment that a newborn must
make at birth is the establishment of respirations. List
the factors that are responsible for the initiation of
breathing after birth.

a. Rooting

b. Grasp

c. Extrusion

d. Glabellar (Myerson)

e. Tonic neck

f. Moro

g. Stepping (walking)

h. Babinski

i. Truncal incurvation (Galant)

j. Magnet

k. Crossed extension

13. During the first 6–8 hours after birth, newborns experience a transitional period characterized by three phases of instability. Indicate the timing/duration and typical behaviors for each phase of this transitional period.

First period of reactivity

Period of decreased responsiveness

Second period of reactivity

14. When assessing a newborn boy at 12 hours of age, the nurse notes a rash on his abdomen and thighs composed of reddish macules, papules, and small vesicles. The nurse would:
    a. document the finding as erythema toxicum.
    b. isolate the newborn and his mother until infection is ruled out.
    c. apply an antiseptic ointment to each lesion.
    d. request nonallergenic linen from the laundry.

15. A breastfed full-term newborn girl is 12 hours old and is being prepared for early discharge. Which of the following assessment findings, if present, could delay discharge?
    a. Dark green-black stool, tarry in consistency
    b. Yellowish tinge in sclera and on face
    c. Swollen breasts with a scant amount of thin discharge
    d. Blood-tinged mucoid vaginal discharge

16. As part of a thorough assessment, the newborn should be checked for hip dislocation and dysplasia. Which of the following techniques would be used?
    a. Check for syndactyly bilaterally
    b. Stepping or walking reflex
    c. Magnet reflex
    d. Ortolani maneuver

17. When assessing a newborn after birth, the nurse notes flat, irregular, pinkish marks on the bridge of the nose, nape of neck, and over the eyelids. The areas blanch when pressed with a finger. The nurse would document this finding as:
    a. milia.
    b. nevus vasculosus.
    c. telangiectatic nevi.
    d. nevus flammeus.

III. CLINICAL JUDGMENT AND NEXT-GENERATION NCLEX® EXAMINATION-STYLE QUESTIONS

1. When caring for newborns, especially during the transition period following birth, the nurse recognizes that newborns are at increased risk for cold stress.

   a. Explain the basis for this risk.

   b. State the danger that cold stress poses for the newborn.

   c. Identify one nursing diagnosis and one expected outcome related to this danger.

   d. Describe care measures the nurse should implement to prevent cold stress from occurring.

2. After a long and difficult labor, baby boy James was born with a caput succedaneum and significant molding over the occipital area. Low forceps were used for the birth, resulting in ecchymotic areas on both cheeks. James's parents tell the nurse that they are very concerned that James may have experienced brain damage. Describe what the nurse should tell the parents of James about these assessment findings.

3. During the first 24 hours of life, it is essential that the nurse monitor a newborn's breathing pattern for signs of distress. Create a checklist that could be used by a nurse to determine if a newborn is exhibiting eupnea (normal breathing pattern) or dyspnea (respiratory distress).

4. Susan and Allen are first-time parents of a baby girl. They ask the nurse about their baby's ability to see and hear things around her and to interact with them.

   a. Specify what the nurse should tell these parents about the sensory capabilities of their healthy full-term newborn.

   b. Name four stimuli Susan and Allen could provide for their baby that would help foster her development.

5. Tonya and Sam, an African-American couple, express concern that their new baby girl has several bruises on her back and buttocks. They ask if their baby was injured during birth or in the nursery. Describe the appropriate response of the nurse to this couple's concern.

6. *NGN Item Type: Extended multiple response exercise*

   A newborn, at 5 hours old, wakes from a sound sleep and becomes very active and begins to cry. Which of the following signs if exhibited by this newborn would indicate expected adaptation to extrauterine life? Select all that apply.

   a. Increased mucus production

   b. Passage of meconium

   c. Heart rate of 160 beats per minute

d. Respiratory rate of 24 breaths per minute and irregular

e. Retraction of sternum with inspiration

f. Expiratory grunting with nasal flaring

g. Blue mucus membranes

h. Axillary temperature of 38.0°C

7. Jaundice in the newborn can represent a normal physiologic response or indicate pathology. Compare and contrast each type of jaundice identified below in terms of causation, characteristics, and significance.

a. Physiologic (nonpathologic) jaundice

b. Pathologic (nonphysiologic) jaundice

c. Breastfeeding-associated jaundice

d. Breast-milk jaundice

23 Nursing Care of the Newborn and Family

I. LEARNING KEY TERMS

FILL IN THE BLANKS: Insert the term that corresponds to each of the following descriptions of newborns and their care.

1. _____ Assessment method used to rapidly assess the newborn's transition to extrauterine existence at 1 and 5 minutes after birth; it is based on five signs that indicate his or her physiologic state, namely: _____,

   _____, _____,

   _____, and _____.

2. _____ Device used to suction mucus and secretions from the newborn's mouth and nose immediately after birth and when needed.

3. _____ Automatic sensor usually placed on the upper quadrant of the abdomen immediately below the right or left costal margin; it is attached to the radiant warmer and monitors the newborn's skin temperature.

4. _____ Inflammation of the newborn's eyes from gonorrheal or chlamydial infection contracted by the newborn during passage through the mother's birth canal. _____ ointment is usually instilled into the newborn's eyes within 1–2 hours after birth to prevent this infection.

5. _____ Medication administered intramuscularly to the newborn to prevent hemorrhagic disease of the newborn; it is administered in a dose of 0.5–1 mg using a 25-gauge, 5/8- to 7/8-inch needle.

6. _____ Scale currently used to assess and estimate a newborn's gestational age at birth.

7. _____ Term that describes an infant whose birthweight falls between the 10th and 90th percentiles as a result of growing at a normal rate during fetal life regardless of length of gestation.

8. _____ Term that describes an infant whose birthweight falls above the 90th percentile as a result of growing at an accelerated rate during fetal life regardless of length of gestation.

9. _____ Term that describes an infant whose birthweight falls below the 10th percentile as a result of growing at a restricted rate during fetal life regardless of length of gestation.

10. _____ Infant born between 34 0/7 and 36 6/7 weeks of gestation; this infant has risk factors because of his or her physiologic immaturity that require close attention by nurses working with them.

11. _____ Infant born before the completion of 37 weeks of gestation, regardless of birth weight.

12. _____ Infant born between 39 0/7 and 40 6/7 weeks of gestation.

13. _____ Infant born after completion of week 42 of gestation.

14. _____ Infant born after completion of week 42 of gestation and showing the effects of progressive placental insufficiency.

15. _____ Infants born from 37 0/7 to 38 6/7 weeks of gestation; a recent increase in the birth of these infants is associated with elective inductions and elective cesarean births that are scheduled before 39 weeks.

16. _____ Pinpoint hemorrhagic areas acquired during birth that may extend over the upper trunk and face; they are benign if they disappear within 2–3 days of birth and no new lesions appear.

17. _____ Yellowish discoloration of the integument and sclera that first appears after the first 24 hours of life, peaks at 3–5 days in term infants, and resolves after 1–2 weeks.

18. _____ Acts as a laxative to promote stooling, which helps rid the body of bilirubin.

19. _____ Device used for noninvasive monitoring of bilirubin via cutaneous reflectance measurements; it allows for repetitive estimation of bilirubin and works well on both dark- and light-skinned newborns.

20. _____ Common method used to reduce the level of circulating unconjugated bilirubin or to keep it from increasing; it uses light energy to change the shape and structure of unconjugated bilirubin and convert it to molecules that can be excreted.

21. _____ Blood glucose concentration less than adequate to support neurologic, organ, and tissue function during the early newborn period; the precise level at which this occurs in every neonate is not known although intervention is usually required if the blood glucose level falls below 40–45 mg/dL.

22. _____ Newborn respiratory rate of 30 breaths per minute or lower.

23. _____ Newborn respiratory rate of 60 breaths per minute or higher.

24. _____ The most important single measure in the prevention of neonatal infection.

25. _____ An alternative device for phototherapy in the treatment of hyperbilirubinemia; it involves a fiberoptic panel attached to an illuminator.

26. _____ Surgical procedure that involves removing the prepuce (foreskin) of the glans penis.

II. REVIEWING KEY CONCEPTS

1. Outline the specific measures nurses should use when caring for newborns to ensure a safe and protective environment.

2. Describe the approach you would use to ensure accuracy when performing each of the following measurements on a newborn.

    a. Weight

    b. Length

    c. Head circumference

    d. Chest circumference

3. Preparing parents for the discharge of their newborn requires informing them about the essential aspects of newborn care. Identify three points that you would emphasize when teaching parents about each of the following aspects of newborn characteristics and care.

    a. Vital signs: temperature and respirations

    b. Elimination: urinary and bowel

    c. Positioning and holding

    d. Safety

    e. Hygiene: bathing, cord care, and skin care

4. Maintaining a patent airway and supporting respirations to ensure an adequate oxygen supply in the newborn are essential focuses of nursing care management of the newborn, especially in the early postbirth period.

    a. State the four conditions that are essential for maintaining an adequate oxygen supply in the newborn.

b. List four signs that the nurse who is assessing a newborn would recognize as indicative of abnormal breathing.

5. A newborn male is estimated to be at 40 weeks of gestation following an assessment using the New Ballard scale. Which of the following would be a Ballard scale finding consistent with this newborn's full-term status? Select all that apply.
   a. Apical pulse rate of 120 beats per minute, regular, and strong
   b. Popliteal angle of 160 degrees
   c. Weight of 3200 g, placing him at the 50th percentile
   d. Thinning of lanugo with some bald areas
   e. Testes descended into the scrotum
   f. Elbow does not pass midline when arm is pulled across the chest

6. A newborn male has been designated as large for gestational age. His mother was diagnosed with gestational diabetes late in her pregnancy. The nurse should be alert for signs of hypoglycemia. Which of the following assessment findings would be consistent with a diagnosis of hypoglycemia?
   a. Hyperthermia
   b. Jitteriness
   c. Loose, watery stools
   d. Laryngospasm

7. A radiant warmer will be used to help a newborn girl to stabilize her temperature. The nurse implementing this care measure should do which of the following?
   a. Undress and dry the infant before placing her under the warmer.
   b. Set the control panel between 35° C and 38° C.

c. Place the thermistor probe on her abdomen just below her umbilical cord.
d. Assess her rectal temperature every hour until her temperature stabilizes.

8. A newborn male has been scheduled for a circumcision using a Gomco device. Essential nursing care measures following this surgical procedure would include which one of the following?
   a. Administer oral acetaminophen every 6 hours for a maximum of 4 doses in 24 hours.
   b. Apply petroleum jelly or A&D ointment to the site with every diaper change.
   c. Check the penis for bleeding every 15 minutes for the first 4 hours.
   d. Teach the parents to remove the yellowish exudate that forms over the glans using a diaper wipe.

9. The provider has ordered that a newborn receive a hepatitis B vaccination prior to discharge. In fulfilling this order, the nurse should do which of the following? Select all that apply.
   a. Confirm that the mother is hepatitis B positive before the injection is given.
   b. Obtain parental consent prior to administering the vaccination.
   c. Inform the parents that the next vaccine in the series would need to be given in 1–2 months.
   d. Administer the injection into the vastus lateralis muscle.
   e. Use a 1-inch, 23-gauge needle.
   f. Insert the needle at a 45-degree angle.

III. CLINICAL JUDGMENT AND NEXT-GENERATION NCLEX® EXAMINATION-STYLE QUESTIONS

1. Apgar scoring is a method of newborn assessment used in the immediate postbirth period, at 1 and 5 minutes. Indicate the Apgar score for each of the following newborns.

   a. Baby boy at 1 minute after birth:
      Heart rate—160 beats/min
      Respiratory effort—good, crying vigorously
      Muscle tone—active movement, well flexed
      Reflex irritability—cries with stimulus to soles of feet
      Color—body pink, feet and hands cyanotic
         Score:
         Interpretation:

b. Baby girl at 5 minutes after birth:
   Heart rate—102 beats/min
   Respiratory effort—slow, irregular with weak cry
   Muscle tone—some flexion of extremities
   Reflex irritability—grimace with stimulus to soles of feet
   Color—pale
      Score:
      Interpretation:

2. Baby girl Saanvi was just born.

   a. Outline the protocol that the nurse should follow when assessing Saanvi's physical status during the first 2 hours after her birth.

   b. State the nurse's legal responsibility regarding identification of June and her mother after birth.

   c. Cite the priority nursing care measures that the nurse must implement to ensure Saanvi's well-being and safety during the first 2 hours after birth.

   d. Describe the emotional and physiologic benefits of early contact between the mother and her newborn.

3. Baby boy Tim is 24 hours old. The nurse is preparing to perform a physical examination of this newborn before his discharge.

   a. List the actions the nurse should take in order to ensure safety and accuracy. Include the rationale for the actions identified.

   b. Identify the major points that should be assessed as part of this physical examination.

   c. Support the premise that Tim's parents should be present during this examination.

4. Baby girl Tayanna has an accumulation of mucus in her nasal passages and mouth, making breathing difficult.

   a. State the nursing diagnosis represented by the assessment findings.

147

b. List the steps that the nurse should follow when clearing Susan's airway using a bulb syringe.

5. Susan and James are taking their newly circumcised (6 hours postprocedure) baby home. This is their first baby and they express anxiety concerning care of both the circumcision and the umbilical cord.

   a. State one nursing diagnosis related to this situation.

   b. State one expected outcome related to the nursing diagnosis identified.

   c. Specify the instructions that the nurse should give to Susan and James regarding assessment of both sites and the care measures required to facilitate healing.

6. Andrew and Marion are parents of a newborn, 30 hours old, who has developed hyperbilirubinemia. They are very concerned about the color of their baby and the need to put the baby under special lights. "A relative was yellow just like our baby and later died of liver cancer!"

   a. Describe how the nurse should respond to Andrew and Marion's concern.

   b. Describe the blanch test as a method of assessment for jaundice.

   c. Identify the expected assessment findings and physiologic effects related to hyperbilirubinemia.

   d. List the precautions and care measures required by the newborn undergoing phototherapy in order to prevent injury to the newborn yet maintain the effectiveness of the treatment. State the rationale for each action identified.

7. A newborn male has just been circumcised. Explain ways to assess newborn pain, including tools, and why it would be appropriate to use it at this time.

8. The nurse is preparing to administer erythromycin ophthalmic ointment 0.5% to a newborn after birth. The newborn is a male and was born 1.5 hours prior via planned cesarean birth. He is 8 lbs 5 oz, and in no signs of distress. He is currently skin-to-skin with his mother.

Use an X to indicate which of the following nursing interactions are Indicated (appropriate or necessary or Not Indicated (not appropriate or contraindicated)

Nursing Actions	Indicated	Not Indicated
Maintain skin-to-skin and administer the ointment at 4 hours of life.		
Explain that it is not recommended because he was born by cesarean.		
Cleanse eyes if secretions are present.		
Squeeze an ointment ribbon of 1–2 inches into the lower conjunctival sac.		
Wipe away excess ointment after 1 minute.		
Apply the ointment from inner to outer canthus.		

24 Newborn Nutrition and Feeding

I. LEARNING KEY TERMS

FILL IN THE BLANKS: Insert the term that corresponds to the following descriptions of breast structures and the breastfeeding process.

1. _____ Structures in the breast that are composed of alveoli, milk ductules, and myoepithelial cells.

2. _____ Milk-producing cells.

3. _____ Breast structure that transports milk from the alveoli to the nipple.

4. _____ Sebaceous glands found on the areola that secrete an oily substance to provide protection against the mechanical stress of sucking and the invasion of pathogens; the odor of the secretion can be a means of communication with the infant.

5. _____ Reflex that occurs when the infant cries, suckles, or rubs against the breast.

6. _____ Cells surrounding alveoli; these cells contract in response to oxytocin, resulting in the milk ejection reflex or let-down.

7. _____ Rounded, pigmented section of tissue surrounding the nipple.

8. _____ The process of milk production.

9. _____ The lactogenic hormone secreted by the anterior pituitary gland in response to the infant's suck and emptying of the breast.

10. _____ Posterior pituitary hormone that triggers the let-down reflex.

11. _____ and _____ Nipple types that do not protrude when stimulated.

12. _____ Plastic device that can be placed over the nipple and areola to keep clothing off the nipple and put pressure around the base of the nipple to promote protrusion of the nipple.

13. _____ A technique for manually displacing areolar interstitial fluid inward, softening the areola and making it easier for the infant's mouth to grasp the nipple and areola and latch.

14. _____ Very concentrated, clear yellowish fluid that is high in protein and antibodies; it is present in the breasts before the formation of milk.

15. _____ The ideal food for human infants.

16. _____ Newborn behaviors that indicate hunger and a desire to eat such as hand-to-mouth movements, rooting, and mouth and tongue movements.

17. _____ or _____ Reflex triggered by the contraction of myoepithelial cells. Colostrum, and later milk, is ejected toward the nipple.

18. _____ Reflex stimulated when a hungry baby's lower lip is touched. The baby opens its mouth and begins to suck.

19. _____ Placing the baby onto the breast with the mouth open wide and the tongue down. The nipple and some of the areola should be in the baby's mouth, making a seal between the mouth and the breast to create adequate suction for milk removal.

20. _____ Breast response that occurs around the third to the fifth day, when the "milk comes in" and blood supply to the breasts increases. The breasts become tender, swollen, hot and hard, and even shiny and red.

21. _____ Breastfeeding position in which the mother holds the baby's head and shoulders in her hand with the baby's back and body tucked under her arm.

22. _____ Breastfeeding position in which the baby's head is positioned in the crook of the mother's arm and the mother and baby are "tummy to tummy."

23. _____ Health care professional who specializes in breastfeeding and may be available to assist a new mother with breastfeeding while in the hospital or after discharge.

24. _____ Infection of the breast manifested by a swollen, tender breast and sudden onset of flulike symptoms.

25. _____ Designed to resemble human milk as closely as possible.

26. _____ Procedure sometimes performed to correct a tight frenulum to promote less painful, more effective breastfeeding.

27. _____ Process whereby the infant is gradually introduced to drinking from a cup and eating solid food while breastfeeding or bottle-feeding is reduced by gradually decreasing the number of feedings.

28. _____ Lower fat milk that is initially released with breastfeeding.

29. _____ Milk that is denser in calories from fat and is necessary for optimal growth and contentment between feedings.

30. _____ Jaundice (hyperbilirubinemia) that occurs in breastfeeding infants as a result of insufficient feeding and infrequent stooling.

31. _____ Jaundice (hyperbilirubinemia) that occurs in breastfed newborns between 5 and 10 days of age; they are typically thriving, gaining weight, and stooling normally. A brief interruption of breastfeeding for 12–24 hours may be recommended.

II. REVIEWING KEY CONCEPTS

1. A nurse has been asked to participate in a women's health seminar for women of childbearing age in the community. Her topic is "Breastfeeding: The Goals for *Healthy People 2020* and Beyond." Outline the points that this nurse should emphasize to help women appreciate the benefits of breastfeeding and seriously consider breastfeeding when they have a baby.

2. It is important that a breastfeeding woman alter the position she uses for breastfeeding as one means of preserving nipple and areolar integrity. Describe four breastfeeding positions the nurse should demonstrate to a woman who is breastfeeding her newborn.

3. Infants exhibit feeding cues as they recognize and express their hunger.

    a. Identify feeding cues of the infant.

    b. State why the new mother should be guided by these cues when determining the timing of feeding sessions.

4. Proper latch (latch-on) is essential for effective breastfeeding and preservation of nipple and areolar tissue integrity.

    a. Indicate the steps the nurse should teach a breastfeeding woman to follow to ensure a proper latch-on.

    b. When observing a woman breastfeeding, it is essential that the nurse determine the effectiveness of the latch-on. State the signs a nurse should look for that would indicate a proper latch-on.

    c. Describe the way a woman should remove her baby from her breast after feeding is completed.

5. During a home visit, the mother of a 1-week-old infant son tells the nurse that she is very concerned about whether her baby is getting enough breast milk. The nurse would tell this mother that at 1 week of age a well-nourished newborn should exhibit which of the following?
    a. Weight gain sufficient to reach his birthweight
    b. A minimum of three bowel movements each day
    c. Approximately 10–12 wet diapers each day
    d. Breastfeeding at a frequency of every 4 hours or about 6 times each day

6. A woman is trying to calm her fussy baby daughter in preparation for feeding. She exhibits a need for further instruction if she does which of the following?
    a. Swaddles the baby
    b. Dims lights in the room and turns off the television
    c. Gently rocks the baby and talks to her in a low voice
    d. Attempts to get the baby to latch on immediately

7. The nurse should teach breastfeeding mothers about breast care measures to preserve the integrity of the nipples and areola. Which of the following should the nurse include in these instructions?
   a. Cleanse nipples and areola twice a day with mild soap and water.
   b. Apply vitamin E cream to nipples and areola at least four times each day before a feeding.
   c. Insert plastic-lined pads into the bra to absorb leakage and protect clothing.
   d. Place a nipple shell into the bra if nipples are sore.

8. A breastfeeding woman asks the nurse about what birth control she should use during the postpartum period. Which is the best recommendation for a safe, yet effective method during the first 6 weeks after birth?
   a. Combination oral contraceptive that she used before she was pregnant
   b. Barrier method using a combination of a condom and spermicide foam
   c. Resume using the diaphragm she used prior to getting pregnant
   d. Complete breastfeeding—baby only receives breast milk for nourishment

9. A woman has determined that formula-feeding is the best feeding method for her. Instructions the woman should receive regarding this feeding method should include which of the following?
   a. Provide the infant with supplemental vitamins along with the iron-fortified formula.
   b. Sterilize water by boiling, then cool and mix with formula powder or concentrate.
   c. Expect a 2-week-old newborn to drink approximately 30–60 mL of formula at each feeding.
   d. Microwave refrigerated formula for about 2 minutes before feeding the newborn.

10. A nurse is evaluating a woman's breastfeeding technique. Which of the following actions would indicate that the woman needs further instruction regarding breastfeeding to ensure success? Select all that apply.
    a. Washes her breasts and nipples thoroughly with soap and water twice a day
    b. Massages a small amount of breast milk into her nipple and areola before and after each feeding
    c. Lines her bra with a thick plastic-lined pad to absorb leakage
    d. Positions baby supporting back and shoulders securely and then brings her breast toward the baby, putting the nipple in the baby's mouth
    e. Feeds her baby every 2–3 hours
    f. Inserts her finger into the corner of her baby's mouth between the gums before removing her baby from the breast

11. A new breastfeeding mother asks the nurse how to prevent nipple soreness. The nurse tells this woman that the key to preventing sore nipples would be which of the following?
    a. Limiting the length of breastfeeding to no more than 10 minutes on each breast until the milk comes in
    b. Applying lanolin to each nipple and areola after each feeding
    c. Using correct breastfeeding technique
    d. Using nipple shells to protect the nipples and areola between feeding

III. CLINICAL JUDGMENT AND NEXT-GENERATION NCLEX® EXAMINATION-STYLE QUESTIONS

1. Elise and her husband, Mark, are experiencing their first pregnancy. During one of their prenatal visits, they tell the nurse that they are as yet unsure about the method they want to use for feeding their baby. "Everyone has an opinion—some say breastfeeding is best, yet others tell us that bottle-feeding is more convenient, especially because the father can help. What should we do?"

   a. Identify one nursing diagnosis and one expected outcome appropriate for this situation.

   b. Discuss why it is important for the pregnant couple to make this decision together.

   c. Indicate why is it preferable to make this decision during the prenatal period rather than waiting until the baby is born.

   d. Describe how the nurse could use the decision-making process to assist Elise and Mark to choose the method that is best for them.

2. Chantel is a 26-year-old gravida 2, para 1 mother who delivered a newborn female 26 hours ago. She is a first-time breastfeeding mother and is anxious about successfully breastfeeding. She states that she was not planning on breastfeeding before the arrival of her newborn, and therefore did not attend any prenatal breastfeeding classes. **Indicate which nursing response listed in the far-left column is most appropriate for each of Chantel's questions. Note that not all responses will be used.**

Nurse's Responses	Mother's Statements	Appropriate Nurse's Response for each Question
"This is a normal finding, particularly in the first few days. It happens because baby is latching."	"Every time I breastfeed, I get cramps and my flow seems to get heavier. Is there something wrong with me?"	
"Unfortunately, breastfeeding is not considered an effective method of contraception. While the lactational amenorrhea method may be effective, let's talk about other effective contraception methods so you know all of your options."	"Everyone keeps talking about this let-down that is supposed to happen. What is it and how will I know I have it?"	
"This is one of the major benefits of breastfeeding, you can trust the process and know that it is working."	"How can I possibly know if my baby is getting enough if I cannot tell how many ounces he gets with each feeding?"	
"If your cramps get worse during breastfeeding, please let your provider know immediately. This can be a sign of retained placental fragments."	"It is only the first day that I am breastfeeding and my nipples already feel sore. What can I do to relieve this soreness and prevent it from getting worse?"	
"It is important to keep track of her urine and stool output to tell if she is getting enough milk. A feeding diary can help with this."	"I am so glad I do not have to worry about getting pregnant again as long as I am breastfeeding. I hate using birth control and my friend told me I do not have to as long as I am breastfeeding."	
"Let-down is when the milk is ejected from the breast. You may feel a warm rush or tingling, and you may experience milk leaking from the opposite breast."		
"Next time she breastfeeds, I would like to observe her latch. Some mild discomfort can be normal in the first few sucks but making sure she has a good latch is critical to preventing sore nipples."		
"Let-down is typically painful for the first week, but you can tell that it is happening due to increased thirst and uterine cramping."		

3. Jordyn is 2 days old. She last fed 5 hours ago. Her mother tells the nurse that Jordyn is so sleepy that she just does not have the heart to wake her.

a. Identify one nursing diagnosis and one expected outcome appropriate for this newborn.

b. Discuss the approach the nurse should take with regard to this situation.

4. Alice has decided that for personal and professional reasons, bottle-feeding with a commercially prepared formula is the feeding method that is best for her. She tells the nurse that she hopes she made a good decision for her baby. "I hope she will be well nourished and feel that I love her even though I am bottle-feeding."

a. Describe how the nurse should respond to Alice's concern.

b. State three guidelines for bottle-feeding technique that the nurse should teach Alice to ensure the safety and health of her baby.

5. Prior to discharge, a nurse is evaluating a woman's ability to breastfeed and her newborn's response to breastfeeding.

a. Identify the factors that the nurse should assess before and during breastfeeding to ensure that this mother and newborn are ready to breastfeed at home.

b. After determining that breastfeeding is progressing well, the woman is discharged. One week later the nurse calls the woman to discuss breastfeeding. Write several questions this nurse should ask to determine whether breastfeeding is continuing to progress normally.

25 The High-Risk Newborn

I. LEARNING KEY TERMS

MATCHING: Match each term with its definition.

1. _____ Birth injury in which the upper nerve plexus is damaged resulting in an immobilized, limp arm with an intact grasp reflex.

2. _____ Birth injury in which the lower plexus is damaged resulting in wrist drop and relaxed fingers yet arm movement is not restricted.

3. _____ Infant whose birthweight is <2500 g, regardless of gestational age.

4. _____ Infant whose birthweight is <1500 g.

5. _____ Infant whose birthweight is <1000 g.

6. _____ Infant born before completion of 37 weeks of gestation.

7. _____ Infants born between 34 0/7 and 36 6/7 weeks of gestation.

8. _____ Infant born between 39 0/7 weeks and 40 6/7 weeks of gestation.

9. _____ An infant born after 42 weeks of gestational age.

10. _____ Infant whose birthweight falls above the 90th percentile on intrauterine growth curves.

11. _____ Infant whose rate of intrauterine growth was restricted and whose birthweight falls below the 10th percentile on intrauterine growth curves.

12. _____ The presence of microorganisms or their toxins in the bloodstream.

13. _____ Cessation of respirations of 20 seconds or more.

14. _____ Surface-active phospholipid secreted by the alveolar epithelium; it reduces the surface tension of fluids that line the alveoli and respiratory passages, resulting in uniform expansion and maintenance of lung expansion at low intraalveolar pressure.

15. _____ The environmental temperature at which oxygen consumption and metabolic rate are minimal but adequate to maintain the body temperature.

16. _____ Death that occurs in the first 27 days of life; it is described as early if it occurs in the first week of life and late if it occurs at 7–27 days.

17. _____ Method that can be used to provide maternal or paternal skin-to-skin contact with the newborn and to reduce stress in the infant.

18. _____ Growth restriction in which the weight, length, and head circumference are all affected.

19. _____ Presence of a bacterial infection in the newborn with symptoms usually manifesting within 72 hours of birth; infection is acquired in the perinatal period.

20. _____ Noninvasive method used to treat high levels of circulating bilirubin in newborn infant.

21. _____ Usually occurs in the first 24 hours of life; is most often the result of hemolytic disease of the newborn (HDN).

22. _____ Common condition that occurs in infants of diabetic mothers (IDM) within minutes to hours after birth; signs and symptoms are variable and infant may be asymptomatic or may have tremors, poor feeding, or respiratory distress.

a. Late preterm infant
b. Kangaroo care
c. Surfactant
d. Early-onset/congenital sepsis
e. Neutral thermal environment
f. Neonatal death
g. Apnea
h. Sepsis
i. Premature or preterm infant
j. Large for gestational age
k. Small for gestational age
l. Full-term infant
m. Erb's palsy
n. Klumpke palsy
o. Low birthweight (LBW)
p. Very low birthweight (VLBW)
q. Extremely low birthweight (ELBW)
r. Postterm infant
s. Symmetric intrauterine growth restriction
t. Phototherapy
u. Hyperbilirubinemia
v. Hypoglycemia

FILL IN THE BLANKS: Insert the term that corresponds to each of the following descriptions.

23. _____ Acronym used to designate certain maternal infections during early pregnancy that are known to be associated with various congenital malformations and disorders.

24. _____ Neonatal infection with this virus can result in disseminated infection, localized CNS disease, or localized infection of the skin, eye, or mouth.

25. The single most effective measure to reduce healthcare-associated infections in high risk infants is _____.

26. _____ Group of disorders caused by fetal exposure to alcohol, which can result in growth restriction, dysmorphic facial features, and CNS involvement.

27. _____ Disorder that occurs when the blood groups of the mother and newborn are different; the most common of these are Rh incompatibility and ABO incompatibility.

28. _____ Condition in which the fetus produces large numbers of immature erythrocytes to replace those hemolyzed as a result of severe Rh incompatibility. _____ The most severe form of this condition; it is characterized by marked anemia with hypoxia, cardiac decompensation, cardiomegaly, hepatosplenomegaly, and generalized edema.

29. The administration of _____ should be given to all unsensitized mothers within 72 hours after birth.

30. _____ The term used to describe the set of behaviors exhibited by infants exposed to narcotics in utero.

31. _____ The most accurate sampling medium used to determine presence of drugs to which the newborn has been exposed in utero.

32. _____ A group of disorders caused by a metabolic defect that results from the absence or deficiency of a substance essential to cellular metabolism, usually an enzyme. Examples include phenylketonuria and galactosemia.

33. _____ In this disorder the infant is placed on a low phenylalanine diet and this diet is maintained throughout life to prevent severe cognitive impairment.

34. _____ Disorder in which the affected infant does not properly convert galactose into glucose resulting in cataracts, profoundly stunted growth, *E. coli* sepsis, and eventual death if treatment is not implemented early in infancy.

35. _____ Treatment of this disorder involves the lifelong administration of thyroid hormone replacement therapy.

36. _____ The bone most often fractured at birth,

37. _____ Nerve injury occurring at birth in which the diaphragm does not expand adequately, often resulting in respiratory distress.

38. _____ Cooling of the infant's head or entire body to reduce severity of neurologic injury in hypoxic ischemic encephalopathy.

39. _____ Complex, multicausal disorder that affects the developing blood vessels in the eyes; it is often associated with oxygen tensions that are too high for the level of retinal maturity, initially resulting in vasoconstriction and continuing problems after the oxygen is discontinued. Scar tissue formation and consequent visual impairment may be mild or severe.

40. _____ Acute inflammatory disease of the gastrointestinal mucosa commonly complicated by perforation; intestinal ischemia, colonization by pathogenic bacteria, and formula feeding all play an important role in its development.

41. _____ is an energy conserving technique for infants learning to nipple feed who may become excessively fatigued, cyanotic, or listless.

42. _____ Chronic lung disease with a multifactorial etiology. Pathologic process related to alveolar damage from lung disease, prolonged exposure to mechanical ventilation, high peak inspiratory pressures and oxygen, and immature alveoli and respiratory tract.

43. _____ Respiratory dysfunction in neonates and is primarily a disease related to developmental delay in lung maturation.

44. _____ Combined findings of severe pulmonary hypertension, right-to-left shunting, and shunting through the ductus arteriosus.

II. REVIEWING KEY CONCEPTS

1. The clinical manifestations of perinatal drug exposure may occur in any one or all of the following categories: CNS, gastrointestinal, respiratory, and autonomic nervous system signs. List some common signs of each category:
   Central nervous system
   Gastrointestinal
   Respiratory
   Autonomic nervous system

2. Explain the relationship between neonatal hypoglycemia and intrauterine hyperinsulism in the infant of a diabetic mother (IDM).

3. What measures should the nurse emphasize when managing the care of pregnant women with gestational diabetes to reduce the risk for fetal congenital anomalies?

4. Explain the pathogenesis of Rh incompatibility and ABO incompatibility.

5. The nursing care management of a newborn whose mother is HIV positive would most likely include which of the following? Select all that apply.
   a. Isolating the newborn in a special nursery
   b. Implementing standard precautions immediately after birth
   c. Telling the mother that she should not breastfeed
   d. Wearing gloves for routine care measures such as feeding
   e. Initiating treatment with antiviral medication(s) as soon as the newborn is confirmed to be HIV positive
   f. Administering chemoprophylaxis against Pneumocystis carinii pneumonia in HIV-exposed infants.

6. The preterm infant is vulnerable to a number of complications related to immaturity of body systems. Identify the potential problems and their physiologic basis for each of the areas listed:
   Respiratory function
   Cardiovascular function

Thermoregulation
Central nervous system function
Nutritional status
Renal function
Hematologic status
Immune status and infection prevention

7. Preterm infants are at increased risk for developing respiratory distress. The nurse should assess for signs that would indicate that the newborn is having difficulty breathing. Which of the following are signs of respiratory distress? Select all that apply.
   a. Use of abdominal muscles to breathe
   b. Tachypnea
   c. Periodic breathing pattern
   d. Suprasternal retraction
   e. Nasal flaring
   f. Acrocyanosis

8. When caring for a preterm infant born at 30 weeks of gestation, the nurse should recognize which of the following as the newborn's primary nursing diagnosis?
   a. Risk for infection related to decreased immune response
   b. Ineffective breathing pattern related to surfactant deficiency and weak respiratory muscle effort
   c. Ineffective thermoregulation related to immature thermoregulation center
   d. Imbalanced nutrition: less than body requirements related to ineffective suck and swallow

9. The nurse is caring for a newborn whose mother had gestational diabetes. His estimated gestational age is 41 weeks, and his birthweight is 4800 g. When assessing this newborn, the nurse should be alert for which of the following?
   a. Fracture of the femur
   b. Hypercalcemia
   c. Blood glucose level less than 40 mg/dL
   d. Signs of a congenital heart defect

III. CLINICAL JUDGMENT AND NEXT-GENERATION NCLEX® EXAMINATION-STYLE QUESTIONS

1. Anne, a preterm newborn who weighs 3 lb. and 12 oz (1800 g) at 34 weeks of gestation, is admitted to the neonatal intensive care unit (NICU) after her birth for observation and supportive care. Anne's nutritional needs are a critical concern in her care. Oral formula feedings are being considered.

   a. State the assessment data that the nurse should document after each of Anne's feedings to indicate feeding method effectiveness.

   b. The nurse determines that Anne's suck is weak and she becomes too fatigued during oral feedings to obtain sufficient nutrients and fluid. The nurse consults with the practitioner and a decision is made to provide intermittent gavage feedings with occasional oral feedings. Describe the guidelines the nurse should follow when inserting the gavage tube.

c. State the priority nursing diagnosis for Anne.

d. Discuss the principles the nurse should follow before, during, and after a gavage feeding to ensure safety and maximum effectiveness.

e. Outline the protocol that should be followed when advancing Anne to full oral feeding.

2. The nurse is preparing to insert a gavage tube and feed a preterm newborn. As part of the protocol for this procedure, the nurse should consider the determination of optimal feeding tube placement. Describe current evidence-based guidelines for ensuring safety of feeding tube placement in infants.

3. The NICU is a stressful environment for preterm infants and their families.

a. Identify the common sources of stress facing infants and their families in an intensive care environment.

Infant stressors

Family stressors

b. Nurses working in the NICU and parents must be aware of infant behavioral cues and adjust stimuli accordingly. List infant behavioral cues that indicate readiness for interaction and stimulation and behavioral cues that signal a need for a time-out.

Approach behaviors (readiness)

Avoidance behaviors (need for a time-out)

c. Identify specific measures that can be used to protect infants from overstimulation and yet provide appropriate stimulation to meet the developmental and emotional needs of infants.

d. Specify the guidelines that should be followed regarding infant positioning.

4. Marion is beginning her 43rd week of pregnancy.

a. Support this statement: Perinatal mortality is significantly higher in the postterm neonate.

b. State the assessment findings that are typical of a postterm infant.

c. Discuss the two major complications that can be experienced by a postterm infant.

5. A 26-week neonate who is medically stable is receiving intravenous total parenteral nutrition. Minimal enteral (trophic) feedings with maternal breast milk are being considered. Describe the concept of these trophic feedings in preterm infants and the reported advantages and disadvantages.

6. Anita and Juan are the parents of a 2-day-old preterm newborn boy. Their baby, who is 27 weeks' gestation and weighs 1 kg, is in the NICU and will be in the hospital for several weeks. The nurse caring for this baby recognizes that he must also provide supportive care for Anita and Juan. **Choose the most likely options for the information missing from the statement below by selecting from the lists of options provided.**

When an infant is very premature and sick, while <u>1</u> is necessary due to the infant's physiologic instability, parents can feel <u>2</u> due to the infant's condition. <u>3</u> may occur, where parents prepare themselves for the infant's death, but still hope for his recovery. Nurses can help facilitate bonding by preparing the parents before seeing their infant for the first time. Parents are encouraged to visit the infant as soon as possible. Feelings of guilt, anxiety, helplessness, and anger are <u>4</u>.

Options for 1	Options for 2	Options for 3	Options for 4
bonding	detached	anticipatory grief	signs of concern
physical separation	separation anxiety	delayed grief	abnormal responses
emotional separation	attached	chronic grief	normal responses

159

26 21st Century Pediatric Nursing

I. LEARNING KEY TERMS

MATCHING: Match each term with its corresponding definition.

1. _____ Analyzing and translating published clinical research into everyday nursing practice.

2. _____ Interaction with patients in which boundaries are blurred and the nurse's personal needs may be served rather than the patient's.

3. _____ Complex developmental process based on rational and deliberate thought.

4. _____ Creating opportunities and means for family members or caregivers to show current abilities and acquire new ones to meet the child's needs.

5. _____ Therapeutic care that minimizes the psychologic and physical distress experienced by children and their families.

6. _____ The philosophy that recognizes the family as the constant in a child's life that service systems must support and enhance.

7. _____ Meaningful interaction with caring, well-defined boundaries separating the nurse from the patient.

8. _____ Body mass index equal to or greater than the 95th percentile for children of the same age and gender.

9. _____ Describes the interaction of professionals with families in such a way that families maintain or acquire a sense of control over their family lives and acknowledge positive changes that result from helping behaviors that foster their own strengths, abilities, and actions.

10. _____ Ensuring parents/caregivers are aware of developmental needs at each stage of developmental growth.

11. _____ Significant yet preventable health problem for children.

12. _____ Opportunities to reduce differences in current health status among members of different groups and to ensure equal opportunities and resources to enable all children to achieve their fullest health potential.

13. _____ Most common cause of death and disability among children.

14. _____ Accounts for approximately 50% of all acute conditions.

15. _____ Involves ensuring that families are aware of all available health services, adequately informed of treatments and procedures, involved in the child's care, and encouraged to change or support existing health care practices.

16. _____ Symptoms severe enough to limit activity or require medical attention.

17. _____ The number of deaths during the first year of life per 1000 live births.

18. _____ A form of self-violence which is the third-leading cause of death among children and adolescents 10–19 years old.

a. Clinical reasoning

b. Enabling

c. Family-centered care

d. Early childhood caries

e. Evidence-based practice

f. Obesity

g. Atraumatic care

h. Anticipatory guidance strategies

i. Therapeutic relationship

j. Nontherapeutic relationships

k. Child health promotion

l. Empowerment

m. Advocacy

n. Injuries

o. Respiratory illness

p. Acute illness

q. Suicide

r. Infant mortality rate

II. REVIEWING KEY CONCEPTS

1. Which of the following category of children sees the most dramatic time of physical, motor, cognitive, emotional, and social development occur?
   a. Infancy
   b. Toddlers
   c. Preschoolers
   d. School-age children

2. Lifestyle interventions showing promise in preventing obesity and decreasing occurrence of obesity if targeted at children aged:
   a. Beginning at 6 months of age
   b. One to three years of age
   c. Three to five years of age
   d. Six to 12 years of age

3. Which of the following most accurately reflects the American Academy of Pediatrics (AAP) view on screen time:
   a. For infants less than 12 months of age no screen time is advised.
   b. It is important the parent or caregiver view the information on the screen with the child.
   c. After the age of 5, there is no screen time limit.
   d. Parents of school-age children do not have to participate in screen-time viewing.

4. Which of the following statements about nutrition in childhood is most accurate?
   a. Children establish lifelong eating habits during the first 5 years of life.
   b. Iron-fortified formula is the preferred form of nutrition for all infants.
   c. During adolescence, parental influence regarding nutrition increases.
   d. Most children's eating preferences and attitudes related to food are established by family influences and culture.

5. List three factors that contribute to increasing the morbidity of any disorder in children.

6. Two basic concepts in the philosophy of family-centered pediatric nursing care are:
   a. enabling and empowerment.
   b. empowerment and bias.
   c. enabling and curing.
   d. empowerment and self-control.

7. An example of atraumatic care would be to:
   a. eliminate or minimize distress experienced by a child in a health care setting.
   b. restrict visiting hours to adults only.
   c. perform invasive procedures only in the treatment room.
   d. permit only traditional clinical practices.

8. Which of the following is most accurate about bicycle associated injuries?
   a. Bicycle helmets can greatly reduce the risk of head injury.
   b. Children ages 8–12 are at the greatest risk of bicycling fatalities.
   c. The majority of bicycling deaths are from liver or splenic lacerations.
   d. The wearing of bicycle helmets has increased significantly.

9. List the first four leading causes of death in infancy which typically occur in the perinatal period.

10. Which of the following most accurately reflects violence in children?
    a. Lower homicide rates have been found among minority groups.
    b. The presence of a gun in a home increases the risk of suicide by about tenfold.
    c. Youth violence is a high-priority concern in the United States.
    d. The problem of childhood homicide is extremely rare.

11. Define quality of care.

12. List the six domains of the National Strategy for Quality Improvement in Healthcare.

CLINICAL JUDGMENT AND NEXT-GENERATION NCLEX® EXAMINATION-STYLE QUESTIONS

1. The pediatric nurse is providing injury prevention teaching to a group of parents at the hospital's daycare center. The nurse discusses the different kinds of injuries according to their developmental stage which could occur. Which type of injury is most common in mobile toddlers? Select all that apply.

   a. Falls

   b. Suffocation

c. Aspirations

d. Burns

e. Tricycle accidents

f. Collision with objects

2. The Nursing Professional Development Specialist (nurse educator) for the pediatric medical-surgical unit is conducting a session on family-centered care for the new graduate nurses. Which of the following actions are supportive of the philosophy of family-centered care? Select all that apply.

a. Offering personal opinions about health care decisions.

b. Recognizing the child and family for their uniqueness.

c. Continuing a connection with the family after discharge via social media.

d. Purchasing needed items (toys, clothes, gift cards, gas cards) for the child and family.

e. Encouraging and providing family members the opportunities to be active participants in the child's care.

f. Having open and honest conversations between the family, child (when appropriate), and healthcare team members.

g. Offering appropriate resources for support and networking to the child and family.

3. Identify at least one health teaching strategy which could be implemented by pediatric nurses regarding current childhood health problems to parents and children.

27 Family, Social, Cultural, and Religious Influences on Child Health Promotion

I. LEARNING KEY TERMS

MATCHING: Match each term with its corresponding definition.

1. _____ Establishment of the rules or guidelines from behavior.

2. _____ A refinement of the practice of sending the child to his or her room; based on the premise of removing the reinforcer and using the strategy of unrelated consequences.

3. _____ A set of rules governing conduct.

4. _____ Used to describe families and how the family unit responds to events both within and outside the family.

5. _____ Family situation in which each parent is awarded custody of one or more of the children, thereby separating siblings.

6. _____ Family situation in which the children reside with one parent, with both parents acting as legal guardians and both participating in child rearing.

7. _____ What an individual considers it to be; an institution where individuals, related through biology or enduring commitments, and representing similar or different generations and genders, participate in roles involving mutual socialization, nurturance, and emotional commitment.

8. _____ The descriptive term that accommodates a variety of family styles, including communal families, single-parent families, and same-sex partner families.

9. _____ Refers to the interactions of family members, especially the quality of those relationships and interactions.

10. _____ Placement in an approved living situation away from the family of origin.

11. _____ Family unit a person is born into.

12. _____ Blood relationships.

13. _____ Refers to the composition of the family.

14. _____ Grouping individuals who share common characteristics unique in comparison to others in a society, resulting in a distinctive, cultural behavior.

15. _____ A unique awareness, belief, practice, and experience starting in childhood and is rooted over time.

16. _____ Grouping of people by their outward, physical appearance.

17. _____ A specific set of beliefs enacted through a practice.

a. Family
b. Family theory
c. Discipline
d. Limit setting
e. Time-out
f. Divided, or split, custody
g. Joint custody
h. Consanguineous
i. Foster care
j. Family of origin
k. Household
l. Family function
m. Family structure
n. Ethnicity
o. Spirituality
p. Race
q. Religion

FILL IN THE BLANKS: Insert the term that best corresponds to each of the following descriptions related to family

1. _____ Explains how families react to stressful events and suggests factors that promote adaptation to stress.

2. _____ Addresses family change over time.

3. _____ Consists of a married couple and their biologic children.

4. _____ Reconstituted family, includes at least one stepparent, stepsibling, or half-sibling.

5. _____ Parents continuing the parenting role while terminating the spousal unit.

6. _____ Initially takes place within the family unit, in which the children fulfill a set of roles and respond to the roles of their parents and other family members.

7. _____ Status an individual may attain as a result of divorce, separation, death of a spouse, or birth or adoption of a child.

8. _____ Children who are raised by grandparents or other family members at some time in their lives.

9. _____ A major factor that influences a family's adaptability.

10. _____ The emphasis is on the interaction between the members; a change in one family member creates a change in other members, which in turn results in a new change in the original member.

II. REVIEWING KEY CONCEPTS

1. Which of the following descriptions would *not* be correct using the current definition of the term *family?*
   a. The family is what the patient considers it to be.
   b. The family may be related or unrelated.
   c. The family members are always related by legal ties or genetic relationships and live in the same household.
   d. The family members share a sense of belonging to their own family.

2. Parenting practices differ between small and large families. Which one of the following characteristics is found in small families?
   a. Able to adjust to a variety of changes and crises.
   b. Adolescents identify more strongly with their parents and rely more on their parents for advice.

   c. More emphasis is placed on the group and less on the individual.
   d. Older siblings often administer discipline.

3. Ignoring a child's bad behavior will hopefully extinguish or minimize the bad behavior occurrence. For ignoring the bad behavior to be effective which of the following is most appropriate for the parent to do?
   a. Give in to the bad behavior every so often.
   b. Be aware of the "response burst" phenomenon.
   c. Offer the parents and child a "cooling-off" period of time and then implement consequences.
   d. Use a pattern of intermittent or occasional enforcement of limits for the child.

4. Areas of concern for parents of adoptive children include:
   a. the initial attachment process.
   b. telling the children that they are adopted.
   c. identity formation of the children during adolescence.
   d. appropriate disciplinary tactics.
   e. a, b, c, d.

5. Which of the following is not an important consideration for parents when telling their children about the decision to divorce?
   a. Initial disclosure should include both parents and siblings.
   b. Time should be allowed for discussion with each child individually.
   c. Initial disclosure should be kept simple and reasons for divorce should not be included.
   d. Parents should physically hold or touch their child to provide feelings of warmth and reassurance.

6. The clinic nurse is explaining the strategy of consequences to use with children when they misbehave to the parents of a set of twins. Which of the following indicates a need for further parental teaching?
   a. Unrelated – those consequences imposed deliberately.
   b. Logical – those consequences directly related to the rules.
   c. Natural – those consequences that occur without intervention.
   d. Reflective – those consequences decided upon by the child.

7. Which of the following is a major cause of acute and chronic stress in children?
   a. Poverty.
   b. School environment.
   c. Divorce.
   d. Parental education level.

8. The nurse is reviewing the importance of role learning for children. The nurse understands children's roles are primarily shaped by which members?

a. Siblings.
b. School friends.
c. Parents.
d. Grandparents.

9. Which of the following would allow integration of spiritual practices into the plan of care for the child and family?
   a. Explain your religious practices to the child and family in conversations with them.
   b. Provide compassionate passive listening.
   c. Sit with and support the child and family during times of spiritual questioning.
   d. Provide appropriate answers to the parent's questions, the children do not really have the cognitive function to understand this concept.

10. Identify the useful functions of limit setting and discipline as they relate to children and child-rearing.

11. Discuss the rationale for children needing limit setting.

MATCHING: Match the different types of parenting styles.

12. _____ Parents who exert little or no control over their children's actions.

13. _____ These parents direct their children's behavior and attitudes by emphasizing the reason for rules and negatively reinforcing deviations.

14. _____ Parents who try to control their children's behavior and attitudes through unquestioned mandates.

a. Authoritarian
b. Permissive
c. Authoritative

III. CLINICAL JUDGMENT AND NEXT-GENERATION NCLEX ® EXAMINATION-STYLE QUESTIONS

1. The nurse is caring for a 12-year-old cystic fibrosis patient admitted for a pulmonary exacerbation who is now ready for discharge. The patient's parents have not been able to visit often due to work- and travel-related issues but call once or twice daily for an update from the providers. Using concepts related to family strengths and functioning style, which are the most appropriate actions for the nurse to implement?

   Use an X for the nursing actions listed below that are Indicated (appropriate or necessary), Contraindicated (could be harmful), or Non-Essential (makes no difference or not necessary) for the patient's care at this time.

Nursing Action	Indicated	Contraindicated	Non-Essential
Continue empowering this family through active participation in the child's care.			
Determine the type of parenting style used by these parents.			
Offer the parents support and resources for possible future hospitalizations.			
Appreciate the family's strengths and uniqueness, use these to facilitate the discharge process.			

Chapter **27** **Family, Social, Cultural, and Religious Influences on Child Health Promotion**

28 Developmental and Genetic Influences on Child Health Promotion

I. LEARNING KEY TERMS

MATCHING: Match each term with its corresponding definition.

1. _____ An effective way to prevent neonatal hypothermia.

2. _____ An increase in competence and adaptability; aging; most often used to describe a qualitative change.

3. _____ The processes by which developing individuals become acquainted with the world and the objects it contains.

4. _____ Processes whereby early embryonal cells and structures are systematically modified and altered (from broad, global patterns) to achieve specific and characteristic physical and chemical properties.

5. _____ The most widely accepted theory of personality development, which emphasizes a healthy personality and was advanced by Erikson; uses the biologic concepts of critical periods and epigenesis, describing key conflicts or more problems that the individual strives to master during critical periods in personality development.

6. _____ Term used by Freud to describe any sensual pleasure.

7. _____ According to Chess and Thomas (1999), a term defined as the manner of thinking, behaving, or reacting that is characteristic of an individual; the way in which a person deals with life.

8. _____ The rate of metabolism when the body is at rest.

9. _____ The work of the child.

10. _____ The most accurate measure of general development; the radiologic determination of osseous maturation.

11. _____ A personal, subjective judgment of one's worthiness derived from and influenced by the social groups in the immediate environment and individuals' perceptions of how they are valued by others.

12. _____ Limited times during a process of growth when the organism is more susceptible to positive or negative influences.

13. _____ A vital component of self-concept, referring to the subjective concepts and attitudes that individuals have toward their own bodies.

14. _____ The directional pattern of growth and development that proceeds from near to far.

15. _____ The term that includes all the notions, beliefs, and convictions that constitute an individual's self-knowledge and influence that individual's relationships with others.

16. _____ The directional trend of growth and development that proceeds from head to tail.

a. Maturation

b. Differentiation

c. Kangaroo care

d. Cephalocaudal

e. Proximodistal

f. Sensitive period

g. Skeletal age

h. Basal metabolic rate

i. Temperament

j. Psychosexual development

k. Psychosocial development

l. Cognition

m. Self-concept

n. Body image

o. Self-esteem

p. Play

II. REVIEWING KEY CONCEPTS

1. Categorizing growth and behavior into approximate age stages:
   a. helps to account for individual differences in children.
   b. can be applied to all children with some degree of precision.
   c. provides a convenient means to describe the majority of children.
   d. determines the speed of each child's growth.

2. Which of the following is an example of a cephalocaudal directional trend in development?
   a. Head growth precedes limb growth.
   b. Fingers and toes develop after embryonic limb buds.
   c. Infants manipulate fingers after they are able to use the whole hand as a unit.
   d. Infants begin to have fine muscle control after gross random muscle movement is established.

3. An average healthy term infant who weighs 7 pounds at birth can be expected to weigh approximately. _____ pounds by 12 months of life.
   a. 14
   b. 18
   c. 21
   d. 24

4. Which of the following is considered fixed and precise in the development of children?
   a. The pace and rate of development
   b. The order of development
   c. Physical growth—in particular, height
   d. Growth during the vulnerable period

5. Behavior that meets with approval and pleases or helps others is considered good is indicative of which moral development stage?
   a. Preconventional level.
   b. Conventional level.
   c. Principled level.
   d. Formal operational level.

6. If the height of a 2-year-old is measured as 88 cm, his height at adulthood would be estimated as:
   a. 132 cm.
   b. 176 cm.
   c. 172 cm.
   d. 190 cm.

7. Growth and development patterns occur in a predictable and universal but in a time unique to each individual. Which of the following is the first pattern to develop?
   a. Proximodistal pattern.
   b. Differentiation pattern.
   c. Cephalocaudal pattern.
   d. Maturational pattern.

8. Which of the following is the most prominent feature of childhood and adolescence?
   a. physical growth.
   b. neurologic maturation.
   c. psychosocial development.
   d. temperament maturation.

9. The nurse determines that a 7-month-old infant who weighs 10 kg needs about:
   a. 500 kcal per day.
   b. 750 kcal per day.
   c. 1050 kcal per day.
   d. 1500 kcal per day.

10. The basal metabolic rate (BMR) is highest in the:
    a. adolescent.
    b. infant over 6 months of age.
    c. school-age child.
    d. infant under 6 months of age.

11. The energy requirement to build tissue:
    a. fluctuates randomly.
    b. fluctuates based on need.
    c. steadily decreases with age.
    d. steadily increases with age.

12. Body temperature in young children and infants responds to:
    a. crying.
    b. exercise.
    c. emotional upset.
    d. a, b, and c.

13. A mother asks whether her 13-month-old child's sleep behavior is abnormal because he usually sleeps through the night and takes two short naps a day. The nurse's response should indicate that the infant probably:
    a. has a normal sleep pattern.
    b. has periods of sleeplessness at night.
    c. does not have colic.
    d. is at risk for having sleep problems in later life.

FILL IN THE BLANKS: Insert the term that describes the child's temperament.

14. _____ These children are highly active, irritable, and irregular in their habits. They require a more structured environment and adapt slowly to new routines, people, and situations.

15. _____ These children typically react negatively and with mild intensity to new stimuli. They are inactive and moody.

16. _____ These children are even tempered, are regular and predictable in their habits, and have a positive approach to new stimuli.

17. Personality development as viewed by Freud focuses on:
    a. the significance of sexual instincts.
    b. the suppression of psychosexual instincts.
    c. direct observations of adults.
    d. retrospective studies of children.

18. Erikson's theory provides a framework for:
    a. clearly indicating the experience needed to resolve crises.
    b. emphasizing pathologic development.
    c. coping with extraordinary events.
    d. explaining children's behavior in mastering developmental tasks.

19. Erikson's stage of trust vs. mistrust corresponds to Freud's:
    a. anal stage.
    b. oral stage.
    c. phallic stage.
    d. guilt stage.

20. For adolescents, their struggle to fit the roles they have played and those they hope to play is best outlined by:
    a. Freud's latency period.
    b. Freud's phallic stage.
    c. Erikson's identity vs. role confusion stage.
    d. Erikson's intimacy vs. isolation stage.

21. The best-known theory regarding cognitive development was developed by:
    a. Sullivan.
    b. Kohlberg.
    c. Erikson.
    d. Piaget.

22. An important prerequisite for all other mental activity is the child's awareness that an object exists even though it is no longer visible. According to Piaget, this awareness is called:
    a. object permanence.
    b. logical thinking.
    c. egocentricity.
    d. reversibility.

23. The predominant characteristic of Piaget's preoperational period is egocentricity, which according to him, means:
    a. concrete and tangible reasoning.
    b. selfishness and self-centeredness.
    c. inability to see another's perspective.
    d. ability to make deductions and generalize.

24. The stages of moral development that allow for prediction of behavior but not for individual differences are outlined in the moral development theory according to:
    a. Fowler.
    b. Holstein.
    c. Gilligan.
    d. Kohlberg.

25. Which of the following psychosocial developmental stages best describes when children learn to compete and cooperate with others, they learn the rules, it is a decisive period in their social relationships with others?
    a. Autonomy vs. shame and doubt.
    b. Initiative vs. guilt.
    c. Industry vs. inferiority.
    d. Identity vs. role confusion.

MATCHING: Match each type of play with the corresponding example of that type of play.

26. _____ Coloring a picture alone.

27. _____ Using the telephone, predominant form of play in preschool children, also known as pretend play

28. _____ Not playful but focusing their attention momentarily on anything that strikes their interest; daydreaming.

29. _____ Play where infants take pleasure in relationships with people.

30. _____ Children watch what other children are doing but make no attempt to enter into the play activity.

31. _____ Organized play.

32. _____ Play demonstrated by repeating an action over and over again.

33. _____ A nonsocial stimulating experience that stimulates the child's senses and gives pleasure.

34. _____ Children play together but there is no organization.

35. _____ Characteristic play of toddlers, each child plays beside but not with the other child.

a. Sense-pleasure play

b. Skill play

c. Unoccupied behavior

d. Dramatic play

e. Social-affective play

f. Onlooker play

g. Solitary play

h. Parallel play

i. Associative play

j. Cooperative play

36. Which of the following best describes the rate of speech development in children?
   a. Infants often learn sign language before vocal language.
   b. Speech precedes gestures.
   c. The first parts of speech typically used are adjectives and adverbs.
   d. At all stages of language development, comprehension vocabulary is about equal to expressed vocabulary.

MATCHING: Match the following genetic terms with the appropriate definition.

37. _____ Agent that causes a birth defect when present in the prenatal environment.

38. _____ Occurs when a single anomaly leads to a cascade of anomalies (e.g., Pierre Robin).

39. _____ A nonrandom pattern of malformations for which a cause has not been established (e.g., VACTERL).

40. _____ A recognized pattern of anomalies resulting from a single specific cause (e.g., trisomy 21).

a. Syndrome

b. Association

c. Sequence

d. Teratogen

41. Identify possible nursing interventions to assist families with children diagnosed with a genetic disorder which may facilitate their ability to manage stress, restore balance, and adapt to this new situation.

FILL IN THE BLANK USING THE CORRECT CONGENITAL MALFORMATION TERM

42. _____ are abnormal formations of organs or body parts resulting from an abnormal developmental process, with most occurring before 12 weeks of gestation.

Chapter **28** **Developmental and Genetic Influences on Child Health Promotion**

43. _____ result from abnormal organization of cells into a particular tissue type.

44. _____ result from the breakdown of previously normal tissue.

45. _____ are often caused by extrinsic mechanical forces on normally developing tissue.

III. CLINICAL JUDGMENT AND NEXT-GENERATION NCLEX® EXAMINATION-STYLE QUESTIONS

1. It is important for nurses to recognize minor anomalies and dysmorphology which may suggest a genetic disorder. Choose the most likely options for the information missing from the statements below by selecting from the list of options provided.

   A _____ option 1 _____ is important to obtain before the initial genetics consult. If a nurse identifies

   a _____ option 2 _____ - _____ that could be indicative of additional congenital anomalies. If

   _____ option 3 _____ or _____ - anomalies are identified this could be suspicious of an underlying syndrome requiring further evaluation.

Options for 1	Options for 2	Options for 3
chromosomal analysis	minor anomaly	one or more
ultrasound	major anomaly	two or more
family health history	congenital anomaly	three or more
immunization history	fetal anomaly	four or more

2. Parents of a 2-year-old child with Down syndrome are considering genetic testing before getting pregnant again. Discuss information the nurse could provide to assist and instruct the family regarding genetic testing.

3. Identify and discuss the significance of nursing interventions to assist families with children with a genetic disorder.

29 Communication, History, and Physical Assessment of the Child and Family

I. LEARNING KEY TERMS

MATCHING: Match each term with its corresponding description.

1. _____ An essential parameter of nutritional status; the measurement of height, weight, head circumference, proportions, skinfold thickness, and arm circumference.

2. _____ The capacity to understand what another person is experiencing from within that person's frame of reference.

3. _____ Specific reason for the child's visit to the clinic or hospital.

4. _____ Produced as air passes through narrowed passageways, regardless of the cause.

5. _____ Specific review of each body system.

6. _____ This type of murmur occurs when there is no anatomic cardiac defect exists, but a physiologic abnormality (e.g., anemia) is may be present.

7. _____ Appears translucent, light pearly pink, or gray.

8. _____ Lateral curvature of the spine.

9. _____ This murmur occurs when a cardiac defect with or without a physiologic abnormality exists.

10. _____ The area of most intense pulsation.

11. _____ This technique is used for palpating organs and large blood vessels and for detecting masses.

12. _____ Bowel sounds.

13. _____ The amount of elasticity in the skin; determined by grasping the skin on the abdomen or arm between the thumb and index finger, pulling it taut, and quickly releasing it.

14. _____ An extra digit.

15. _____ Used to identify any areas of tenderness, muscle tone, and superficial lesions, such as cysts.

16. _____ Fusion of digits.

17. _____ Result from the passage of air through fluid or moisture.

18. _____ A person's standing height.

19. _____ Occurs when one eye deviates from the point of fixation; sometimes called "cross eye."

20. _____ A patient's length measured while the patient is lying down or supine.

21. _____ The ability to visually fixate on one visual field with both eyes simultaneously.

22. _____ This type of murmur occurs when there is noanatomic or physiologic abnormality.

a. Empathy

b. Chief complaint

c. Wheezes

d. Review of systems

e. Anthropometry

f. Recumbent length

g. Stature

h. Tissue turgor

i. Innocent murmur

j. Syndactyly

k. Organic murmur

l. Polydactyly

m. Functional murmur

n. Deep palpation

o. Tympanic membrane

p. Binocularity

q. Strabismus

r. Crackles

s. Superficial palpation

t. Peristalsis

u. Point of maximum intensity

v. Scoliosis

II. REVIEWING KEY CONCEPTS

1. A mother has brought her daughter to the clinic as a new patient. Her daughter is 12-years-old and, requires a physical examination so that she can play volleyball. Which of the following techniques used by the nurse to establish effective communication during the interview process is not correct?
   a. The nurse introduces himself or herself and asks the names of all family members present.
   b. After the introduction, the nurse is careful to direct questions about the child to her mother because she is the best source of information.
   c. After the introduction and explanation of her role, the nurse begins the interview by saying to the child, "Tell me about your volleyball team."
   d. The nurse chooses to conduct the interview in a quiet area with few distractions.

2. While assessing the child, the nurse communicates with the child's family. Which of the following does the nurse recognize as *not* productive in obtaining information?

   a. Obtaining input from the child, verbal and nonverbal
   b. Observing the relationship between parents and child
   c. Using broad, open-ended questions
   d. Avoiding the use of guiding statements to direct the focus of the interview

3. Anticipatory guidance should:
   a. view family weakness as a competence builder.
   b. focus on problem resolution.
   c. base interventions on needs identified by the nurse.
   d. empower the family to use information to build parenting ability.

4. T F Children are alert to their surroundings and attach meaning to gestures.

5. T F Active attempts to make friends with children before they have had an opportunity to evaluate an unfamiliar person may increase their anxiety.

6. T F When communicating with small children the nurse should assume a position that is at eye level with the child.

MATCHING: Match each development stage with its corresponding description of appropriate communication guidelines to be used.

7. _____ Children focus communication on themselves; experiences of others are of no interest to them.

8. _____ Children primarily use and respond to nonverbal communication.

9. _____ Children require explanations and reasons why procedures are being done to them.

10. _____ Children are often willing to discuss their concern with an adult outside the family and often welcome the opportunity to interact with a nurse.

a. Infancy
b. Early childhood
c. School-age years
d. Adolescence

11. Which of the following best describes the appropriate use of play as a communication technique in children?
    a. Small infants have little response to activities that focus on repetitive actions like patting and stroking.
    b. Few clues about intellectual or social developmental progress are obtained from the observation of children's play behaviors.
    c. Therapeutic play has little value in reduction of trauma from illness or hospitalization.
    d. Play sessions serve as a tool to reduce the trauma of illness and hospitalization.

12. List the components of a complete pediatric health history.

13. In eliciting the chief complaint, it would be inappropriate for the nurse to:
    a. limit the chief complaint to a brief statement restricted to one or two symptoms.

    b. use labeling-type questions such as "How are you? Are you sick?" to facilitate information exchange.
    c. record the chief complaint in the child's or parent's own words.
    d. use open-ended neutral questions to elicit information.

14. Which component of the pediatric health history is illustrated by the following statement? "Nausea and vomiting for 3 days. Started with abdominal cramping after eating hamburger at home. No pain or cramping at present. Unable to keep any foods down but able to drink clear liquids without vomiting. No temperature elevation; no diarrhea."
    a. Chief complaint
    b. Past history
    c. Present illness
    d. Review of systems

15. Head circumference in children should be measured up until what age and what circumstance?
    a. Until 18 months of age when the anterior fontanel should close.
    b. Until 24 months of age and in any child whose head size is questionable.
    c. Up to 36 months of age and in any child whose head size is questionable.
    d. There is no specific time frame needed.

16. The nurse knows that the best description of the sexual history for a pediatric health history:
    a. includes a discussion of plans for future children.
    b. allows the patient to introduce sexual activity history.
    c. includes a discussion of contraception methods only when the patient discloses current sexual activity.
    d. alerts the nurse to the need for sexually transmitted infection screening.

17. When assessing respirations in a 3-month-old, the nurse would assess respirations by observing which muscle group?
    a. Thoracic muscles
    b. Abdominal muscles
    c. Intercostal muscles
    d. Accessory muscles

18. The dietary history of a pediatric patient includes:
    a. a 12-hour dietary intake recall.
    b. a more specific, detailed history for the older child.
    c. financial and cultural factors that influence food selection.
    d. criticism of parents' allowance of nonessential foods.

19. To effectively establish a setting for communication, the nurse, upon entering the room with a child and his mother, introduces herself and explains the purpose of the interview. The child is included in the interaction as the nurse asks his name and age and what he is expecting at his visit today. The nurse next tells them both, "The child is 25 pounds overweight, and his diet and exercise plan must be dreadful for him to be in such appalling shape." Which aspect of effective communication has the nurse disregarded that will most significantly impact the exchange of information during this interview?
    a. Assurance of privacy and confidentiality
    b. Preliminary acquaintance
    c. Directing the focus away from the complaint of fatigue to one of obesity
    d. Injecting her own attitudes and feelings into the interview

20. A mother brings her 11-month-old daughter to the clinic because she is "sleeping poorly and tugging at her ear when she is awake." Based on the information provided, the nurse can correctly record which of the following?
    a. Chief complaint
    b. Present illness
    c. Past medical history
    d. Symptom analysis

21. Which of the following provides resources to help families build healthy meals and be active.
    a. 12-hour recall of food intake
    b. 24-hour recall of food intake
    c. MyPlate Kids Place
    d. Clinical examination

22. The nurse is measuring a 20-month-old child's length. The most accurate method to obtain this measurement is with the child:
    a. sitting on the mom's lap.
    b. laying on a recumbent measuring board.
    c. laying on the exam table paper.
    d. standing with head and shoulders against a tape measure on the wall.

23. In examining pediatric patients, the normal head-to-toe sequence is often altered to accommodate the patient's developmental needs. With this approach, the nurse will:
    a. increase the stress and anxiety associated with the assessment of body parts.
    b. record the findings according to the normal sequence.
    c. hinder the trusting nurse–child relationship.
    d. decrease the security of the parent–child relationship.

24. A father brings his 12-month-old son in for the child's regular well-infant examination. The nurse knows that the best approach to the physical examination for this patient will be to:
    a. have the infant sit on the parent's lap to complete as much of the examination as possible.
    b. place the infant on the examining table with parent out of view.
    c. perform examination in head-to-toe direction.
    d. completely undress the child and leave him undressed during the examination.

25. Of the following behaviors, the behavior that indicates to the nurse that a child may be reluctant to participate and cooperate during a physical examination is:
    a. talking to the nurse.
    b. making eye contact with the nurse.
    c. allowing physical touching.
    d. sitting on parent's lap, playing with a doll.

26. The Centers for Disease Control and Prevention (CDC) recommend that the World Health Organization (WHO) growth standards be used to monitor growth for infants and children between the ages of _____ and _____ years old. The CDC and WHO growth charts are used for children . years old and older.

27. The assessment method that provides the best information about the physical growth pattern of a preschool-age child is to:
   a. record child's height and weight measurements on the standardized growth reference chart.
   b. keep a flow sheet for height, weight, and head circumference increases.
   c. obtain a history of sibling growth patterns.
   d. measure the height, weight, and head circumference of the child.

28. T F Normally height is less if measured in the afternoon than in the morning.

29. T F Growth is a continuous but uneven process, and the most reliable evaluation lies in comparison of growth measurements over a given time period (e.g., over a year).

30. T F Growth measurements during the physical examination should be age-specific and include length, height, weight, skinfold thickness, and arm and head circumference.

31. Head circumference is:
   a. measured in all children up to the age of 24 months.
   b. about equal to chest circumference at about 12 months of age.
   c. about 8–9 cm smaller than chest circumference during childhood.
   d. measured slightly below the eyebrows and pinna of the ears.

32. In infants and small children, the _____ pulse should be taken because it is the most reliable. This pulse should be counted for _____ because of the possibility of irregularities in rhythm.

33. What method would be considered most accurate and is recommended for screening temperature in infants under 1 month of age?
   a. Rectal.
   b. Temporal.
   c. Tympanic.
   d. Axillary.

34. When assessing a 7-year-old's lymph nodes, the nurse uses the distal portions of the fingers and gently but firmly presses in a circular motion along the occipital and postauricular node areas. The nurse records the findings as "tender, enlarged, warm lymph nodes." The nurse knows that the:
   a. findings are within normal limits for the child's age.
   b. assessment technique was incorrect and should be repeated.
   c. findings suggest infection or inflammation close to their location.
   d. recording of the information is complete because it includes temperature and tenderness.

35. Which of the following observations would not be recorded as part of the child's general appearance during a well-child examination?:
   a. Behavior, interactions with parents.
   b. Hygiene, cleanliness.
   c. Facial expressions.
   d. Vital signs.

36. Normal findings on examination of the pupils may be recorded as PERRLA, which means: _____

37. Which of the following assessments is an expected finding in the child's eye examination?
   a. Opaque red reflex of the eye
   b. Ophthalmoscopic examination reflecting veins that are darker in color and about one-fourth larger in size than the arteries
   c. Strabismus in the 12-month-old infant
   d. Five-year-old who reads the Snellen eye chart at the 20/40 level

38. When palpating the abdomen of a 7-year-old who is complaining of pain, what is the most appropriate nursing action?
   a. Palpate the painful area first.
   b. Palpate the painful area last.
   c. Palpate for rebound tenderness.
   d. Use percussion instead of palpation.

39. At what age should blood pressure readings begin to be measured annually on children?
   a. At 1 year of age.
   b. At 2 years of age.
   c. At 3 years of age.
   d. At 5 years of age.

40. Closure of the pulmonic and aortic valves:
   a. S_1.
   b. S_2.
   c. S_3.
   d. S_4.

41. In performing an examination for scoliosis, the nurse understands that which of the following is an incorrect method?
   a. The child should be clothed in a gown that opens in the back with underwear exposing the iliac crests and posterior and anterior superior iliac spines.
   b. The child should stand erect with the nurse observing from behind.
   c. The child should squat down with hands extended forward so that the nurse can observe for asymmetry of the shoulder blades.
   d. The child should bend forward from the waist so that the back is parallel to the floor and the nurse can observe from behind.

42. If strabismus is not detected and corrected by what age, the condition known as amblyopia or blindness from disuse of the eye may develop.:
    a. One to two years of age.
    b. Three to five years of age.
    c. Four to six years of age.
    d. By eight years of age.

43. Which of the following organs normally descends during inspiration as the diaphragm moves downward?
    a. Spleen
    b. Liver
    c. Kidney
    d. Appendix

III. CLINICAL JUDGMENT AND NEXT-GENERATION NCLEX® EXAMINATION-STYLE QUESTIONS

1. Which of the following would be appropriate therapeutic communication techniques to use when interviewing a child and their parents upon arrival to the pediatric medical-surgical unit? Select all that apply.

   a. Speak with the parents first if the child appears shy.

   b. Allow the parents to direct the conversation to provide them with a sense of control.

   c. Communicate at eye level with children.

   d. Allow an older child to serve as an interpreter for their family.

   e. Use broad open-ended questions to gather more information.

   f. Use careful listening which relies on the use of clues and verbal leads to gather information and move the conversation along.

Chapter **29 Communication, History, and Physical Assessment of the Child and Family**

2. Growth measurements are essential in assessing children's health status. Linear growth is one of those measurements. Which of the following would be appropriate nursing actions for obtaining linear growth in children? Use an X for the nursing actions listed below which are Indicated (appropriate or necessary), Contraindicated (could be harmful), or Non-Essential (makes no difference or not necessary).

Nursing Actions	Indicated	Contraindicated	Non-Essential
All children should be measured at least twice, three times is preferred, using the mean value of measurements.			
Use a tape measure to measure the infant's length if a length board is unavailable.			
Children between 24 and 36 months of age can be measured using recumbent length or height with a stadiometer depending on the cooperation of the child.			
When using the stadiometer, it is important to place the headboard just above the crown of the head.			
The linear growth measurement should be read to the last completed millimeter or 1/16 inch.			

30 Pain Assessment and Management in Children

I. LEARNING KEY TERMS

MATCHING: Match each term with its corresponding definition or description.

1. _____ Vocalization of sounds associated with pain, changes in facial expression, and unexpected or unusual body movements.

2. _____ Distraction, relaxation, and guided imagery to help decrease pain perception.

3. _____ A behavior pain measurement tool recommended for use with children in critical care settings.

4. _____ Eutectic mixture of local anesthetics.

5. _____ This occurs when the dose of an opioid needs to be increased to achieve the same analgesic effects that were previously achieved at a lower dose.

6. _____ A multidimensional pain instrument to assess patient and parental perceptions of the pain experience in a manner appropriate for the cognitive-developmental level of children and adolescents.

7. _____ A multidimensional pain instrument for children and adolescents that is used to assess three dimensions of pain: location, intensity, and quality.

8. _____ Uses descriptors along a line that provides a highly subjective evaluation of a pain or other symptom.

9. _____ A pain assessment tool that uses six cartoon faces ranging from a smiling face for "no pain" to a tearful face for "worst pain." The child is asked to choose a face that describes their pain.

10. _____ Interval scale that includes five categories of behavior: facial expression (F), leg movement (L), activity (A), cry (C), and consolability (C).

11. _____ A Likert-style pain scale for children 8 years and older that uses numbers 0–10 to denote intensity of pain.

12. _____ Pain that persists for 3 months or more beyond the expected period of healing.

13. _____ Drugs which may be used alone or with opioids to control pain symptoms and opioid side effects.

14. _____ Often used for postoperative pain and may include NSAIDs, local anesthetics, nonopioids, and opioid analgesics to achieve optimum relief and minimize side effects.

15. _____ Often found to lower postoperative pain, lower analgesic requirement, lower hospital stay, lower complications after surgery, and minimize the risks for peripheral and central nervous system sensitization that can lead to persistent pain.

16. _____ This is considered a` normal, natural, physiologic state of "neuroadaptation."

17. _____ Pain that is episodic and recurs.

a. COMFORT scale

b. Coanalgesic drugs or adjuvant analgesics

c. Distress behaviors

d. Chronic pain

e. Nonpharmacologic techniques

f. Pediatric Pain Questionnaire (PPQ)

g. Wong-Baker Faces Pain Rating Scale

h. Adolescent Pediatric Pain Tool (APPT)

i. Visual Analog Scale (VAS)

j. FLACC Pain Assessment Tool

k. Numeric Rating Scale (NRS)

l. EMLA

m. Tolerance.

n. Physical dependence

o. Preemptive analgesia

p. Multimodal or balanced analgesia

q. Recurrent pain

1. What information would be important to include when teaching parents about nonpharmacologic strategies for pain management in children?
   a. Nonpharmacologic strategies are used to supplement pharmacologic strategies.
   b. Gently suggesting to the parents not to stay with the child during a painful procedure.
   c. It may take time to identify a nonpharmacologic strategy that works well for their child.
   d. Using nonpharmacologic strategies basically "tricks" the child into believing they will not have pain.

2. When using patient-controlled analgesia (PCA) with children, the:
   a. drug of choice is meperidine.
   b. parent should control the dosing.
   c. nurse should control the dosing.
   d. drug of choice is morphine.

3. The anesthetic cream EMLA is applied:
   a. before invasive procedures.
   b. as preoperative oral sedation.
   c. for chronic cancer pain.
   d. postoperatively.

4. For postoperative or cancer pain control, analgesics should be administered:
   a. as needed.
   b. around the clock.
   c. before the pain escalates.
   d. after the pain peaks.

5. The most common side effect from opioid therapy is:
   a. respiratory depression.
   b. pruritus.
   c. nausea and vomiting.
   d. constipation.

6. T F Younger children may require higher doses of opioids to achieve the same analgesic effect.

7. T F Dilaudid has a longer duration of action than morphine and is associated with less nausea and pruritus than morphine.

8. T F Nonopioids, including acetaminophen (Tylenol, paracetamol) and NSAIDs (ibuprofen) are suitable for mild to moderate pain.

9. T F Self-report measures of pain are most often used for children older than 4 years of age.

10. T F For continuous pain control, such as for postoperative or cancer pain, a preventive schedule of medication around the clock (ATC) would be considered effective.

11. T F Using a PCA for children as young as 5-years-of age who can understand the concept of pushing a button to obtain pain relief would be appropriate.

12. T F Infants do not feel pain.

13. T F Parenteral and oral dosages of opioids are not the same.

14. _____ is very common in children and adolescents with chronic or recurrent pain.

15. T F Behavioral or observational measures of pain are generally used for children from neonate to 4 years old or for children of any age who are unable to report pain due to neurocognitive or communication challenges.

16. Most children _____ years and older are able to use the 0–10 numeric rating scale because of its easy use.

17. This measure provides a more comprehensive evaluation of the influence of pain on physical functioning and is known as the _____ which assesses the child's ability to perform everyday physical activities and has established psychometric properties with different populations.

18. The Noncommunicating Children's Pain Checklist is a pain measurement tool specifically designed for children with _____ .

19. The two most common types of chronic pain conditions in children are _____ and

_____ .

20. List the five classifications of complementary and alternative medicine (CAM) therapies and give an example of each.

FILL IN THE BLANK WITH THE APPROPRIATE PATIENT CONTROLLED ANALGESIA (PCA) TERM.

21. _____ are infused only according to the preset amount and lockout interval (time between doses).

22. _____ delivers a constant amount of analgesic and prevents pain from returning during those times, such as sleep.

23. _____ are typically used to give an initial loading dose to increase blood levels rapidly and to relieve breakthrough pain.

1. **When caring for a 1-month-old male infant status post pyloromyotomy, the parents are concerned about the infant's pain level because of the incisions. They ask how it will be determined if their child is experiencing pain from the surgery?**

    Use an X for the health teaching to the parents who are concerned about pain listed below that is Indicated (appropriate or necessary), Contraindicated (could be harmful), or Non-Essential (makes no difference or not necessary) regarding whether the infant is experiencing pain and how the nurses will know.

Health Teaching	Indicated	Contraindicated	Non-essential
It is important to observe the infant for distress behaviors such as crying, changes in facial expressions, unexpected or unusual body movements.			
There are specific pain assessment tools which can be used to assess pain by examining various behaviors of infants.			
Infant do not really feel pain because their nerves and pain receptors are not fully developed yet.			
Healthcare personnel can use different techniques such as rocking them or cuddling to relax them in addition to pain medication. There really is not a good way to determine if they are in pain or not, once they start crying hard, healthcare personnel can administer the ordered pain medication.			

2. Which pain assessment scale is useful for measuring pain in children with communication challenges or children with cognitive impairment who may not have be able to communicate they are in pain? Why is this the most effective way of measuring pain in these children?

31 | The Infant and Family

I. LEARNING KEY TERMS

MATCHING: Match each term with its corresponding definition or description.

1. _____ Between ages 4 and 8 months, the infant progresses through the first stage of separation-individuation and begins to have some awareness of self and mother as separate beings.

2. _____ Not an instinctual ability but a learned acquired process.

3. _____ The unexpected and abrupt death of an infant under 1 year of age that remains unexplained after a complete postmortem examination, including an investigation of the death scene and a review of the case history.

4. _____ A sign of inadequate growth resulting from inability to obtain or use calories required for growth.

5. _____ A major accomplishment of cognitive development that develops at approximately 9–10 months of age; the realization that objects continue to exist after they leave one's visual field.

6. _____ The process of giving up one method of feeding for another; usually refers to relinquishing the breast or bottle for a cup.

7. _____ Fusion of two ocular images that begins to develop at 6 weeks and should be well established by age 4 months.

8. _____ Paroxysmal abdominal pain manifested by a duration of more than 3 hours and by drawing up of the legs to the abdomen in an infant under the age of 3 months.

9. _____ Behaviors that demonstrate attachment to one person becomes prominent between 6 and 8 months-of-age. Infants cannot discriminate between familiar and unfamiliar people.

10. _____ An acquired condition that occurs as a result of cranial molding during infancy; incidence has increased dramatically since implementation of the Back to Sleep campaign.

11. _____ Usually observed in children under 1 year of age, report of a sudden, brief but resolved episode.

12. _____ The most desirable complete diet for the infant during the first 6 months.

13. _____ Begins to develop by age 7–9 months but may not be fully mature until 2 or 3 years of age, thus increasing the infant's and younger toddler's risk of falling.

a. Binocularity

b. Object permanence

c. Stranger fear/anxiety

d. Brief resolved unexplained event (BRUE)

e. Weaning

f. Parenting

g. Failure to thrive

h. Separation anxiety

i. Colic

j. Sudden infant death syndrome (SIDS)

k. Human milk

l. Positional plagiocephaly

m. Stereopsis (depth perception)

II. REVIEWING KEY CONCEPTS

1. An infant is brought to the clinic for their 1-year well-child visit. The infant weighed 7 lbs. 8 oz. at birth. Based on normal growth and development what would an appropriate weight be at this visit?
   a. 12 lbs. 8 oz.
   b. 14 lbs. 8 oz.
   c. 22 lbs. 1 oz.
   d. 23 lbs. 10 oz.

2. The age at which most infants can roll from back to abdomen is:
   a. 3 months.
   b. 6 months.
   c. 9 months.
   d. 12 months.

3. The child's anterior fontanel usually closes by:
   a. 3–6 months.
   b. 7–9 months.
   c. 12–18 months.
   d. 24 months.

4. At what age can an infant sit well unsupported?
   a. Four months
   b. Six months
   c. Eight months
   d. Ten months

5. Which of the following assessment findings would be considered most abnormal?
   a. The infant who displays head lag at 3 months of age
   b. The infant who displays head lag at 6 months of age
   c. The infant who begins to roll from front to back at 4 months
   d. The infant who begins to roll from front to back at 6 months

6. At what age would the neat pincer grasp typically be seen in an infant following normal growth and development patterns?
   a. 2 months
   b. 4 months
   c. 6 months
   d. 10 months

7. Which of the following would be appropriate guidance to give parents or caregivers about the introduction of solid foods to an infant?
   a. It is acceptable to introduce foods by mixing them with the formula in the bottle.
   b. New foods should be introduced at intervals of 4–7 days to allow for identification of food allergies.
   c. Solid foods are typically introduced between 6 and 8 months-of-age.
   d. Cow's milk may be introduced between 9 and 10 months of age if the child is receiving an iron supplement.

8. If a mother is concerned about the fact that her 14-month-old infant is not walking, the nurse would particularly want to evaluate whether the infant:
   a. pulls up to the furniture.
   b. uses a pincer grasp.
   c. transfers objects.
   d. has developed object permanence.

9. Colic is said to be more common in the infant who:
   a. is between 3 and 6 months of age.
   b. has a difficult temperament.
   c. has other congenital abnormalities.
   d. has signs of failure to thrive.

10. The nurse should withhold the vaccine if the child:
    a. has a common cold.
    b. is currently taking antibiotics.
    c. has a severe febrile illness.
    d. was born prematurely.

11. What is the third-leading cause of infant mortality in the United States?
    a. Falls
    b. Motor vehicle accidents
    c. SIDS
    d. Accidental poisoning

12. Honey should be avoided in infants younger than 12 months of age because of its association with the occurrence of:
    a. SIDS.
    b. Food allergy.
    c. Infant botulism.
    d. Pertussis.

13. Which of the following information should the nurse include when teaching the parents of a 9-month-old infant about administering liquid iron supplements?
    a. Give with meals.
    b. Administer the liquid iron supplement with whole cow's milk.
    c. Iron supplements may turn stools black or tarry green.
    d. Iron supplements may cause transient diarrhea.

14. T F The incidence of SIDS is associated with receiving the diphtheria, tetanus, and pertussis (DTaP) vaccines.

15. T F Maternal smoking during pregnancy has been implicated as a contributor to SIDS.

16. T F Parents should be advised to position an infant on his or her abdomen to prevent SIDS.

17. T F The nurse should encourage the parents to sleep in the same bed as the infant being monitored for apnea of infancy in order to detect subtle clinical changes.

18. T F Car seats have an expiration date.

19. T F An infant who does not pull to a standing position by 11–12 months old should be further evaluated for possible developmental dysplasia of the hip.

20. T F The intramuscular influenza vaccine is administered as two separate doses 4 weeks apart in first-time recipients younger than 9 years old.

MATCHING: Match each term with its corresponding definition or description.

21. _____ This vaccine is administered in early fall and is repeated yearly for ongoing protection; may be given to infants as young as 6 months.

22. _____ Vaccine protects against a number of serious infections caused by *Haemophilus influenzae* type b, especially bacterial meningitis, epiglottitis, bacterial pneumonia, septic arthritis, and sepsis.

23. _____ Vaccine protects against Streptococcal pneumococci, which are responsible for a number of bacterial infections in children under 2 years; these include generalized infections such as septicemia and meningitis or localized infections such as otitis media, sinusitis, and pneumonia.

24. _____ This vaccine is administered at 2, 4, and 6 months to protect from pertussis, diphtheria, and tetanus.

25. _____ Vaccine is administered to protect against severe diarrhea in infants and young children.

26. _____ Vaccine given to protect against muscle paralysis.

27. _____ Given to prevent severe liver disease.

28. _____ A relatively mild infection in children, recommended for all children at 12–15 months of age and at age of school entry or 4–6 years of age.

29. _____ Also known as the rubeola vaccine and is given at 12–15 months of age.

30. _____ Is spread by the fecal-oral route and from person-to-person contact, by ingestion of contaminated food or water

31. _____ Is recommended for children at 12–15 months of age and is typically given in combination with measles and rubella.

32. _____ Recommended for any susceptible child between ages 12 and 15 months with a second vaccine is recommended for children at 4 to 6 years of age, also known as the vaccine to prevent chickenpox.

a. Inactivated poliovirus vaccine (IPV)

b. Hib

c. Prevnar 13

d. DTaP

e. Influenza vaccine

f. Rotavirus vaccine

g. Hep A

h. Hep B

i. Varicella

j. Measles

k. Mumps

l. Rubella

III. CLINICAL JUDGMENT AND NEXT-GENERATION NCLEX® EXAMINATION-STYLE QUESTIONS

1. Place the following social development milestones of an infant in the order in which they occur.

Developmental Milestone	Order of Occurrence (earliest to latest)
Object permanence.	
Recognizes self in a mirror.	
Develops a social smile.	
Points to body parts.	

2. At a one-month-old well child visit, the nurse provides anticipatory guidance regarding sudden infant death syndrome (SIDS) to the parents. Which of the following would be appropriate to discuss with the parents of this infant? Place an X in the preventive teaching box below that would be Indicated (appropriate or necessary), Contraindicated (could be harmful), or Non-Essential (not necessary or makes no difference).

Preventive Teaching	Indicated	Contraindicated	Non-Essential
Room sharing is not indicated as long as the parents have a baby monitor/camera to observe the baby.			
The infant's head position can be alternated during sleep time to prevent plagiocephaly (flat spot on the infant's head).			
Soft bedding, stuffed animals, and crib bumper pads should not be used.			
A pacifier is a SIDS protective factor and does not interfere with breast feeding.			
All infants should be placed supine to sleep unless a medical condition prohibits this position of sleeping and places them at greater risk of death than the risk of death from SIDS.			

3. A 2-month-old infant presents for their well-child visit. The nurse determines that the child is exclusively breast fed. What would the nurse discuss regarding the infant's nutritional needs? Choose the most likely option for the information missing from the statements below by selecting from the list of options provided.

The nurse recognizes exclusively breast-feeding infants require _____ option 1 _____ IU of _____ option 1 _____ _____ daily to prevent rickets. Also, these infants may also need a supplement of _____ option 2 _____. Infants do not need additional fluids, especially _____ option 3 _____ or _____ option 3 _____ which may result in hyponatremia.

Options for 1	Options for 2	Options for 3
200 IU, Vitamin D	Vitamin B	Water, iron fortified formula
400 IU, Vitamin B	Fluoride	Iron fortified formula, juice
400 IU, Vitamin D	Iron	Low fat milk, water
800 IU, Vitamin B	Multivitamin	Water, juice

32 The Toddler and Family

I. LEARNING KEY TERMS

MATCHING: Match each term with its corresponding description.

1. _____ The need to maintain sameness and reliability.

2. _____ The destruction of teeth resulting from the process of bathing the teeth in a cariogenic environment for a prolonged period; now considered to be an infectious disease of childhood.

3. _____ Imitating household activities

4. _____ Soft bacterial deposits that adhere to the teeth and cause dental decay and periodontal disease.

5. _____ A necessary assertion of self-control in the toddler.

6. _____ The manifestation of decreased nutritional needs along with a decreased appetite, usually seen around 18 months of age.

7. _____ The retreat from one's present pattern of functioning to past levels of behavior.

8. _____ Characterized by the child playing alongside, but not with, other children.

9. _____ The developmental stage in which the toddler relinquishes dependence on others.

10. _____ One of the major tasks of toddlerhood.

a. Autonomy
b. Negativism
c. Ritualism
d. Domestic mimicry
e. Physiologic anorexia
f. Parallel play
g. Regression
h. Plaque
i. Early childhood caries
j. Toilet training

II. REVIEWING KEY CONCEPTS

1. Which of the following is the current recommendation by the American Academy of Pediatrics (AAP) regarding car seat safety?
   a. All infants and toddlers should be rear facing until they reach the age of 1 year or height recommended by the car seat manufacturer.
   b. All infants and toddlers should be rear facing as long as possible until they reach the highest weight or height recommended by the car seat manufacturer.
   c. All infants and toddlers who have outgrown their car seats may be switched to a booster seat in the back seat of the car.
   d. Manual shoulder belts are appropriate to use for toddlers.

2. The nurse is assessing fine motor development in a 3-year-old. Which of the following is the expected drawing skill for this age?
   a. Holds the writing instrument with his or her fist
   b. Can draw a complete stick figure
   c. Can copy a triangle
   d. Draws a circle

3. The usual number of words acquired by the age of 2 years is about:
   a. 50.
   b. 100.
   c. 300.
   d. 500.

4. Which of the following types of play increases in frequency as the child moves through the toddler period?
   a. Parallel play
   b. Imitative play
   c. Tactile play
   d. Solitary play

5. Which of the following statements is *false* in regard to toilet training?
   a. Bowel training is usually accomplished after bladder training.
   b. Nighttime bladder training is usually accomplished after bowel training.
   c. The toddler who is impatient with soiled diapers is demonstrating readiness for toilet training.
   d. Fewer wet diapers signal that the toddler is physically ready for toilet training.

6. Which of the following strategies is appropriate for parents to use to prepare a toddler for the birth of a sibling?
   a. Explain the upcoming birth as early in the pregnancy as possible.
   b. Move the toddler to their own new room close to the birthdate of the new sibling.
   c. Provide a doll for the toddler to imitate parenting.
   d. Tell the toddler that a new playmate will come home soon.

7. The best approach for extinguishing a toddler's attention-seeking behavior of a temper tantrum with head banging is to:
   a. ignore the behavior.
   b. provide time-out.
   c. offer a toy to calm the child.
   d. protect the child from injury.

8. What is the initial action in the emergency treatment of poisoning in a child?
   a. Locate the poison and take it to the emergency room.
   b. Prevent absorption of the poison.
   c. Terminate exposure to the poison.
   d. Assess/treat the child.

9. Regression in toddlers occurs when there is:
   a. stress.
   b. a threat to their autonomy.
   c. disruption of established routines.
   d. a, b, and c.

10. What is the recommended amount of 100% fruit juice for toddlers 1–3 years-of-age?
    a. 4 ounces/day
    b. 8 ounces/day
    c. 12 ounces/day
    d. There is no recommended amount.

11. Which of the following methods is most effective for plaque removal?
    a. Brushing and flossing
    b. Annual fluoride treatments
    c. Allowing the child to brush his or her own teeth
    d. Using a large stiff toothbrush

12. A mother of an 18-month-old asks the nurse whether she can begin to introduce low-fat milk like the rest of the family drinks. The nurse answers the mother based on the knowledge low-fat milk can safely be introduced at what age?
    a. Now would be an appropriate time.
    b. 24 months.
    c. 30 months.
    d. 36 months.

13. Physiologic anorexia in toddlers is characterized by:
    a. strong taste preferences.
    b. extreme changes in appetite from day to day.
    c. heightened awareness of social aspects of meals.
    d. weight loss and thinner appearance.

14. Healthy ways of serving food to toddlers include:
    a. Requiring the child to sit at a table for meals.
    b. Permitting nutritious grazing between meals.
    c. Discouraging between-meal snacking.
    d. Providing rewards for foods consumed.

15. The use of screen time for other than video-chatting is discouraged in children younger than _____ months of age.

16. Which of the following should the nurse expect of an 18-month-old child with normal growth and development patterns?
    a. Has slowed physical growth and enjoys associative play.
    b. Is able to separate easily from parent and enjoys a variety of foods.
    c. Has a vocabulary of 900 words and has all their deciduous teeth.
    d. May experience physiologic anorexia and usually takes an afternoon nap.

17. A 2-year-old female is brought to clinic by her parents for a well-child check. They are extremely concerned their daughter is not meeting her developmental milestones. Which of the following finds would be of concern?
    a. Their daughter is not really saying any words yet.
    b. Their daughter does not share her toys well with other children at daycare.
    c. Their daughter just started walking independently.
    d. Their daughter uses her fingers to feed herself.

18. Development of _____ is the major gross motor skill of the toddler years.

19. _____ are often an indication of the child's inability to control their emotions.

20. _____ refers to a natural jealousy and resentment toward a new child in the family or toward other children in the family when a parent turns his or her attention from them and interacts with their brother or sister.

III. CLINICAL JUDGMENT AND NEXT-GENERATION NCLEX® EXAMINATION-STYLE QUESTIONS

1. Place the following fine motor skills of a toddler in the order in which they occur.

Developmental Milestone	Order in which they occur (earliest to latest)
Uses a spoon well.	
Turns pages of a book one at a time.	
Scribbles spontaneously.	
Draws/copies circles.	

2. A mother brings her 2-year-old son in for his well-child visit. The mother asks if her 2-year-old son is ready for toilet training. Which of the following would indicate signs of toilet-training readiness? Select all that apply.

a. Myelination of the spinal column is usually complete between 18 and 24 months.

b. The child should be able to assist in taking off clothes (pants/underpants).

c. The child should be able to sit for at least 10–12 minutes without fussing.

d. The child is waking up dry from naps.

e. The child does not mind having a soiled diaper.

f. The child can tell you when they need to "go potty."

3. Toddlers are characteristically known to be ritualistic and finicky eaters which may concern parents. Which of the following suggestions would be appropriate anticipatory guidance for parents to promote optimal nutrition for growth and development of toddlers? Select all that apply.

a. Attempt to provide a regular mealtime daily using favorite dishes, cups, and utensils of the toddler which may contribute to their desire and need for predictability and ritualism.

b. Toddlers should have three regular meals and two nutritious snacks per day.

c. Once a toddler reaches 2 years of age, they can begin drinking low-fat milk with a daily milk intake of 24–30 ounces/day.

d. It is recommended toddlers have one cup of fruit per day.

e. The recommended portion size of food for toddlers is 1 tablespoon of solid food per year of age or ¼ to ¼ an adult size portion.

f. It is important the toddler has some "down time" before meals to allow them to settle before having to sit for meals.

33 The Preschooler and Family

I. LEARNING KEY TERMS

MATCHING: Match each term with its corresponding definition or description.

1. _____ Imitating the behavior of significant others.
2. _____ Infectious disease that has declined greatly since the advent of immunizations and the use of antibiotics and antitoxins.
3. _____ Group activities that have no rigid organization or rules; typical of the preschool period.
4. _____ Serious form of physical abuse caused by violent shaking of infants and young children.
5. _____ The infliction of harm on a child caused by a parent or other person who fabricates or induces illness in the child.
6. _____ Ascribing lifelike qualities to inanimate objects.
7. _____ The result of a preschooler's transductive reasoning; the belief that thoughts are all powerful.
8. _____ Failure to meet the child's need for affection, attention, and emotional nurturance.
9. _____ Articulation problems that occur when children are pressured to produce sounds ahead of their developmental level.
10. _____ Imitating the behavior of significant others.
11. _____ A type of speech pattern that occurs normally in children during the preschool period, when children are using their rapidly growing vocabulary faster than they can produce the words.
12. _____ The use, persuasion, or coercion of any child to engage in sexually explicit conduct.
13. _____ Deliberate infliction of bodily injury on a child, usually by the child's caregiver.
14. _____ Preschool-aged children have difficulty understanding the concept of tomorrow, yesterday, or next week.
15. _____ The deprivation of necessities such as food, clothing, shelter, supervision, medical care, and education.
16. _____ Behavior that attempts to hurt a person or destroys property; differs from anger.
17. _____ The superego; development in this area is a major task for the preschooler.
18. _____ Intentional bodily injury or neglect, emotional abuse or neglect, and/or sexual abuse of children, usually by adults.
19. _____ A feeling of accomplishment in one's activities; a psychosocial developmental task of the preschool period.
20. _____ Occur between early manifestations of a disease and its overt clinical syndrome.
21. _____ An invented companion that serves many purposes in the preschooler's development.

a. Sense of initiative
b. Conscience
c. Concept of time
d. Modeling
e. Magical thinking
f. Animism
g. Associative play
h. Modeling
i. Imaginary playmates
j. Aggression
k. Stuttering (stammering)
l. Dyslalia
m. Communicable disease
n. Prodromal symptoms
o. Child maltreatment
p. Physical neglect
q. Emotional neglect
r. Abusive head trauma
s. Physical abuse
t. Munchausen syndrome by proxy
u. Sexual abuse

II. REVIEWING KEY CONCEPTS

1. A 4-year-old male is admitted to the hospital with a bacterial cellulitis in which he will require 10 days of IV antibiotics. He tells the nurse he has to be in the hospital because he was "mean to his sister and wished she would go away." What is the nurse's best interpretation of the child's comment.
   a. This is animism and a common occurrence at this age.
   b. Suggestive of maladaptive behavior
   c. This is magical thinking and a common occurrence at this age.
   d. A sign of stress.

2. The average annual weight gain during the preschool years is _____ kg or _____ lb.

3. Which of the following statements about the average preschooler's physical proportions is *true*?
   a. Preschoolers have a squat and potbellied frame.
   b. Preschoolers have a slender but sturdy frame.
   c. The muscle and bones of the preschooler have reached full maturity.
   d. Sexual characteristics can be differentiated in the preschooler.

4. A 3-year-old female is hospitalized for an ASD (atrial septal defect) repair. Her parents need to go home for a few hours to see her other siblings and will be back about 6 pm. The child asks the nurse when her mommy and daddy will be back. The nurse's best response is:
   a. "Your mommy and daddy will be back at 6:00 pm."
   b. "Your mommy and daddy will be back after you eat dinner."
   c. "Your mommy and daddy will be back later this evening."
   d. "Your mommy and daddy will be back in 4 hours."

5. The moral and spiritual development of the preschooler is characterized by:
   a. concern for why something is wrong.
   b. actions that are directed toward satisfying the needs of others.
   c. thoughts of loyalty and gratitude.
   d. a very concrete sense of justice and fairness.

6. T   F   During the preschool period, the separation-individuation process is completed.

7. T   F   Stuttering affects boys more frequently than girls, and has been shown to have a genetic link, which usually resolves during childhood.

8. T F Preschoolers can independently brush and floss their teeth.

9. T   F   To help preschoolers overcome their fears it is important to actively involve them in finding practical ways to deal with the frightening experience.

10. _____ _____ includes the use of about three or four words to convey a meaning.

11. When educating the preschool child about injury prevention, the parents should:
    a. set a good example.
    b. help children establish safety habits.
    c. be aware that pedestrian/motor vehicle injuries increase in this age group.
    d. do all of the above.

12. Which of the following gross motor skills would be expected for a 5-year-old child?
    a. Ride a tricycle
    b. Hop on one foot
    c. Jump rope
    d. Throw a ball reliably

13. The nurse is assessing fine motor development in a 4-year-old. Which of the following is the expected skill for this age?
    a. Can tie their shoes.
    b. Can copy a square.
    c. Can print a few letters.
    d. Can use scissors successfully.

14. Which of the following is the priority action needed in abusive situations of children?
    a. Reporting of the incident to the proper authorities.
    b. Removing the child to prevent further injury.
    c. Providing a safe place to speak with the child.
    d. Reinforcing to the child they have done nothing wrong and are not to blame.

15. Parents tell the nurse they are concerned. They found their 4-year-old daughter and a male cousin of the same age inspecting each other closely as they used the bathroom. What is the most appropriate response by the nurse?
    a. Discipline the children placing them in a time-out for bad behavior.
    b. Suggest further evaluation as this is not normal behavior.
    c. Neither condone nor condemn the behavior.
    d. Do not allow the children to play unsupervised.

16. The nurse needs to flush the saline lok of a 4-year-old admitted with nephrotic syndrome. The nurse approaches the child and the child states "Are you going to give my IV a drink? It is thirsty." This is an example of:
    a. Animism
    b. Magical thinking
    c. Transductive reasoning
    d. Telegraphic speech

17. During the preschool period, the emphasis of injury prevention should be placed on which of the following?
    a. Limitation of physical activities
    b. Teaching about safety and potential hazards.
    c. Disciplining for unsafe behaviors
    d. Strict parental supervision of children.

18. Which of the following is most descriptive of the nutritional requirements during the preschool years?
    a. The average daily intake of preschoolers should be about 2500 calories.
    b. The quality of food consumed is more important than the quantity.
    c. Preschoolers have very different eating habits than toddlers.
    d. Larger portions of each food item being served should be offered to the preschooler.

III. CLINICAL JUDGMENT AND NEXT-GENERATION NCLEX® EXAMINATION-STYLE QUESTIONS

1. **Place the following language skills of the preschool years in the order in which they occur.**

Language Developmental Milestones of Preschoolers	Order in which they occur (earliest to latest)
Uses sentences with 6–8 words, can follow 3 commands in succession.	
Vocabulary of about 900 words. Uses sentences with 3–4 words.	
Questioning is at its peak. Tells exaggerated stories, obeys prepositional phrases.	

2. **Which of the following represent developmental concepts displayed during the preschool years? Select all that apply.**

    a. Egocentrism is still rather prevalent during the preschool years.

    b. Preschoolers are beginning to understand the concept of time.

    c. Preschoolers are very "literal."

    d. Imaginary friends may appear during the preschool years.

    e. The task of conservation is mastered by the preschooler.

34 The School-Age Child and Family

I. LEARNING KEY TERMS

MATCHING: Match each term with its corresponding definition.

1. _____ An effective disciplinary technique for school-age children.

2. _____ Any recurring activity that intends to cause harm, distress, or control toward another in which there is a perceived imbalance of power between the aggressor (s) and the victim.

3. _____ Previously well-behaved children who may engage in lying, stealing, and cheating.

4. _____ The principal oral problem in children and adolescents; if untreated can result in total destruction of the involved teeth.

5. _____ Elementary school children who are left to care for themselves before or after school without supervision of an adult.

6. _____ Repeated bowel movements into bed or clothing at least one time per month for a period of at least 3 months, is not due directly to a physiologic condition or substance.

7. _____ Making judgments based on what they reason.

8. _____ An awareness of oneself regarding personal attributes and the idea of self in relation to others.

9. _____ Repeated urination into bed or clothing at least twice a week for a period of at least 3 months that is not due directly to a physiologic condition or substance.

10. _____ Signals the beginning of the development of secondary sex characteristics.

11. _____ Exarticulation; "knocked out."

12. _____ Making judgments based on what they see.

13. _____ An important factor in gaining independence from parents; one of the most influential socializing agents in the school-age years.

a. Conceptual thinking

b. Self-concept

c. Puberty

d. Latchkey children

e. Dental caries

f. Avulsed tooth

g. Perceptual thinking

h. Antisocial behavior

i. Reasoning

j. Bullying

k. Encopresis

l. Peer group identification

m. Enuresis

Copyright © 2023 Elsevier Inc. All rights reserved.

Chapter **34** The School-Age Child and Family

1. The middle childhood is also referred to as "school age" or the "school years." What ages does this period represent?
   a. 5–13 years
   b. 4–14 years
   c. 6–12 years
   d. 6–16 years

2. Which of the following would be an appropriate health promotion intervention to promote during the school-age years?
   a. Education on the need for an increased caloric intake during this time.
   b. Discourage questions on sex education until the adolescent stage.
   c. Education that sleep requirements will significantly increase toward the end of the school-age years.
   d. Education on the importance of good dental hygiene because these are the years in which permanent teeth erupt.

3. T F In middle childhood, the amount of sleep depends on various components, such as age, activity, and state of health.

4. T F The school environment can be a source of stress for school-age children.

5. T F School-aged children develop thought processes which allow them to see things from another's point of view.

6. T F During the middle years, the immune system develops little immunity to pathogenic microorganisms.

7. T F Middle childhood is the period of development where children learn the value of doing things with others and the benefits derived from division of labor in the accomplishment of goals.

8. T F Physical maturity correlates well with emotional and social maturity during the middle years.

9. Generally, the earliest age at which puberty begins is age _____ for girls and age _____ for boys, but it can be normal for either sex after the age of _____ years.

10. _____ is when children can use thought processes to experience events and actions.

11. Middle childhood is the time when children:
    I. learn the value of doing things with others.
    II. acquiring a sense of initiative.
    III. achieving a sense of industry and accomplishment.
    IV. expand interests and engage in tasks that can be carried to completion.
    a. I, II, III, and IV
    b. I, III, and IV
    c. I and IV
    d. II and III

12. When describing play by the school-aged child to a group of nursing students, the instructor would emphasize the need for which of the following?
    a. Rules
    b. Recreation
    c. Physical activity
    d. Ritualism

13. During the school-age years, children learn valuable lessons from peers. How is this accomplished?
    a. The child learns to appreciate the varied points of view that are within the peer group.
    b. The child becomes sensitive to the social norms and pressures of the group.
    c. The child's interactions among peers lead to the formation of intimate friendships between same-sex peers.
    d. All of the above are correct.

14. Children's self-concepts are composed of:
    a. their own critical self-assessment.
    b. their idea of self in relation to others.
    c. their body image awareness.
    d. all of the above.

15. A 9-year-old girl often comes to the school nurse complaining of stomach pains. Her teacher says she seems to be having some trouble concentrating in class and has become a bit aggressive in the classroom. The school nurse should recognize this as which?
    a. A possible physical problem needing medical intervention.
    b. Signs of stress
    c. Normal school-age behaviors
    d. Lack of adequate sleep

16. A group of 7-year-old girls have formed a "girls only" club. It is only open to girls who still like to play with dolls. How should this behavior be interpreted?
    a. Poor peer relationships.
    b. Encouragement for bullying.
    c. Appropriate social development.
    d. Immaturity for this age group.

17. T F Previously well-behaved children may engage in lying, stealing, and cheating during the school-age years.

18. T F The rear vehicle seat is the safest place for children younger than 13 years old.

19. Bullying which uses force and most often used by boys is referred to as _____ _____ and bullying using methods such as gossip, rumors, and exclusion and used mainly by girls is referred to as _____ _____.

20. T F Falls from bicycles are the cause of a significant number of head injuries in school-age children.

III. FILL IN THE BLANK WITH THE CORRECT SCHOOL-AGE DISORDER WITH BEHAVIORAL COMPONENTS

1. _____ this disorder usually occurs after exposure to an extremely traumatic experience or catastrophic event. The traumatic experience is typically life threatening to self or a significant other, without professional support the victim may develop severe depression, aggression, or psychosis.

2. _____ refers to severe deviations in ego functioning and is generally reserved for psychotic disorders that appear in children younger than 15 years old and fortunately is a relatively rare illness in children.

3. _____ is a psychophysiologic disorder with a sudden onset that usually can be traced to a precipitating environmental event. The disorder is observed with equal frequency in both sexes in childhood.

4. _____ this disorder is often unrecognized, and children do not receive suitable treatment recognition. The child finds it difficult to control worry, with comorbid symptoms of restlessness or feeling keyed up or on edge, being easily fatigued, difficulty concentrating or the mind going blank, irritability, muscle tension, and sleep disturbance.

5. _____ is often times not recognized and the symptoms being experienced are "just a stage of development" and will resolve with maturation. Additionally, it is difficult to detect because children may be unable to express their feelings and tend to act out their problems and concerns rather than identify them verbally. It is important to assess the risk of suicide in this disorder.

6. _____ this disorder is seen in children who resist going to school or who demonstrate extreme reluctance to attend school for a sustained period as a result of severe anxiety or fear of school-related experiences. Children can develop symptoms as a protective mechanism to avoid facing the situation that distresses them. Physical symptoms are prominent and may affect any part of the body; anorexia, nausea, vomiting, diarrhea, dizziness, headache, leg pains, and abdominal pains are most common.

7. _____this disorder refers to developmentally inappropriate degrees of inattention, impulsiveness, and hyperactivity. The behaviors exhibited by the child are not unusual aspects of child behavior. Treatment depends on the child's age and severity of symptoms. Evidence supports behavioral therapy as the first-line treatment, but other approaches include family education and counseling, medication, proper classroom placement, environmental manipulation, and psychotherapy for the child.

IV. CLINICAL JUDGMENT AND NEXT-GENERATION NCLEX® EXAMINATION-STYLE QUESTIONS

1. The nurse is reviewing the medical record for a 12-year-old child who is being seen for concerns about school attendance. The physician has noted the child has "school phobia."
What behaviors may be noted in a child experiencing this phenomenon? Select all that apply.

   a. Anxious to attend school.

   b. Demonstrates negative behaviors before school.

   c. No symptoms usually present on weekends.

d. Reports of feeling bored at school.

e. Difficulty concentrating in class.

2. The nurse is reviewing behavioral techniques to use for an 8-year-old child with attention deficit hyperactivity disorder (ADHD) with the child's parents. Use an X to indicate whether the nursing actions listed below are Effective (helped to meet expected quality patient outcome), Ineffective (did not help to meet expected quality patient outcome), or Unrelated (not related to the quality patient outcome) for the child's care at this time.

Nursing Action	Effective	Ineffective	Unrelated
Encouraging free time at a time of day that the child chooses.			
Providing structured responsibilities during the child's routine.			
Make organizational charts to allow for more choices and responsibility for actions.			
Children receiving medication for ADHD need regularly scheduled appointments for medication effectiveness, side effects, and to monitor development and health status.			
Attempt to provide a consistent routine for the child.			

35 The Adolescent and Family

I. LEARNING KEY TERMS

MATCHING: Match each term with its corresponding definition.

1. _____ The masculinizing hormones; secreted in small and gradually increasing amounts up to about 7 or 9 years of age, then followed by a rapid increase in both sexes, the level of androgens in males increasing over that in females with the onset of testicular function.

2. _____ The process of developing a reasonable picture of oneself that includes integrating one's past and present experiences with a sense of where one is headed in the future.

3. _____ This is considered a form of modern-day slavery.

4. _____ Pattern of sexual arousal or romantic attraction toward persons of the same sex, opposite sex or both sexes.

5. _____ Repeated episodes of binge eating, no purging involved.

6. _____ The initial appearance of menstruation; occurs about 2 years after the appearance of the first pubescent changes.

7. _____ The feminizing hormone; found in low quantities during childhood; increasing in quantity in early puberty.

8. _____ Temporary breast enlargement and tenderness; common during mid-puberty in boys.

9. _____ Eating disorder characterized by binge eating and purging followed by self-deprecating thoughts, a depressed mood, and awareness that the eating pattern is abnormal.

10. _____ A period of transition between childhood and adulthood—a time of rapid physical, cognitive, social, and emotional maturation.

11. _____ The first period of puberty; occurs about 2 years immediately before puberty, when the child is developing preliminary physical changes that herald sexual maturity.

12. _____ Eating disorder characterized by a refusal to maintain a minimally normal body weight; severe weight loss in the absence of obvious physical causes.

13. _____ The maturational, hormonal, and growth process that occurs when the reproductive organs begin to function and the secondary sex characteristics develop.

14. _____ This event which is the initial indication of puberty and includes the appearance of breast buds.

15. _____ An increase in body weight resulting from an excessive accumulation of body fat relative to lean body mass.

a. Puberty
b. Prepubescence
c. Adolescence
d. Estrogen
e. Androgens
f. Sex-trafficking
g. Menarche
h. Gynecomastia
i. Thelarche
j. Obesity
k. Anorexia nervosa
l. Bulimia
m. Identity formation
n. Binge eating disorder
o. Sexual orientation

II. REVIEWING KEY CONCEPTS

1. The normal age range for menarche is usually

   _____ to _____ years,

   with the average age being _____ years,

   _____ months for non-Hispanic white

   girls and _____ years _____
   months for African American girls.

2. A nurse is reading a journal article about adolescents and major causes of injuries in this age group. The nurse demonstrates understanding of this information by identifying which situation as the major cause of adolescent injuries?
   a. Drowning
   b. Motor vehicle crashes
   c. Violence
   d. Suicide

3. The adolescent growth spurt is characterized as beginning:
   a. sooner in boys.
   b. between the ages of 9.5 and 14.5 years in boys.
   c. sooner in girls.
   d. between the ages of 10.5 and 16 years in girls.

4. Girls may be considered to have _____

   _____ if breast development has not

   occurred by age _____.

5. The first pubescent change in boys is:
   a. appearance of pubic hair.
   b. testicular enlargement with thinning, reddening, and increased looseness of the scrotum.
   c. penile enlargement.
   d. temporary breast enlargement and tenderness.

6. Which of the following is the psychosocial task is to be developed during adolescence?
   a. intimacy
   b. independence
   c. initiative
   d. identity

7. On the average, girls gain _____

   to _____ inches in height and

   _____ to _____ pounds dur-

   ing adolescence, whereas boys gain _____

   to _____ inches and _____ to

   _____ pounds.

8. Which of the following best describes the formal operational thinking that occurs during adolescence?
   a. Thought process includes thinking in concrete terms.
   b. Thought process includes information obtained from the environment and peers.
   c. Their thoughts are influenced by experience.
   d. They become increasingly capable of scientific reasoning and formal logic.

9. Which of the following is the recommended amount of sleep for adolescents?
   a. 7 hours/night
   b. 9 hours/night
   c. 10 hours/night
   d. 11 hours/night

10. According to Piaget, adolescents tend to be in what stage of cognitive development?
    a. Concrete operations
    b. Conventional thought
    c. Principled reasoning
    d. Formal operational thought

11. When interviewed by the school nurse, a 13-year-old adolescent female states she has a boyfriend and that her parents do not talk about sex with her. She says is confused about the facts and wants to know the truth. Which approach would be the most appropriate to address this adolescent's concerns?
    a. Explain that a discussion about sex is best handled by her parents, and she should go home and ask them.
    b. Offer to provide her some brochures to help her better understand how her body works.
    c. Sit down with her and openly discuss her concerns and questions in an honest, straightforward manner.
    d. Refer the adolescent to a local health department for sexual counseling and pregnancy prevention.

12. T F Adolescents are capable of abstract thinking and scientific reasoning.

13. Compared with school-age children, adolescent peer groups are:
    a. more likely to include peers of the opposite sex.
    b. less autonomous.
    c. less likely to influence members' socialization roles.
    d. more likely to require parental supervision.

14. T F Excess intake of calories, sugar, fat, cholesterol, and sodium is common among adolescents and may lead to an increased risk of obesity and chronic diseases.

15. T F Suicidal ideation is common in adolescents.

16. T F Motor vehicle crashes are the single greatest source of intentional injury and death in young people.

17. T F Health promotion for adolescents consists mainly of teaching and guidance to avoid risk-taking activities and health-damaging behaviors.

18. T F Growth in height in girls typically ceases 2–2.5 years after menarche begins and around ages 18–20 for boys.

19. Concern for pubertal delay in boys may be considered if there is no enlargement of the testes or scrotal changes by age _____.

III. CLINICAL JUDGMENT AND NEXT-GENERATION NCLEX® EXAMINATION-STYLE QUESTIONS

1. A nurse is developing a health promotion pamphlet to be distributed to 16-year-old adolescents at a high school health fair. Which health topics/safety concerns should the nurse

   a. include in the pamphlet? Select all that apply.

   b. Strategies for dealing with stress and promoting emotional well-being.

   c. Risk of body art.

   d. Strategies for preventing violence, injury prevention, and risk reduction.

   e. Good nutrition.

   f. Bicycle safety.

2. Adolescents should receive a tuberculin skin test if which of the following have occurred? Select all that apply.

   a. They have been exposed to active tuberculosis (TB).

b. Have lived in a homeless shelter.

c. Have been incarcerated.

d. Have lived in or come from an area with a high prevalence of TB.

e. Work in a health care setting.

3. The nurse is interviewing a 17-year-old female who presents for their annual physical examination. Which of the following strategies would help the nurse in therapeutically communicating with the adolescent? Select all that apply.

a. Use open-ended questions with the adolescent.

b. Interview the adolescent with their parents to obtain an accurate health history.

c. Maintain a nonjudgmental attitude and avoid assumptions.

d. Begin the interview with the most sensitive issues.

e. Include personal experiences to relate to the adolescent.

f. Be open and honest by explaining the limits of confidentiality.

36 Impact of Chronic Illness, Disability, or End-of-Life Care for the Child and Family

I. LEARNING KEY TERMS

MATCHING: Match each term with its corresponding description.

1. _____ A principle in the care of children with chronic or complex conditions that refers to establishing a normal pattern of living.

2. _____ Actions carried out by a person other than the patient to end the life of the patient suffering from a terminal illness.

3. _____ Coping mechanisms that result in movement away from adjustment; maladaptation to the crisis.

4. _____ This focuses on providing optimal symptom management, helping families align medical interventions with their goals for their child, assisting with complex decision making, and supporting the family and health care team caring for children throughout the trajectory of their illness.

5. _____ Care provided by an interprofessional group in the patient's home or an inpatient facility.

6. _____ Coping mechanisms that result in movement toward adjustment and resolution of the crisis.

7. _____ Can be used to convey the discharge from an acute or chronic care facility to home for children with complex health care needs.

8. _____ The behavioral reaction that occurs when death is the expected or possible outcome of a disorder.

9. _____ A process of recognizing, promoting, and enhancing competence.

10. _____ Behaviors aimed at reducing the tension caused by a crisis.

11. _____ A defense mechanism that is a necessary cushion to prevent disintegration and is a normal response to grieving for any type of loss.

a. Coping mechanisms

b. Normalization

c. Approach behaviors

d. Transition

e. Avoidance behaviors

f. Anticipatory grief

g. Palliative care

h. Euthanasia

i. Hospice

j. Denial

k. Empowerment

II. REVIEWING KEY CONCEPTS

1. Which of the following can be used to assist families in coping with stress they may be experiencing due to their child's chronic illness, disability, or end-of-life care decisions?
   a. Providing communication when asked by parents.
   b. Engaging only family members in conversations.
   c. Establishing therapeutic relationships with the child and their family.
   d. Provide personal experiences which are relevant to the situation.

2. Which of the following situations does not support a therapeutic nurse–patient–family relationship?
   a. The nurse is planning to read the patient their favorite story.
   b. During shift report, the nurse is criticizing parents for not visiting their child.
   c. The nurse is discussing with a fellow nurse the emotional draw to a certain patient.
   d. The nurse is working with a family to find additional resources to assist the family after discharge.

3. List a major goal in working with the family of a child with a chronic or complex illness.

4. Discuss the impact of a child's chronic illness as it relates to single-parent families. How can nursing assist in this situation?

5. Which of the following factors is more characteristic of a father's pattern than a mother's pattern of adjusting to a chronically ill child? The father is more likely to:
   a. hide their feelings and display an outward confidence.
   b. report a periodic crisis pattern.
   c. forfeit personal goals.
   d. seek immediate professional counseling.

FILL IN THE BLANK WITH THE APPROPRIATE PARENTAL RESPONSE WHICH MAY OCCUR DURING THE ADJUSTMENT PHASE OF A CHILD DIAGNOSED WITH A CHRONIC OR COMPLEX ILLNESS

6. _____ This may occur when the parents act as if the disorder does not exist or attempt to have the child overcompensate for it.

7. _____ This may occur when the parents detach themselves emotionally from the child but usually provide adequate physical care or constantly nag and scold the child.

8. _____ The parents fear letting the child achieve any new skill, avoid all discipline, and cater to every desire to prevent frustration.

9. _____ is when the parents place necessary and realistic restrictions on the child, encourage self-care activities, and promote reasonable physical and social abilities.

10. List the three common phases of families' responses to the diagnosis of a chronic illness or disability.

11. When the parent of a child who is dying tells the nurse the child is in pain even when the child appears comfortable, the nurse should be sure that:
    a. as needed (prn) pain control measures are instituted on admission.
    b. pain control is administered on a regular schedule, and extra doses for breakthrough pain are available to maintain comfort of the child.
    c. parents understand that pain is a physical process and is difficult to control.
    d. parents understand that the child is probably in less pain than he or she appears to be.

12. Pain control is often a concern of dying children and their parents. Which of the following strategies should the nurse use to help them deal with this fear?
    a. Assure the parents that the pain will be completely relieved.
    b. Use heavy sedation to help the child cope with this phase.
    c. Educate the parents that their child's pain will be assessed frequently and medications adjusted as necessary to achieve a level of comfort.
    d. Give pain medications intravenously only when the child is near death.

13. List at least five physical signs of approaching death.

14. Anticipatory grieving is characterized by:
    a. pangs of severe emotion.
    b. denial.
    c. excessive loneliness.
    d. unusual sleep disturbances.

15. Several nurses express to their nurse manager they would like to attend the funeral of a child for whom they had cared. They say they felt especially close to the child and family. The nurse manager recognizes attending the funeral serves what purpose?
    a. It is improper because it increases burnout.
    b. It is inappropriate because it is unprofessional.
    c. It is proper because families expect this expression of concern.
    d. It is appropriate because it can assist in the resolution of personal grief.

16. Which of the following would be a characteristic of parental overprotection for children with special needs or chronic illnesses?
    a. Encouraging independence of the child.
    b. Provides consistent discipline and limit-setting.
    c. Promotes decision making by the child when appropriate.
    d. Continually helps the child even when the child is capable.

17. What is the minimum support and guidance recommended for family members to assist with the resolution of their loss?
    a. A written questionnaire
    b. An online survey
    c. Meeting with the family at the time of death
    d. A follow-up telephone call or meeting

18. Which of the following techniques is perhaps the most supportive measure the nurse can use with the bereaved family?
    a. Cheerfulness
    b. Interpretation
    c. Listening
    d. Reassurance

III. CLINICAL JUDGMENT AND NEXT-GENERATION NCLEX® EXAMINATION-STYLE QUESTIONS

1. Which of the following characterizes a preschooler's concept of death? Select all that apply.

   a. May feel that their thoughts or actions have caused the death.

   b. They understand the universality and inevitability of death.

   c. Most preschooler's do not understand that death is permanent.

   d. They have the most difficulty dealing with death.

   e. They may recognize the fact of physical death.

2. Which of the following would be appropriate nursing actions to assist a school-age child with a chronic illness in meeting their expected developmental milestones. For each nursing action, use an X to indicate whether it was Effective (helped to meet expected quality patient outcomes), Ineffective (did not help to meet expected quality patient outcomes), or Unrelated (not related to the quality patient outcomes).

Nursing Action	Effective	Ineffective	Unrelated
Provide the child with developmentally appropriate information about their condition.			
Encourage increased responsibility for own care and management of the disease or condition.			
Encourage socialization in clubs as appropriate.			
Encourage independence in as many areas as possible.			
Help with decision making and other skills necessary to manage personal plans.			

Chapter **36** Impact of Chronic Illness, Disability, or End-of-Life Care for the Child and Family

3. What are common symptoms dying children may experience? (Select all that apply.)
   a. Decrease in secretions.
   b. Eupnea.
   c. Muscle weakness.
   d. Difficulty in swallowing.
   e. Periods of apnea.

4. Describe why adolescents, more than any other age group, have more difficulty coping with death, particularly their own.

37 Impact of Cognitive or Sensory Impairment on the Child and Family

I. LEARNING KEY TERMS

MATCHING: Match each term with its corresponding description.

1. _____ Refers to a person whose hearing disability precludes successful processing of linguistic information through audition, with or without a hearing aid.

2. _____ General term that encompasses both partial sight and legal blindness.

3. _____ Refers to a person who, generally with the use of a hearing aid, has residual hearing sufficient to enable successful processing of linguistic information through audition.

4. _____ A disability that may range in severity from slight to profound hearing loss; one of the most common disabilities in the United States.

5. _____ Most common inherited cause of cognitive impairment, caused by an abnormal gene on the lower end of the long arm of the X chromosome.

6. _____ Systematic program of therapy, exercises, and activities intended to address developmental delays and subsequently assist children in achieving their full potential.

7. _____ Where there has been the loss or damage to some or all of their hair cells or auditory nerve fibers.

8. _____ Important in prenatal care, may help decrease occurrence of neural tube defects.

9. _____ A unit of loudness measured at various frequencies; used to express the degree of hearing impairment.

10. _____ Most common chromosomal abnormality of a generalized syndrome.

11. _____ Occurs with a loss of intensity of sound.

12. _____ Most common eye infection.

13. _____ The measurement of an individual's hearing impairment by means of an audiometer.

14. _____ Complex neurodevelopmental disorders of unknown etiology with alterations in social interactions, social communication bcx and unusually restricted, repetitive behavior, interest, or activities.

15. _____ This is measured by the intelligence quotient (IQ) test.

16. _____ A general term that encompasses any type of intellectual disability.

a. Cognitive impairment

b. Autism spectrum disorders

c. Conjunctivitis

d. Down syndrome

e. Folic acid supplements

f. Early intervention programs

g. Fragile X syndrome

h. Hearing impairment

i. Severe to profound hearing loss (deaf)

j. Slight to moderate hearing loss

k. Decibel

l. Hearing threshold level

m. Intellectual functioning

n. Conductive hearing loss

o. Sensorineural hearing loss

p. Visual impairment

II. REVIEWING KEY CONCEPTS

1. The nurse is discussing sexuality with the parents of an adolescent girl who has a mild to moderate cognitive impairment. Which of the following is the most appropriate to include in the discussion?
   a. Sterilization is recommended for any adolescent with cognitive impairment.
   b. Sexual drive and interest are very limited in individuals with cognitive impairment.
   c. Individuals with cognitive impairment need a well-defined, concrete code of sexual conduct.
   d. Sexual intercourse rarely occurs unless the individual with cognitive impairment is sexually abused.

2. Trisomy 21 is also known as:
   a. Jacob syndrome.
   b. Turner syndrome.
   c. Down syndrome.
   d. Klinefelter syndrome.

3. Prenatal testing and genetic counseling for Down syndrome should be offered to all women:
   a. Regardless of family history.
   b. With a family history of the disorder and who are of advanced maternal age.
   c. With no family history of the disorder and who are of advanced maternal age.
   d. Who become pregnant in their adolescent years.

4. Autism spectrum disorder is usually diagnosed during the _____ years and is more common in _____ than _____.

5. Because the disorder is hereditary, parents of a child with fragile X syndrome should optimally receive _____ _____.

6. Which of the following is a primary goal in caring for a child with cognitive impairment?
   a. Developing vocational skills.
   b. Promoting optimum development.
   c. Finding appropriate out-of-home care.
   d. Helping child and family adjust to future care.

7. In the initial screening of an infant with a suspected hearing impairment, the nurse should be alert for:
   a. Absent cry.
   b. Consistent lack of the startle reflex.
   c. A louder than usual cry.
   d. Absence of babble or voice inflections by age 4 months.

8. In the assessment of a child to identify whether a hearing impairment has developed, the nurse would look for:
   a. A loud monotone voice.
   b. Consistent lack of the startle reflex.
   c. A high level of social activity.
   d. Attentiveness, especially when someone is talking.

9. Which of the following lip reading strategies could enhance communication with a child who is hearing impaired?
   a. Touching the child lightly to signal presence of a speaker
   b. Speaking to the child at a 90-degree angle
   c. Avoid using facial expressions as this may confuse the message.
   d. Repeat the message in the exact same way several times.

10. If a child has a penetrating injury to the eye, the nurse should:
    a. Apply an eye patch.
    b. Attempt to remove the object.
    c. Irrigate the eye.
    d. Take the child to the emergency department.

11. Understanding autism spectrum disorders (ASDs) is essential for those who care for children. Which of the following is a goal of treatment for children with ASD?
    a. Assisting the family with long-term placement as most children cannot remain at home.
    b. Introduce new situations quickly for the child with ASD.
    c. Cuddling or holding the child with ASD to provide comfort when their routines are disrupted.
    d. Provide a structured environment.

12. The American Academy of Pediatrics has recommended that pediatric health care providers administer two ASD screenings at ages _____ and _____ months using a valid screening tool.

13. Identify strategies the nurse can use during hospitalization with a child who has lost their sight.

14. Which of the following statements is correct about eye care and sports?
    a. Glasses may interfere with the child's ability in sports.
    b. Eye protection gear must be worn for golfing.
    c. Corrective lenses improve visual acuity allowing children to compete more effectively in sports.
    d. Contact lenses are better for sports because they require less care.

15. T F Delayed developmental milestones may be indicative of cognitive impairment.

1. A mother brings her 2-month-old infant in for a well-child visit. The mother discusses with the nurse she is concerned about her infant's hearing. Which of the following would the nurse include as possible signs of hearing impairment? Select all that apply.

   a. Lack of a blink reflex to a loud sound.

   b. No babbling by 7 months of age.

   c. Responds to loud noises as opposed to voice.

   d. Greater response to facial expression and gestures than to verbal response.

   e. Lack of a fencer reflex.

2. The parents of a 4-year-old child recently diagnosed with cognitive impairment ask the nurse for guidance on promoting optimal development for their child. Which of the following nursing actions would be appropriate. Use an X for the health teaching to the parents who are concerned about optimal development for their child below that is Indicated (appropriate or necessary), Contraindicated (could be harmful), or Non-Essential (makes no difference or not necessary) regarding anticipatory guidance for optimal development.

Health Teaching	Indicated	Contraindicated	Non-Essential
Encourage the need for play and exercise.			
Initially it may be beneficial to avoid individuals who may not understand cognitive development.			
Focus should be on the development of verbal skills as physical skills are often delayed and require additional intervention.			
Limit-setting measures should be simple and consistent, with behavior modification as a very effective discipline strategy.			
Seek out opportunities for social interaction such as early intervention programs and appropriate preschool programs			

38 Family-Centered Care of the Child During Illness and Hospitalization

I. LEARNING KEY TERMS

MATCHING: Match each term with its corresponding description.

1. _____ An effective, nondirective modality for helping children deal with their concerns and fears; often helpful to the nurse in gaining insights into children's needs and feelings.

2. _____ Provides an expressive outlet for creative ideas and interests. An effective tool for managing a child's stress at home and during hospitalization.

3. _____ Technique for emotional release, allowing children to reenact frightening or puzzling hospital experiences.

4. _____ The major stress from middle infancy throughout the preschool years, especially for children ages 6–30 months, also called anaclitic depression.

5. _____ One of the most traumatic hospital experiences for the child and parents.

6. _____ Health care professionals with extensive knowledge of child growth and development and of the special psychosocial needs of hospitalized children.

a. Separation anxiety

b. Play

c. Emergency admission

d. Child life specialists

e. Dramatic play

f. Therapeutic play

II. REVIEWING KEY CONCEPTS

1. A major stress from middle infancy throughout the preschool years is known as _____ _____ and occurs from approximately _____ _____ to _____ _____ of age.

MATCHING: Match each phase of separation anxiety with the behaviors that are typical of that phase.

2. _____ Withdraws from others; crying stops, much less active, and depression is evident.

3. _____ Becomes more interested in surroundings; appears the child has adjusted to the loss, interacts with caregivers; resigned to the situation; rarely seen in hospitalized children; occurs in prolonged parental absences.

4. _____ Cries; screams; refuse the attention of anyone else and are inconsolable in their grief continuous crying.

5. T F Preschoolers may demonstrate separation anxiety by refusing to eat, experiencing difficulty in sleeping, crying quietly for their parents, continually asking when the parents will visit, or withdrawing from others.

a. Protest

b. Despair

c. Detachment

6. T F Parents of a hospitalized child may experience a sense of helplessness and question the skill level of the staff.

7. What age group is more likely to experience increased stress to hospitalization and loss of peer group contact?
   a. Preschooler
   b. Middle school-age child
   c. Adolescent
   d. Early school-age child

8. A toddler is most likely to react to short-term hospitalization with feelings of loss of control that result from altered routines; this is often manifested by:
   a. Regression.
   b. Withdrawal.
   c. Formation of new superficial relationships.
   d. Self-assertion and anger.

9. Which of the following risk factors make a child more vulnerable to the stressors of hospitalization?
   a. Male gender
   b. Strong support network
   c. Female gender
   d. Passive temperament

10. Describe at least three posthospital stay behaviors commonly observed in young children.

11. Siblings who visit their brother or sister in the hospital have an increased tendency to exhibit which of the following behaviors?
    a. Denial
    b. Anger
    c. Sadness
    d. Acceptance

12. To help the parents deal with the issues related to separation while their child is hospitalized, the nurse should suggest that parents:
    a. Quietly leave while the child is distracted or asleep.
    b. Make the surroundings familiar with the child's toys from home.

c. Encourage infrequent parental visits to help decrease the child's frequency of disappointment.
d. Visit over one extended time if rooming-in is impossible.

13. One technique used during hospitalization that can minimize the disruption in the routine of the school-age child who is not critically ill is:
    a. Stop school activities.
    b. Wear hospital scrubs.
    c. Encourage self-care.
    d. Watch television.

14. Preparing children for painful procedures usually increases their:
    a. Cooperation.
    b. Fear.
    c. Stress.
    d. Misconceptions.

15. Whenever performing a painful procedure on a child, the nurse should attempt to:
    a. Perform the procedure in the playroom.
    b. Perform the procedure in the child's hospital room.
    c. Perform the procedure quickly.
    d. Request the parents leave during the procedure.

16. Which of the following reactions to surgery is most typical of an adolescent's reaction to fear of bodily injury?
    a. Concern about the pain
    b. Concern about the procedure itself
    c. Concern about the scar
    d. Understanding explanations literally

17. Identify three factors that affect parents' reactions to their child's illness.

18. Describe techniques for modifying procedural techniques for children in each age group which may assist in minimizing fear of bodily injury.

III. CLINICAL JUDGMENT AND NEXT-GENERATION NCLEX® EXAMINATION-STYLE QUESTIONS

1. Play is considered children's "work." Which of the following are functions of play for the hospitalized child? Select all that apply.

   a. To provide the parents with a "break" from the stress of the hospitalization.

   b. Gives the child choices and control of the situation.

   c. Provides diversion for the child.

   d. Should be limited according to the child's disease process.

   e. Helps the child feel more secure in a strange environment.

2. The nurse is providing care to a newly admitted 4-year-old experiencing an asthma exacerbation. Which of the following nursing actions would the nurse include to promote optimal support for the family and child during hospitalization? Use an X for the nursing actions listed below which are Indicated (appropriate or necessary), Contraindicated (could be harmful), or Non-Essential (makes no difference or not necessary).

Nursing Actions	Indicated	Contraindicated	Non-Essential
Encourage parental participation in the child's care, during family-centered rounds, and visitation			
Have the parents bring familiar objects from home to place in child's hospital room			
Refrain from having siblings visit as it may be upsetting to see their sibling ill, especially for younger siblings			
Enabling independence and promoting self-care when appropriate for the child			
Provide the family information about the disease, its treatment, prognosis, and home care			

39 Pediatric Variations of Nursing Interventions

I. LEARNING KEY TERMS

MATCHING: Match each term with its corresponding description.

1. _____ Provides a rapid, safe, and life-saving alternate route for administration of fluids and medications until intravascular access is possible.

2. _____ Designed for patients documented or suspected to be infected or colonized with highly transmissible or epidemiologically important pathogens.

3. _____ Positioning of the child using gravity to remove secretions from the lobes to the larger airways to be expelled.

4. _____ These are designed for the care of all patients to reduce the risk of transmission of microorganisms from both recognized and unrecognized sources of infection.

5. _____ Designed to reduce the risk of transmission of droplets suspended in the air for long periods of time.

6. _____ Designed to reduce the risk of transmission of infectious agents generated from the source person primarily during coughing, sneezing, or talking and during the performance of certain procedures such as suctioning and bronchoscopy.

7. _____ One who is legally under the age of majority but is recognized as having the legal capacity of an adult under circumstances prescribed by state law, such as pregnancy, marriage, high school graduation, living independently, or military service.

8. _____ A simple, continuous, noninvasive method of determining oxygen saturation; used to guide oxygen therapy.

9. _____ These precautions are used to reduce the risk of transmission of microorganisms by direct or indirect contact.

10. _____ A noninvasive measurement of exhaled carbon dioxide which is very sensitive to the mechanics of ventilation.

11. _____ Fever state.

12. _____ Refers to the patient or the patient's legal surrogate receiving sufficient information on which to make an informed health care decision. The information should include the nature of the illness or condition, proposed care, or treatment; potential risks, benefits, and alternatives if treatment is not chosen.

13. _____ Used for repeated blood sampling or medications, long-term chemotherapy, intensive care, or frequent hyperalimentation or antibiotic therapy.

a. Informed consent

b. Emancipated minor

c. Standard Precautions

d. Transmission-based precautions

e. Airborne precautions

f. Droplet precautions

g. Contact precautions

h. Febrile

i. Central venous access device

j. End-tidal carbon dioxide monitoring

k. Pulse oximetry

l. Bronchial (postural) drainage

m. Intraosseous infusion

II. REVIEWING KEY CONCEPTS

1. Which of the following routes is the preferred method of medication administration in children?
   a. Intravenous
   b. Intramuscular
   c. Oral
   d. Otic

2. A 4-year-old attending daycare came home with a fever and runny nose. The child is being cared for at home. What is the principal reason for treating the fever in this child?
   a. Avoid the development of life-threatening complications.
   b. To prevent a bacterial infection from developing.
   c. To relieve discomfort.
   d. To prevent a prolonged illness.

3. A 2-month-old infant is admitted to the hospital with probable respiratory syncytial virus (RSV). The infant's mother is 17 years old, single, and lives with her parents. The father of the infant lives with his parents. Who signs the informed consent for the infant?
   a. The infant's mother
   b. The maternal grandparents
   c. The paternal grandparents
   d. Both maternal and paternal grandparents

4. Identify two age-specific strategies for children undergoing a procedure based on their developmental level.

5. Describe at least one play activity for each of the following procedures.
   a. Ambulation
   b. Range of motion
   c. Injections
   d. Deep breathing
   e. Extending the environment
   f. Soaks
   g. Fluid intake

6. T F When administering eye drops and eye ointment, the eye drops should be administered first, followed by the eye ointment 3 minutes later.

7. T F When administering a medication via the rectum, if the dose ordered is not available, the suppository should be cut lengthwise and inserted with the apex first.

8. T F The angle for injection for a subcutaneous medication is typically 90 degrees.

9. An increased heart rate, increased respiratory rate, and increased blood pressure in the immediate postoperative period of a young child would most likely indicate:
   a. Pain.
   b. Infection.
   c. Shock.
   d. Increased intracranial pressure.

10. The nurse is going over discharge instructions with a mother whose 11-month-old child will be treated with antibiotics for their ear infection. Which of the following is the most accurate measuring device to use for liquid administration of medication?
    a. Medicine cups.
    b. Plastic syringe for po use.
    c. Teaspoons.
    d. Dropper.

11. Which of the following examples of a child's food intake is the best example of adequate documentation?
    a. Child ate about a cup of cereal with ½ cup of milk.
    b. Child ate an adequate breakfast.
    c. Child ate 80% of the breakfast served.
    d. Parent states that child ate an adequate breakfast.

12. After cleft lip surgery, which of the following would be most appropriate to use to protect the operative site:
    a. Arm and leg restraints.
    b. Elbow restraints.
    c. A jacket restraint.
    d. A mummy restraint.

13. The best positioning technique for a lumbar puncture in a child is a:
    a. Side-lying position with neck flexion.
    b. Sitting position.
    c. Side-lying position with modified neck extension.
    d. Side-lying position, head flexed with knees to chest.

14. The most frequently used site for bone marrow aspiration in children is the:
    a. Femur.
    b. Sternum.
    c. Tibia.
    d. Iliac crest.

15. To avoid the complication of necrotizing osteochondritis when performing infant heel puncture, the puncture should be:
    a. No deeper than 4 mm and on the inner aspect of the heel.
    b. No deeper than 2 mm and on the outer aspect of the heel.
    c. No deeper than 2 mm and on the inner aspect of the heel.
    d. No deeper than 4 mm and on the outer aspect of the heel.

16. To obtain a nasal washing for RSV in an infant, the nurse would optimally:
    a. Have the infant cough.
    b. Obtain mucus from the throat.
    c. Insert a suction catheter into the back of the throat.
    d. Instill 1–3 ml of sterile normal saline into a nostril

17. Of the following choices for measuring 1 teaspoon of medication at home, the best device for the nurse to instruct the parent to use at home is the:
    a. Household soup spoon.
    b. Household measuring spoon.
    c. Measuring cup.
    d. Plastic disposable calibrated oral syringe.

18. All of the following techniques for medication administration to an infant are acceptable except:
    a. Adding the medication to the infant's 8 oz. bottle of formula.
    b. Allowing the infant to sit in the parent's lap during administration.
    c. Allowing the infant to suck the medication from an empty nipple.
    d. Inserting the needleless syringe into the side of the mouth while the infant nurses.

19. T F The needle length needed for intramuscular injections will vary depending on the amount of subcutaneous fat a child has. The needle length must be long enough to penetrate the subcutaneous fat and deposit the medication into the body of the muscle.

20. The preferred site for intramuscular injection in an infant is the:
    a. Deltoid muscle.
    b. Ventrogluteal.
    c. Vastus lateralis.
    d. Dorsogluteal.

21. Total parenteral nutrition (TPN) is infused by way of a central intravenous line because:
    a. Other medications need to be infused with the TPN.
    b. Several attempts to administer it peripherally have probably occurred.
    c. There is less risk of infection.
    d. The glucose in the solution is irritating to the smaller veins.

22. The correct process to administer eye drops and eye ointment to an infant or child is to administer _____ _____ first, wait three minutes and then administer _____ _____ to allow the drugs to work effectively.

23. During gavage or gastrostomy feedings the nurse should:
    a. Push the formula gradually through the feeding tube.
    b. Use a parenteral burette to calibrate the feeding times.
    c. Give the infant a pacifier for sucking.
    d. Hang the feeding container from an IV pole.

24. A 3-year-old with cystic fibrosis has a skin-level feeding device and is being cared for at home. The mother calls the skin specialist and says the skin around the skin-level device is moist and beefy red but there is no evidence of foul odor, bleeding, or formula leakage. The nurse is aware this finding is:
    a. A skin infection.
    b. Normal granulation tissue.
    c. A reason to change the skin-level device.
    d. A reason to discontinue using this device.

25. One of the major advantages of the recently developed skin-level devices for feeding children is that the button device:
    a. Does not clog as easily as other devices.
    b. Eliminates the need for frequent bubbling.
    c. Is less expensive than the traditional devices.
    d. Allows the child more mobility.

26. A 7-year-old child is being prepared for bowel surgery. Which of the following is the most appropriate to use for bowel cleansing in this child:
    a. A pediatric Fleet enema.
    b. A commercially prepared hypertonic enema solution.
    c. An oral polyethylene glycol–electrolyte solution.
    d. Plain water enemas.

27. In order to protect the pouch, a young child with an ostomy may need to:
    a. Wear a loose-fitting one-piece outfit.
    b. Begin toilet training at a later than usual age.
    c. Limit activity to avoid skin damage.
    d. Use elbow restraints at all times.

28. Which of the following is a priority intervention for an infant with a temporary colostomy for Hirschsprung disease?
    a. Teaching the parents how to irrigate the colostomy.
    b. Protecting the skin around the colostomy.
    c. Flushing the colostomy with a small amount of water.
    d. Applying elbow restraints to protect the colostomy site.

29. When administering ear drops to a child 3-years-of age and younger pull the pinna _____ and _____, in children older than 3-years-of-age pull the pinna _____ and _____. Eardrops should be administered at _____ _____ to avoid stimulation of vertigo.

30. Parents are being taught how to feed their infant using a newly placed gastrostomy tube (G-tube). Which of the following is essential information for the parents to receive?
    a. The parents should be taught how to verify placement of the G-tube before each feeding.
    b. The parents should be taught how to irrigate the G-tube before each feed.
    c. The parents should be taught to place the infant on their right side after feedings.
    d. The parents should be taught if beefy red tissue develops around the G-tube site that must be reported to the practitioner.

211

1. The nurse is caring for an 8-year-old child who is on fall precautions. Which of the following interventions would be appropriate to include in the child's plan of care? Select all that apply.

   a. Keep the call light and tray table with desired items within reach.

   b. Keep the bed in the highest position with the two side rails up.

   c. Keep personal belongings and clutter contained in one area of the floor.

   d. Ensure that the patient has an appropriate-size gown and nonskid footwear.

   e. Keep lights on at all times, including dim lights while sleeping.

2. The nurse is preparing scheduled vaccine injections for a 4-month-old child. Which of the following principles apply to the administration of IM injections for children? Choose the most likely options for information missing from the statements below by making selections from the list of options provided.

   The site recommended by the CDC and AAP for IM immunization administration is the _____ option 1 _____ _____. Injections can also be given in the _____ option 2 _____ _____ to children and infants as young as 2-months-old as this site is relatively large and free of major nerves and blood vessels. The _____ option 3 _____ _____ can be used in children 18 months of age and older. Usually _____ option 4 _____ ml is the maximum volume administered in a single site to small children and older infants.

Option 1	Option 2	Option 3	Option 4
Deltoid muscle	Deltoid muscle	Deltoid muscle	0.5 ml
Dorsogluteal muscle	Dorsogluteal muscle	Dorsogluteal muscle	1 ml
Vastus lateralis muscle	Vastus lateralis muscle	Vastus lateralis muscle	1.5 ml
Ventrogluteal muscle	Ventrogluteal muscle	Ventrogluteal muscle	2 ml

40 The Child with Respiratory Dysfunction

I. LEARNING KEY TERMS

MATCHING: Match each term with its corresponding description.

1. _____ The most frequent cause of hospitalization in children younger than 2 years old. An acute viral infection with maximum effect at the bronchiolar level.

2. _____ Provides an objective method of evaluating the presence and degree of lung disease, as well as the response to therapy.

3. _____ Cessation of breathing for more than 20 seconds or for a shorter period of time when associated with hypoxemia or bradycardia.

4. _____ A medical emergency that can result in respiratory failure and death if untreated.

5. _____ Involves stimulating the production of sweat with a special device (stimulation with 3-mA electric current), collecting the sweat on filter paper, and measuring the sweat electrolytes; used in the diagnosis of cystic fibrosis.

6. _____ Inability of the respiratory system to maintain adequate gas exchange.

7. _____ A serious obstructive inflammatory process in the upper airway may see dysphagia, toxic appearance, drooling, and high fever.

8. _____ Occurs when food, secretions, vomitus, medications, inert materials, volatile compounds, hydrocarbons, or liquids enter the lung and cause inflammation and a chemical pneumonitis.

9. _____ Upper airway infection characterized by hoarseness and a "barking" cough.

10. _____ A life-threatening event due to potential airway obstruction and inability to adequately oxygenate the body.

11. _____ Usually caused by the Epstein–Barr virus (EBV), it is mildly contagious, and believed to be transmitted by direct contact.

12. _____ Inflammation of the pulmonary parenchyma.

13. _____ An infection of the mucosa and soft tissues of the upper trachea a distinct entity with features of both croup and epiglottitis.

14. _____ Considered to be the cornerstone treatment for children and adolescents with cystic fibrosis.

15. _____ May occur as a result of a strain of group A streptococcus. The clinical manifestations may include pharyngitis and a characteristic erythematous sandpaper-like rash;

16. _____ An acute respiratory tract infection young infants demonstrate a characteristic expiratory whoop but older children may only have a cough.

a. Bacterial tracheitis

b. Croup

c. Infectious mononucleosis

d. Acute epiglottitis

e. Status asthmaticus

f. Pulmonary function tests (PFTs)

g. Bronchiolitis

h. Pneumonia

i. Foreign body aspiration

j. Aspiration pneumonia

k. Respiratory failure

l. Pertussis

m. Sweat chloride test

n. Scarlet fever

o. Airway clearance therapies

p. Apnea

II. REVIEWING KEY CONCEPTS

1. Most respiratory infections in children are caused by:
   a. Pneumococci.
   b. Viruses.
   c. Streptococci.
   d. *Haemophilus influenzae*.

2. The most likely reason that the respiratory infection rate increases drastically in the age range from 3 to 6 months is that the:
   a. Infant's exposure to pathogens is greatly increased during this time.
   b. Viral agents that are mild in older children are extremely severe in infants.
   c. Maternal antibodies have decreased and the infant's own antibody production is immature.
   d. Diameter of the airways is smaller in the infant than in the older child.

3. The primary concern of the nurse when giving tips for how to increase humidity in the home of a child with a respiratory infection should be to make sure the child has:
   a. Continuous contact with the humidification source.
   b. A warm humidification source.
   c. A humidification source that is safe.
   d. A cool humidification source.

4. Which of the following is the best choice for the child with acute respiratory disorder?
   a. IV fluid restriction
   b. Maintenance of patient comfort
   c. Insist that the child play quietly in bed.
   d. Use tidal volumes of 10 ml/kg

5. The best technique to prevent spread of nasopharyngitis is:
   a. Prompt immunization.
   b. Frequent hand washing and use of a tissue or their elbow to cover their mouth or nose when they cough or sneeze.
   c. Mist vaporization.
   d. To ensure adequate fluid intake.

6. Group A β-hemolytic streptococcal (GABHS) infection is usually a:
   a. Serious infection of the upper airway.
   b. Common cause of pharyngitis in children over the age of 15 years.
   c. Brief illness that places the child at risk for serious sequelae.
   d. Disease of the heart, lungs, joints, and central nervous system.

7. In the postoperative period following a tonsillectomy, the child should be:
   a. Placed in the Trendelenburg position.
   b. Encouraged to cough and deep breathe.
   c. Suctioned vigorously to clear the airway.
   d. Positioned to facilitate drainage of secretions.

8. The best pain medication administration regimen for a child in the initial postoperative period following a tonsillectomy is:
   a. At regular intervals for at least the first 24–48 hours.
   b. As needed for at least the first 24–48 hours.

9. Of the foods listed, the most appropriate selection to offer first to an alert child who is in the postoperative period following a tonsillectomy is:
   a. Strawberry ice cream.
   b. Red cherry-flavored gelatin.
   c. An apple-flavored ice pop.
   d. Cold diluted orange juice.

10. Which of the following signs is an early indication of hemorrhage in a child who has had a tonsillectomy?
   a. Continuous swallowing
   b. Decreasing blood pressure
   c. Irritability
   d. Nasal drainage

11. During influenza epidemics, it is generally believed the age group that provides a major source of transmission is the:
   a. Infant.
   b. School-age child.
   c. Adolescent.
   d. Preschool-age child.

12. Which of the following is not a typical clinical manifestation of the influenza virus?
   a. Stridor and lymphadenopathy
   b. Fever and chills
   c. Sore throat and dry mucous membranes
   d. Photophobia and myalgia

13. An infant with bronchiolitis is hospitalized. The causative organism is respiratory syncytial virus (RSV). The nurse knows that a child infected with this virus requires which of the following types of isolation would be appropriate?
   a. Standard and droplet
   b. Droplet and contact
   c. Standard, droplet, and contact
   d. Standard, contact, and airborne

14. An abnormal otoscopic examination would reveal:
   a. Visible landmarks.
   b. A light reflex.
   c. An erythematous bulging tympanic membrane.
   d. A mobile tympanic membrane.

15. Children with mild croup syndrome (no stridor):
   a. Require hospitalization.
   b. Will need to be intubated.
   c. Can be cared for at home.
   d. Are over 6 years old.

16. The nurse should prepare for an impending emergency situation to care for the child with suspected:
    a. Spasmodic croup.
    b. Laryngotracheobronchitis.
    c. Acute spasmodic laryngitis.
    d. Epiglottitis.

17. The nurse should suspect epiglottitis if the child has:
    a. Cough, sore throat, and agitation.
    b. Cough, drooling, and retractions.
    c. Absence of cough in the presence of drooling and agitation.
    d. Absence of cough, hoarseness, and retractions.

18. In the child who is suspected of having epiglottitis, the nurse should:
    a. Have intubation equipment available.
    b. Visually inspect the child's oropharynx with a tongue blade.
    c. Obtain a throat culture.
    d. Prepare to immunize the child for *Haemophilus influenzae*.

19. Since the advent of immunization for *Haemophilus influenzae*, there has been a decrease in the incidence of:
    a. Laryngotracheobronchitis.
    b. Epiglottitis.
    c. Influenza (seasonal).
    d. Croup.

20. A 4-year-old child is 12 hours status post a tonsillectomy. The child is taking some clear liquids; however, the child "spit up" a small amount of fresh red blood. What is the most appropriate action to take?
    a. Notify the health care provider immediately.
    b. Ask the parents to let you know if the child vomits any more.
    c. Give the child pain medication and a popsicle.
    d. Give the child an ice pack to promote vasoconstriction and decrease/stop the bleeding.

21. A toddler has been diagnosed with *S. pneumonia*. Nursing care of the child with pneumonia includes which intervention?
    a. Administration of antibiotics.
    b. Administration of oseltamivir (Tamiflu).
    c. Round-the-clock administration of antitussive agents.
    d. Strict monitoring of intake and output to avoid congestive heart failure.

22. Respiratory syncytial virus (RSV) is:
    a. An uncommon virus that causes severe bronchiolitis.
    b. An uncommon virus that usually does not require hospitalization.
    c. A common virus that usually occurs primarily in winter and early spring.
    d. A common virus that usually does not require hospitalization.

23. The use of palivizumab (Synagis), for RSV is given because:
    a. It helps prevent RSV in high-risk populations.
    b. It is an antiviral agent.
    c. It helps treat patients at low risk for mortality.
    d. It can be used for any infant.

24. Nursing care management of the 6-month-old infant with RSV bronchiolitis should include:
    a. Supplemental oxygen to keep oxygen saturation levels greater than 94%.
    b. IV fluids during the acute phase of the illness.
    c. Appropriate bronchodilation therapy.
    d. Chest physiotherapy (CPT) every 4 hours and as needed.

25. General signs of bacterial pneumonia include:
    a. Low fever and nausea.
    b. Clear breath sounds and brown sputum.
    c. Cough, tachypnea, and fever.
    d. Nasal flaring and tympany with percussion.

26. Which of the following is the most common bacterial pathogen responsible for community-acquired pneumonia in children 5 years or older?
    a. *Haemophilus pneumoniae*
    b. *Mycoplasma pneumoniae*
    c. *Staphylococcal aureus pneumoniae*
    d. *Streptococcal pneumoniae*

27. In an 8-month-old infant admitted to the hospital with pertussis, the nurse should inquire about the:
    a. Living conditions of the infant and family.
    b. Labor and delivery history of the mother.
    c. Immunization status of the infant.
    d. Alcohol and drug intake of the mother.

28. The best test to screen for tuberculosis infection is the:
    a. Chest radiograph.
    b. Tuberculin skin test (TST).
    c. Sputum culture.
    d. DNA blood test.

29. The nurse is caring for a child who has been admitted with a possible diagnosis of tuberculosis. Which laboratory or diagnostic tool would most likely be used to help diagnose this child?
    a. Purified protein derivative test
    b. Sweat sodium chloride test
    c. Blood culture and sensitivity
    d. Pulmonary functions test

30. An 8-year-old child diagnosed with asthma is being taught how to use a spacer with an albuterol inhaler. What is the best way for the nurse to evaluate the child's understanding of how to use the spacer?
    a. Guide the child step by step through the process.
    b. Have the child attach the spacer to the inhaler and use it.
    c. Have the child verbalize how to use the spacer.
    d. Attach the spacer to the inhaler, then have the child to use it.

215

31. Which of the following are common symptoms seen in a foreign body aspiration of children?
    a. Wheezing
    b. Diaphoresis
    c. Drooling
    d. Nasal congestion

32. Which of the following questions would be most important for the nurse to ask the parents of a child admitted to the hospital with a diagnosis of reactive airway disease?
    a. "What brings you to the hospital?"
    b. "What is your ethnic background?"
    c. "Do you have a history of asthma in your family?"
    d. "Were your pregnancy and delivery uneventful?"

33. The nurse examines a 6-year-old child with asthma and finds that there is hyperresonance on percussion. Breath sounds are coarse and loud with sonorous crackles throughout the lung fields. Expiration is prolonged; crackles can be heard. There is generalized inspiratory and expiratory wheezing. The child has these symptoms two times a week, with nighttime episodes a few times per month. He uses a short-acting β agonist daily and his FEV_1 is 80%. Based on these findings, the nurse suspects that there is:
    a. Moderate persistent asthma.
    b. Severe persistent asthma.
    c. Mild persistent asthma.
    d. Mild intermittent asthma.

34. The parents of a newly diagnosed 5-year-old female with CF ask the nurse what time to begin the child's airway clearance therapies (ACT) each day. Which is the nurse's best response?
    a. Do the ACTs 30 minutes before meals.
    b. Do the ACTs before any nebulized aerosol treatments.
    c. Do the ACTs 30 minutes after meals.
    d. Do the ACTs when you notice your daughter has a cold or congestion.

35. What drug is usually given first in the emergency treatment of an acute, severe asthma episode in a young child?
    a. Magnesium sulfate
    b. Theophylline
    c. Atrovent
    d. Albuterol

36. The principal treatment for the pancreatic insufficiency which occurs in cystic fibrosis is the administration of:
    a. Enemas.
    b. Corticosteroids.
    c. Antibiotics.
    d. Enzymes.

37. Cystic fibrosis (CF) may affect single or multiple systems of the body. What is the primary factor responsible for possible multiple clinical manifestations in CF?
    a. Hyperactivity of sweat glands
    b. Hypoactivity of autonomic nervous system
    c. Atrophy in the mucosal walls of all body systems
    d. Increased thickness of mucous gland secretions

38. A 17-year-old female with cystic fibrosis is hospitalized for a "tune-up." Which documentation in the chart would indicate the need for counseling regarding nutrition?
    a. Five to six frothy, foul-smelling stools.
    b. Weight unchanged from 3 days ago.
    c. Consumed 50% of her breakfast this morning.
    d. Eats three snacks a day.

39. An 18-month-old is admitted with acute laryngotracheobronchitis (LTB). The child will most likely be treated with which of the following?
    a. Racemic epinephrine nebulized treatments and corticosteroids
    b. Intravenous (IV) and oxygen
    c. Antibiotics and albuterol
    d. Chest physiotherapy (CPT) and oxygen

40. A quantitative sweat chloride test has been done on a 6-month-old child. What value should be most indicative of cystic fibrosis (CF)?
    a. Less than 18 mEq/L
    b. 18–40 mEq/L
    c. 40–60 mEq/L
    d. Greater than 60 mEq/L

MATCHING: Match each drug used for pediatric emergency care with its appropriate use during resuscitation.

41. _____ Short-acting β-adrenergic agonist used as an inhaled bronchodilator for acute asthma exacerbations.

42. _____ Antibiotic of choice in otitis media when causative organism is a highly resistant pneumococcus.

43. _____ A long-acting β2-agonist (bronchodilator) that is used twice a day (no more frequently than every 12 hours).

44. _____ A potent muscle relaxant that acts to decrease inflammation and improves pulmonary function and peak flow rate among pediatric patients with severe asthma.

45. _____ Common medication for pulmonary tuberculosis infection.

46. _____ Considered first-line therapy in children older than 5 years of age.

47. _____ Leukotriene modifier used to block inflammatory and bronchospasm effects.

48. _____ Anticholinergic used to relieve acute bronchospasm.

49. _____ When nebulized it has been shown to be effective in improving airway hydration and increasing mucus clearance in patients with CF.

50. _____ A monoclonal antibody that blocks the binding of IgE to mast cells; inhibits the inflammation that is associated with asthma, and it is used in patients with moderate to persistent asthma who have confirmed perennial aeroallergen sensitivity.

51. _____ Acts to decrease the viscosity of mucus to improve airway clearance.

52. _____ First-line choice antibiotic for the treatment of acute otitis media.

a. Inhaled corticosteroid

b. Ceftriaxone

c. Magnesium sulfate

d. Singulair

e. Salmeterol

f. Amoxicillin

g. Dornase alfa (Pulmozyme)

h. Albuterol

i. Ipratropium

j. Omalizumab (Xolair)

k. Hypertonic saline

l. Isoniazid

III. CLINICAL JUDGMENT AND NEXT-GENERATION NCLEX® EXAMINATION-STYLE QUESTIONS

1. An 11-month-old infant is experiencing their first acute otitis media (AOM). What should the nurse include in the discharge teaching to the infant's parents? Select all that apply.

   a. A follow-up visit should occur after the antibiotic treatment is completed.

   b. Antibiotic ear drops will be administered in conjunction with the oral antibiotics to decrease pain.

   c. Tylenol should not be given because it may mask symptoms of mastoiditis.

   d. All prescribed medication should be completed even if the infant appears to be feeling better.

   e. Tylenol or Ibuprofen may be administered to assist in controlling the infant's fevers.

Chapter **40** **The Child with Respiratory Dysfunction**

2. An 8-year-old female presents to the clinic with complaints of a sore throat and fever. A throat culture is obtained, and the diagnosis of group A beta-hemolytic streptococcus (GABHS) pharyngitis is confirmed. Which of the following would be appropriate health teaching for the parents and child. Use an X for the health teaching below that is Indicated (appropriate or necessary), Contraindicated (could be harmful), or Non-Essential (makes no difference or not necessary) regarding treatment of GABHS pharyngitis.

Health Teaching	Indicated	Contraindicated	Non-essential
In certain strains of this disease, a characteristic erythematous sandpaper-like rash; known as Scarlet Fever may develop.			
A follow up throat culture is recommended after completion of antibiotic therapy.			
Children who experience a GABHS infection are at increased risk for the development of acute rheumatic fever and acute glomerulonephritis, thus it is imperative to complete the antibiotic therapy prescribed.			
Application of a warm or cold compress to the neck area may provide pain relief, anti-pyretics may also be administered for throat pain and to decrease fevers.			
Children should discard their toothbrush after completion of antibiotic therapy.			
Children are considered contagious until they have received antibiotic therapy for a full 48-hour period of time.			

41 The Child with Gastrointestinal Dysfunction

I. LEARNING KEY TERMS

MATCHING: Match each term with its corresponding description.

1. _____ Inflammation of the blind sac at the end of the cecum, the most common cause of abdominal surgery in childhood.

2. _____ A protrusion of a portion of an organ or organs through an abnormal opening.

3. _____ Characterized by extremely long intervals between defecation.

4. _____ An alteration in the frequency, consistency, or ease of passing stool. It is defined as unsatisfactory defecation due to infrequent stools, difficult stool passage, or perceived incomplete defecation

5. _____ Absence of ganglion cells in the affected intestine resulting in mechanical obstruction from inadequate motility.

6. _____ Transfer of gastric contents into the esophagus occurring throughout the day especially after meals and at night.

7. _____ Symptoms or tissue damage resulting from transfer of gastric contents into the esophagus.

8. _____ Ingestion of excessive amounts of electrolyte-free water develop a concurrent decrease in serum sodium accompanied by central nervous system (CNS) symptoms.

9. _____ Constipation with fecal soiling.

10. _____ Malabsorptive disorder that occurs as a result of decreased mucosal surface area, usually because of extensive resection of the small intestine.

11. _____ A common body fluid disturbance, commonly referred to as volume depletion.

12. _____ Inflammation of the colon and rectum with distal colon and rectum most severely affected.

a. Dehydration

b. Water intoxication

c. Gastroesophageal reflux

d. Hernia

e. Appendicitis

f. Ulcerative colitis

g. Short bowel syndrome

h. Gastroesophageal reflux disease

i. Hirschsprung disease

j. Constipation

k. Obstipation

l. Encopresis

II. REVIEWING KEY CONCEPTS

1. The initial phase of fluid replacement is contraindicated in which type of dehydration because of the risk of water intoxication?
   a. Isotonic.
   b. Hypotonic.
   c. Hypertonic.
   d. It is appropriate in all three types of dehydration.

2. Which of the following clinical manifestations indicates a fluid volume deficit in infants?
   a. Brisk skin turgor.
   b. Urine output less than 1 ml/kg/hr.
   c. Capillary refill less than 2 seconds.
   d. Soft and flat anterior fontanel.

3. Which of the following findings is the most important determinant of the percent of total body fluid loss in infants and younger children?
   a. Weight.
   b. Intake and output.
   c. Fontanel assessment.
   d. Skin turgor.

4. Which of the following clinical manifestations are the most useful in predicting dehydration of 5% or more in children?
   a. Sunken fontanel, abnormal skin turgor, abnormal temperature.
   b. Rapid pulse, dry mucous membranes, absent tears.
   c. Rapid respirations, irritable behavior, prolonged capillary refill.
   d. Abnormal capillary refill, abnormal skin turgor, and abnormal respiratory pattern.

5. Which of the following organisms is the most common cause of diarrhea-associated hospitalization?
   a. Salmonella
   b. Shigella
   c. Campylobacter
   d. Rotavirus

6. Which of the following indicates an insensible fluid loss?
   a. Urine output
   b. Fecal output
   c. Emesis output
   d. Fever

7. Infants and young children are at high risk for fluid and electrolyte imbalance. Which of the following factors contributes to this vulnerability?
   a. Decreased body surface area
   b. Lower metabolic rate
   c. Mature kidney function
   d. Increased extracellular fluid volume

8. _____ dehydration occurs when electrolyte and water deficits are present in balanced proportion.

9. _____ dehydration occurs when the electrolyte deficit exceeds the water deficit. There is a greater loss of extracellular fluid, and plasma sodium concentration is usually _____ than 130 mEq/L.

10. _____ dehydration results from water loss in excess of electrolyte loss. This is often caused by a large _____ of water and/or a large _____ of electrolytes. Plasma sodium concentration is _____ than 150 mEq/L.

11. Which of the following choices most accurately describes dehydration or fluid loss in infants and young children?
    a. As a percentage
    b. In milliliters per kilogram of body weight
    c. By the amount of edema present
    d. By the degree of skin elasticity

12. An infant with moderate dehydration may demonstrate:
    a. Mottled skin color and decreased pulse and respirations.
    b. Decreased urine output, tachycardia, and fever.
    c. Dry mucous membranes and prolonged capillary refill greater than two seconds.
    d. Tachycardia, bulging fontanel, and decreased blood pressure.

13. List eight assessment findings that may be used to determine dehydration in a child.

14. A priority goal in the management of acute diarrhea is:
    a. Determining the cause of the diarrhea.
    b. Preventing the spread of the infection.
    c. Rehydrating of the child.
    d. Managing the fever associated with the diarrhea.

15. To confirm the diagnosis of Hirschsprung disease, the nurse prepares the child for:
    a. Endoscopy.
    b. Sonogram.
    c. Rectal biopsy.
    d. Esophagostomy.

16. The nurse is caring for a child with newly diagnosed Hirschsprung disease. Which of the following does the nurse understand about the infant's condition?
    a. There is a lack of peristalsis in the large intestine resulting in accumulation of abdominal contents causing abdominal distention.
    b. There is excessive peristalsis throughout the large intestine resulting in diarrhea.
    c. There is a small-bowel obstruction resulting in dark, tarry-like stools.
    d. There is inflammation throughout the large intestine, leading to accumulation of abdominal contents and subsequent abdominal distention.

17. A 10-month-old is being admitted to the hospital with acute gastroenteritis and severe dehydration due to vomiting and excessive fluid loss. The health care provider prescribes an antiemetic. Which of the following antiemetic drugs does the nurse anticipate being given?
    a. Ondansetron (Zofran)
    b. Promethazine (Phenergan)
    c. Metoclopramide (Reglan)
    d. Dimenhydrinate (Dramamine)

18. The nurse should instruct parents to administer the prescribed daily proton pump inhibitor to their infant with gastroesophageal reflux at which time to be most effective?
    a. Administers 30 minutes before breakfast.
    b. Administers 30 minutes before any meals.
    c. Administers mid-afternoon.
    d. Administers 30 minutes before dinner.

19. The most common clinical manifestations expected with Meckel diverticulum include:
    a. Fever, vomiting, and constipation.
    b. Weight loss, hypotension, and obstruction.
    c. Painless rectal bleeding, abdominal pain, or intestinal obstruction.
    d. Abdominal pain, bloody diarrhea, and foul-smelling stool.

20. A common occurrence of Crohn disease is:
    a. Growth failure.
    b. Chronic constipation.
    c. Obstruction.
    d. Burning epigastric pain.

21. Which clinical manifestation would be the most suggestive of acute appendicitis?
    a. Abdominal pain relieved by eating
    b. Red, currant jelly-like stools
    c. Ribbon like, foul-smelling stools
    d. Abdominal pain most intense at McBurney point

22. The single most effective strategy to prevent and control hepatitis is _____.

23. A 5-week-old male infant with pyloric stenosis is having excessive vomiting. What is the most likely complication from the excessive vomiting?
    a. Hyperkalemia
    b. Hyperchloremia
    c. Metabolic acidosis
    d. Metabolic alkalosis

MATCHING: Match each viral hepatitis type with its corresponding description.

24. _____ Particularly prevalent in developing countries with poor living conditions, inadequate sanitation, crowding, and poor personal hygiene practices.

25. _____ An acute or chronic infection, humans are the main source of this infection.

26. _____ Non-A, non-B hepatitis with transmission through the fecal-oral route or with contaminated water.

27. _____ Must occur in individuals already infected with HBV.

28. _____ The most common cause of chronic liver disease.

a. Hepatitis A
b. Hepatitis B
c. Hepatitis C
d. Hepatitis D
e. Hepatitis E

29. The definition of *biliary atresia* is:
    a. Persistent jaundice with elevated direct bilirubin levels.
    b. Progressive inflammatory process causing bile duct fibrosis.
    c. Absence of bile pigment.
    d. Hepatomegaly and palpable liver.

30. The most common early symptom of biliary atresia is:
    a. Projectile vomiting.
    b. Bloody stools.
    c. Alcoholic stools.
    d. Jaundice.

31. _____ is often a significant problem in children with biliary atresia that is addressed by drug therapy or comfort measures such as baths in colloidal oatmeal compounds.

32. To assess for the presence of a cleft palate, the nurse should:
    a. Assess the infant's ability to swallow.
    b. Assess the color of the infant's oral mucosa.
    c. Palpate the hard and soft palates with a gloved finger.
    d. Flick the infant's foot and make it cry.

33. One of the major problems for infants born with cleft lip and palate is related to:
    a. Rejection by the mother.
    b. Feeding problems and weight loss.
    c. Apnea and bradycardia.
    d. Aspiration pneumonia.

34. The nurse is caring for a 2-month-old infant whose cleft lip was repaired. Important aspects of this infant's postoperative care include:
    a. Elbow immobilizers, lip irrigations, cleansing the suture line daily.
    b. Petroleum jelly application, elbow immobilizers, pain management.
    c. Lip irrigations, prone position, cleansing suture line after feedings.
    d. Supine position, chest physiotherapy (CPT), elbow immobilizers.

35. A parent of an infant with moderate gastroesophageal reflux asks how to decrease the number and the total volume of emesis. What is the most appropriate recommendation the nurse can make?
    a. There will probably be the need for surgical intervention of tightening the lower esophageal stricture.
    b. Place in supine position to sleep after feeding with HOB elevated.
    c. Thicken feedings with rice cereal.
    d. Reduce the frequency of feeding by encouraging larger volumes of formula.

36. A proximal segment of the bowel telescopes into a more distal segment, pulling the mesentery with it is called:
    a. Intussusception.
    b. Pyloric stenosis.
    c. Tracheoesophageal fistula.
    d. Hirschsprung disease.

37. The nurse would expect to see which of the following clinical manifestations in the child diagnosed with Hirschsprung disease?
    a. History of bloody diarrhea, fever, and vomiting.
    b. Irritability, severe abdominal cramps, and fecal soiling.
    c. Increased serum lipids and positive stool for O&P (ova and parasites).
    d. Bilious vomiting, abdominal distention, and delay in passage of meconium.

38. A 5-month-old infant's intussusception is treated with hydrostatic reduction. The nurse should expect care after the reduction to include:
    a. Administration of antibiotics.
    b. Enema administration to remove remaining stool.
    c. Close observation of stool patterns.
    d. Blood pressure every 4 hours.

39. The nurse observes frothy saliva in the mouth and nose of the neonate who is a few hours old. When fed, the infant swallows normally, but suddenly the fluid returns through the nose and mouth of the infant. The nurse suspects:
    a. Esophageal atresia.
    b. Pyloric stenosis.
    c. Anorectal malformation.
    d. Biliary atresia.

40. A l-month-old infant is brought to the clinic by his mother. The nurse suspects pyloric stenosis because the mother gives a history of:
    a. Diarrhea.
    b. Projectile vomiting.
    c. Fever and dehydration.
    d. Abdominal distention.

41. The parents of a newborn with an umbilical hernia ask about treatment options. The nurse's response should be based on which knowledge.
    a. Taping the abdomen to flatten the protrusion is sometimes helpful but can be painful for the infant.
    b. The defect usually resolves spontaneously by 3–5 years of age.
    c. Radiation treatment is necessary to reduce the hernia.
    d. Surgery is recommended as soon as possible.

42. The assessment finding that most indicative of an anorectal malformation is:
    a. Abdominal distention and vomiting.
    b. A normal-appearing perineum.
    c. Passage of meconium stool after 24 hours.
    d. Failure to pass meconium through the anal opening.

43. The most important therapeutic management for the child with celiac disease is:
    a. Eliminating corn, rice, and millet from the diet.
    b. Adding iron, folic acid, and fat-soluble vitamins to the diet.
    c. Eliminating wheat, rye, barley, and oats from the diet.
    d. Educating the child's parents about the short-term effects of the disease and the necessity of reading all food labels for content until the disease is in remission.

44. The prognosis for children with short bowel syndrome has improved as a result of:
    a. Dietary supplemental vitamin B12 additions.
    b. Improvement in surgical procedures to correct the deficiency.
    c. Improved home care availability.
    d. Total parenteral nutrition and enteral feeding.

45. A common long-term complication after surgical repair of esophageal atresia is:
    a. Feeding difficulties.
    b. Tracheomalacia.
    c. Pneumothorax.
    d. Short bowel syndrome.

46. Describe the 3 phases of parenteral rehydration therapy for the child diagnosed with severe dehydration.

47. Explain the rationale and methodology for oral rehydration management in a child with mild dehydration.

III. CLINICAL JUDGMENT AND NEXT-GENERATION NCLEX® EXAMINATION-STYLE QUESTIONS

1. A nurse is providing postoperative care to an infant who has undergone a cleft lip and palate repair. Which of the following would be appropriate interventions to implement in the postoperative period? Select all that apply.

   a. Pain analgesia as ordered.

   b. Use of an upright position or infant seat.

   c. Sterile water irrigations to the operative site as ordered.

   d. Feeding resumed when tolerated, using a blenderized or soft diet in older children.

   e. Use of elbow immobilizers to protect the operative site.

   f. Application of petroleum jelly to operative site as ordered.

2. The nurse is caring for a 3-year-old who presents with acute intestinal obstruction of unknown etiology. Choose the most likely options for information missing from the statements below by making selections from the list of options provided. _____ Option 1 _____ is the most common cause of intestinal obstruction in children between 3 months and 6 years old. The usual clinical manifestation is _____ option 2 _____ with the passage of _____ option 3 _____ stool. Passage of a _____ colored stool often indicates resolution of the disease process.

Option 1	Option 2	Option 3	Option 4
Gastroesophageal reflux	Crampy abdominal pain	Black and tarry	Black
Hirschsprung disease	Projectile vomiting	Ribbon-like	Brown
Intussusception	Rigid abdomen	Foul-smelling	Meconium
Tracheoesophageal fistula	Visible peristalsis	Currant jelly-like	

42 The Child with Cardiovascular Dysfunction

I. LEARNING KEY TERMS

MATCHING: Match each term with its corresponding description.

1. _____ Abnormally fast heart rhythm.

2. _____ Measurements of pressures and oxygen saturations in heart chambers.

3. _____ Abnormally slow heart rhythm.

4. _____ Refers to abnormalities of the myocardium in which the cardiac muscles' ability to contract is impaired; relatively rare in children.

5. _____ Refers to excessive cholesterol in the blood; believed to play an important role in atherosclerosis development.

6. _____ A general term for excessive lipids (fat) and fatlike substances; believed to play an important role in atherosclerosis development.

7. _____ A treatment strategy to try for supraventricular tachycardia (SVT); performed by applying ice to the face, massaging one carotid artery, or having the child exhale against a closed glottis.

8. _____ A thickening and flattening of the tips of the fingers and toes; thought to be a result of chronic tissue hypoxemia and polycythemia.

9. _____ Often see tachycardia which is pronounced and narrowed pulse pressure. There is poor capillary filling, and the child exhibits confusion, sleepiness, and decreased responsiveness.

10. _____ An invasive diagnostic procedure in which a radiopaque catheter is introduced through a large-bore needle into a peripheral vessel.

11. _____ Slower than normal heart rate.

12. _____ Cardiac arrest represents this type of shock.

13. _____ The inability of the heart to pump an adequate amount of blood to meet the metabolic demands of the body; not a disease; in children, most common in infants; usually secondary to increases in blood volume and pressure from anomalies; result of an excessive workload imposed on normal myocardium.

14. _____ Faster than normal heart rate.

15. _____ An increased number of red blood cells; increases the oxygen carrying capacity of the blood.

16. _____ Includes primarily anatomic abnormalities present at birth that result in abnormal cardiac function, the consequences of which are hypoxemia and heart failure.

17. _____ Refers to an arterial oxygen tension (or pressure) that is less than normal and can be identified by a decreased arterial saturation or a decreased PaO_2.

18. _____ Vital organ function is maintained by intrinsic compensatory mechanism; blood flow is usually normal or increased, but generally uneven or maldistributed in the microcirculation.

19. _____ Disease processes or abnormalities that occur after birth and can be seen in the normal heart or in the presence of congenital heart defects; resulting from factors such as infection, autoimmune responses, environmental factors, and familial tendencies.

20. _____ A reduction in tissue oxygenation that results from low oxygen saturation and PaO_2 and results in impaired cellular processes.

21. _____ A common feature of CHD, and pallor is associated with poor perfusion

a. Congenital heart disease

b. Acquired cardiac disorders

c. Tachycardia

d. Bradycardia

e. Cardiac catheterization

f. Congestive heart failure

g. Hypoxemia

h. Hypoxia

i. Cyanosis

j. Polycythemia

k. Clubbing

l. Hyperlipidemia

m. Hypercholesterolemia

n. Bradydysrhythmias

o. Tachydysrhythmias

p. Cardiomyopathy

q. Vagal maneuvers

r. Hemodynamics

s. Compensated shock

t. Hypotensive shock

u. Irreversible shock

II. REVIEWING KEY CONCEPTS

1. During fetal life, oxygenated blood travels into the left atrium through a structure known as the:
   a. Truncus arteriosus.
   b. Foramen ovale.
   c. Sinus venosus.
   d. Ductus venosus.

2. Which of the following fetal structures is a conduit in which blood is shunted from the pulmonary artery to the descending aorta.
   a. Superior vena cava.
   b. Ductus arteriosus.
   c. Foramen ovale.
   d. Ductus venosus.

3. When an abnormal connection exists between the heart chambers (e.g., a septal defect), blood will necessarily flow from an area of higher pressure (left side) to one of lower pressure (right side). This is called a:
   a. Left-to-right shunt.
   b. Right-to-left shunt.

4. Which of the following is best described as the inability of the heart to pump an adequate amount of blood to the systemic circulation at normal filling pressures?
   a. Pulmonary venous congestion
   b. Congenital heart defect
   c. Congestive heart failure
   d. Systemic venous congestion

5. Coarctation of the aorta should be suspected when the:
   a. Blood pressure is higher in the arms than in the legs.
   b. Blood pressure in the right arm is different from the blood pressure in the left arm.
   c. Apical pulse is greater than the radial pulse.
   d. Point of maximum impulse is shifted to the right.

6. The test in which a transducer is placed behind the heart to obtain images of posterior heart structures or used in patients with poor images from chest approach is the:
   a. Electrocardiogram (EKG)
   b. Echocardiogram (Echo)
   c. Transesophageal echocardiogram (TEE)
   d. Two-dimensional echocardiogram (2-D Echo)

7. A 2-year-old with a known cardiac defect is presenting in congestive heart failure. Which assessment finding would indicate to the nurse possible digoxin toxicity?
   a. Tachycardia
   b. Bradypnea
   c. Bradycardia
   d. Tachypnea

8. List five of the most significant complications following a cardiac catheterization in an infant or young child.

9. If bleeding occurs at the insertion site after a cardiac catheterization, the nurse should apply:
   a. Warmth to the unaffected extremity.
   b. Pressure below the insertion site.
   c. Warmth to the affected extremity.
   d. Pressure above the insertion site.

10. A chest X-ray examination is ordered for a child with suspected cardiac problems. The child's parent asks the nurse, "What will the x-ray show about the heart?" The nurse's response should be based on knowledge that the x-ray film will do which of the following?
    a. Show bones of chest but not the heart
    b. Evaluate the vascular anatomy outside of the heart
    c. Show a graphic measure of electrical activity of the heart
    d. Provide information on size of the heart

11. The goal of treatment for hypertension in children is decreasing systolic and diastolic BP values to below the _____ percentile in children younger than 13 years old and less than _____ mm Hg in adolescents older than 13 years of age.

12. The nurse is teaching a mother how to administer digoxin (Lanoxin) at home to her 4-year-old child. The nurse tells the mother that as a general rule, digoxin should not be administered to the older child whose pulse is:
    a. 108.
    b. 98.
    c. 78.
    d. 58.

13. An infant is receiving Lanoxin elixir 0.028 mg once daily. Lanoxin is available in an elixir concentration of 50 mcg/mL. The correct dose to draw up and administer is:
    a. 0.56 mL.
    b. 0.28 mL.
    c. 0.84 mL.
    d. 1.12 mL.

14. A 12-month-old infant in heart failure is taking enalapril (ACE inhibitor) and spironolactone. The nurse should be especially alert for:
    a. Sodium 142 mEq/L.
    b. Potassium 5.5 mEq/L.
    c. Potassium 3.1 mEq/L.
    d. Sodium 132 mEq/L.

15. The nurse is assessing a 6-month-old with congestive heart failure. Which of the following is a clinical manifestation of systemic congestion which can occur with CHF?
    a. Tachypnea
    b. Bradycardia
    c. Systemic venous hypertension
    d. Intercostal retractions

16. The two main angiotensin-converting enzyme (ACE) inhibitors most commonly used for children with congestive heart failure are:
    a. Digoxin and captopril.
    b. Enalapril and captopril.
    c. Enalapril and furosemide.
    d. Spironolactone and captopril.

17. The electrolyte most commonly depleted with diuretic therapy is:
    a. Sodium.
    b. Chloride.
    c. Potassium.
    d. Magnesium.

18. Meeting the nutritional needs of an infant with congestive heart failure is challenging due to the poor cardiac function, increased respiratory rate and heart rate of the infant. Which of the following measures would most likely ensure the nutritional needs of the infant with congestive heart failure are being met?
    a. The infant should be fed about 30 minutes before napping.
    b. The infant should be fed every 2 hours to promote adequate caloric intake
    c. The infant should be fed every 3 hours to promote adequate rest periods between feedings.
    d. The infant should be given about 45 minutes to complete feeding.

19. The calories are usually modified for an infant with congestive heart failure by:
    a. Feeding every 2 hours.
    b. Increasing the volume of each feeding.
    c. Increasing the caloric density of the formula.
    d. Increasing the feeding duration to 1 hour.

20. A nurse is providing care to an infant diagnosed with a ventricular septal defect (VSD). The infant's parents are confused and ask the nurse for additional information about the defect. Which would be the most appropriate response by the nurse?
    a. "When your health care provider makes rounds, we will make sure to get your questions answered."
    b. "If you like, I can call and ask your health care provider to come back and talk to you."
    c. "It is one of the structures of the fetal heart that sometimes fails to close after birth and can cause heart failure."
    d. "This congenital defect is an opening between the left and right ventricles of the heart that can cause heart failure if not corrected."

21. Prostaglandin is administered to the newborn with a congenital heart defect to:
    a. Keep the ductus arteriosus open.
    b. Close the ductus arteriosus.
    c. Keep the foramen ovale open.
    d. Close the foramen ovale.

22. Dehydration must be prevented in children who are hypoxemic because dehydration places the child at risk for:
    a. Infection.
    b. Cerebral vascular accident.
    c. Fever.
    d. Air embolism.

23. The leading cause of death in the first 3 years after heart transplantation (the greatest risk in the first 6 months) in children is:
    a. Heart failure.
    b. Infection.
    c. Rejection.
    d. Renal dysfunction.

MATCHING

Match each specific disorder with its corresponding type of defect. (Defects may be used more than once.)

24. _____ Patent ductus arteriosus

25. _____ Coarctation of the aorta

26. _____ Ventricular septal defect

27. _____ Subvalvular aortic stenosis

28. _____ Hypoplastic left heart syndrome

29. _____ Atrioventricular canal defect

30. _____ Pulmonic stenosis

31. _____ Tetralogy of Fallot

32. _____ Aortic stenosis

33. _____ Tricuspid atresia

34. _____ Valvular aortic stenosis

35. _____ Truncus arteriosus

36. _____ Atrial septal defect

37. _____ Transposition of the great vessels

a. Defects with decreased pulmonary blood flow

b. Mixed defects

c. Defects with increased pulmonary blood flow

d. Obstructive defects

38. Which of the following congenital heart defects usually has the best prognosis?
    a. Tetralogy of Fallot
    b. Ventricular septal defect
    c. Atrial septal defect
    d. Hypoplastic left heart syndrome

39. Which of the following sets of assessment findings are the most frequent clinical manifestations of an ventricular septal defect in an infant or child?
    a. Decreased cardiac output and low blood pressure
    b. Heart failure and a characteristic murmur
    c. Increased blood pressure and pulse
    d. Dyspnea and bradycardia

40. The nurse is assessing a 6-month-old with congestive heart failure. Which of the following is a clinical manifestation of systemic congestion which can occur with CHF?
    a. Tachypnea
    b. Bradycardia
    c. Hepatomegaly
    d. Intercostal retractions

41. An 18-month-old child is receiving Digoxin, Lasix, and Captopril to assist in medical management of CHF until their scheduled surgery. The provider has added Aldactone as well. Which laboratory value will be most important to monitor for this child?
    a. Serum sodium
    b. Serum potassium
    c. Serum chloride
    d. Serum calcium

42. Which of the following structural defects constitutes the classic form of tetralogy of Fallot?
    a. Pulmonary stenosis, ventricular septal defect, overriding aorta, right ventricular hypertrophy.
    b. Aortic stenosis, ventricular septal defect, overriding aorta, right ventricular hypertrophy.
    c. Aortic stenosis, ventricular septal defect, overriding aorta, left ventricular hypertrophy.
    d. Pulmonary stenosis, ventricular septal defect, aortic hypertrophy, left ventricular hypertrophy.

43. Medical management for a patent ductus arteriosus (PDA) failed and now the physician suggests surgery be performed for the infant's PDA to lessen which complication?
    a. Hypoxemia.
    b. Right to left shunting.
    c. Decreased workload on the left side of the heart.
    d. Pulmonary congestion.

44. An infant who weighs 7 kg has just returned to the intensive care unit following cardiac surgery. The chest tube has drained 40 mL in the past hour. In this situation, what is the first action for the nurse to take?
    a. Notify the surgeon.
    b. Identify any other signs of hemorrhage.
    c. Suction the patient.
    d. Identify any other signs of renal failure.

227

45. An infant who weighs 7 kg has just returned to the intensive care unit following cardiac surgery. The urine output has been 5 mL in the past hour. In this situation, what is the first action the nurse should take?
    a. Notify the surgeon.
    b. Identify any other signs of hypervolemia.
    c. Suction the patient.
    d. Identify any other signs of renal failure.

46. A nurse is providing care to a 7-month-old infant diagnosed with a ventricular septal defect who has developed congestive heart failure. The nurse has identified fluid volume excess as a key problem with the goal of attaining fluid balance. Which intervention is most applicable to the key problem and goal?
    a. Administer digoxin as prescribed.
    b. Administer furosemide as prescribed.
    c. Cluster the infant's care to promote adequate rest.
    d. Auscultate the infant's lungs to monitor for pulmonary edema.

47. Nursing care of the child with Kawasaki disease is challenging because of which occurrence?
    a. The child's irritability
    b. Predictable disease course
    c. Complex aspirin therapy
    d. The child's ongoing requests for food

48. One of the most important factors in preventing bacterial endocarditis is:
    a. administration of antibiotics before dental work to high-risk patients.
    b. surgical repair of the defect.
    c. administration of prostaglandin to maintain patent ductus arteriosus.
    d. administration of antibiotics after dental work to high-risk patients.

49. The most reliable test to provide evidence of recent streptococcal infection in the patient with suspected acute rheumatic fever is the:
    a. Throat culture.
    b. Mantoux test.
    c. Liver enzymes test.
    d. Antistreptolysin O test.

50. Nursing care of the child with Kawasaki disease is challenging because of which occurrence?
    a. The child's irritability
    b. Predictable disease course
    c. Complex aspirin therapy
    d. The child's ongoing requests for food

51. Discharge teaching for a child with Kawasaki disease who received IVIG should include:
    a. Temperature should be taken daily; occurrence of fever should be reported immediately.
    b. Arthritis, especially in the weight-bearing joints, although temporary, may persist for about a week after the initial infusion was completed.
    c. Administer live vaccines such as measles, mumps, and rubella (MMR) vaccine after at least six months from the IVIG infusion.
    d. No special instructions are needed except for cardiology follow-up.

52. An infant with Tetralogy of Fallot is at home, the infant became upset and was crying "hard." The infant has an increase in cyanosis and becomes tachypnea.
    To relieve the cardiac load on the heart, which of the following should the parent do first?
    a. Administer morphine sulfate.
    b. Place the child in knee-chest position.
    c. Place the child in a high-Fowler position.
    d. Administer oxygen.

53. Elevated cholesterol:
    a. Can predict the long-term risk of heart disease for the individual.
    b. Can predict the risk of hypertension in adulthood.
    c. Plays an important role in causing atherosclerosis.
    d. Plays an important role in causing congestive heart failure.

54. Recent concerns regarding the incidence of hypertension in children and adolescents has led to the recommendation that children older than _____ years receive _____ BP screening.

55. An 11-year-old male is in the clinic to receive booster childhood vaccines. The nurse asks the child's mother if they have ever had cholesterol screening performed. The mother replies the child is too young for such screening. The nurse informs the child's mother that universal cholesterol screening is recommended for:
    a. Children aged 3–5 years.
    b. Children aged 9–11 years and adolescents 17–21 years
    c. Adolescents 12 and older.
    d. Not necessary until they reach 21-years of age.

1. Priority nursing responsibilities after cardiac catheterization in children includes which of the following? Select all that apply.

   a. Monitoring IV fluid intake and subsequently oral fluid intake.

   b. Checking pulses below the site of catheterization.

   c. Assessing the temperature and color of the affected extremity.

   d. Checking vital signs including blood pressure every 15 minutes.

   e. Monitoring blood glucose levels in infants.

   f. Checking the dressing for bleeding.

2. A nurse has been recently hired for the pediatric cardiology clinic. It is necessary for this nurse to understand the pathophysiology and hemodynamics of congenital heart defects. Choose the most likely options for the information missing from the table below by selecting from the lists of options provided.

Defect (option 1)	Hemodynamic characteristics (option 2)	Effect on blood flow (option 3)
	Usually a right-to-left shunt, depends on size of VSD and degree of pulmonary stenosis. Includes four defects	3
Patent ductus arteriosus (PDA)	2	3
1	2	Obstructed blood flow
1	2	Mixed pulmonary blood flow

Option 1	Option 2	Option 3
Coarctation of the aorta	Valve fails to develop, no communication between right atrium and right ventricle	Increased pulmonary blood flow
Atrioventricular canal defect	No communication between the systemic and pulmonary circulations	Decreased pulmonary blood flow
Tetralogy of Fallot	Localized narrowing near the insertion of the ductus arteriosus. Increased pressure proximal to the defect and decreased pressure distal to the obstruction	Mixed pulmonary blood flow
Transposition of the great vessels (TOGV)	Continued patency of this vessel allows blood to flow from the higher-pressure aorta to the lower pressure pulmonary artery, which causes a left-to-right shunt	Obstructed blood flow

43 The Child with Hematologic and Immunologic Dysfunction

I. LEARNING KEY TERMS

MATCHING: Match each term with its corresponding definition or description.

1. _____ Nosebleed.

2. _____ The removal of blood from an individual, separation of the blood into its components, retention of one or more of these components, and reinfusion of the remainder of the blood into the individual.

3. _____ The process that stops bleeding when a blood system vessel is injured.

4. _____ Bleeding into the joints.

5. _____ A condition in which the number of red blood cells and/or hemoglobin concentration is reduced below normal; oxygen-carrying capacity of the blood is diminished; less oxygen is available to the tissues.

6. _____ A secondary disorder of coagulation which occurs as a complication of numerous pathological processes.

a. Hemostasis

b. Anemia

c. Apheresis

d. Disseminated intravascular coagulation

e. Epistaxis

f. Hemarthrosis

II. REVIEWING KEY CONCEPTS

1. A common term used in describing an abnormal CBC is shift to the left, which is usually caused by:
   a. An infection.
   b. Anemia.
   c. Hemolysis.
   d. Bleeding.

2. The common childhood anemia that occurs more frequently in toddlers between the ages of 12 and 36 months is _____.

3. At birth, the healthy full-term newborn has maternal stores of iron sufficient to last:
   a. 5–6 months.
   b. 2–3 months.
   c. 8 months.
   d. less than 1 month.

4. Which of the following information should the nurse include when teaching the mother of a 9-month-old infant about administering liquid iron preparations?
   a. Give with meals.
   b. Stop administering if constipation occurs.
   c. Adequate dosage may turn the child's stools a tarry green color.
   d. Allow preparation to be swished and spit out.

5. A child with moderate anemia requires a unit of red blood cells (RBCs). The nurse explains to the child that the transfusion is necessary for which reason?
   a. To decrease the bleeding episodes the child is having
   b. To increase her energy level
   c. To fight off infections
   d. To increase the cardiac demands on the heart

6. A school-age child with sickle-cell anemia is admitted for an acute painful episode. Which of the following interventions would be the most beneficial to provide in the child's plan of care?
   a. Hydration and pain management
   b. Oxygenation and factor VIII replacement therapy
   c. Exchange transfusion and hydration
   d. Correction of alkalosis and reduction of energy expenditure

7. Because of susceptibility to infection from functional asplenia in the child with sickle-cell anemia, which of the following vaccines are strongly recommended?
   a. Pneumococcal, Hib, varicella
   b. MMR, Hib, meningococcal
   c. DTaP, pneumococcal, Hib
   d. Pneumococcal, Hib, meningococcal

8. Which of the following would be an appropriate intervention for a child presenting with an acute case of immune thrombocytopenia?
   a. Intravenous administration of anti-D antibody
   b. Use of nonsteroidal anti-inflammatory drugs (NSAIDs)
   c. Hydroxyurea
   d. Splenectomy

9. Treatment for the child with severe aplastic anemia will most likely include:
   a. Administration of testosterone.
   b. Administration of iron-chelating agents.
   c. Irradiation.
   d. Bone marrow transplant.

10. Primary prophylaxis in hemophilia patients involves the infusion of factor VIII:
    a. Regularly at the emergency room before joint damage occurs.
    b. Regularly at home before the onset of joint damage.
    c. Whenever bleeding into a joint occurs.
    d. When bleeding begins to impair joint function.

11. A child with severe anemia requires a unit of packed red blood cells (PRBCs). The nurse explains to the child that the transfusion is necessary for which reason?
    a. Allow her parents to come visit.
    b. To fight off infections.
    c. To increase her energy level.
    d. To help her not bruise so easily.

12. An acquired hemorrhagic disorder characterized by excessive destruction of platelets and a discoloration caused by petechiae beneath the skin with normal bone marrow is _____.

13. T F Thalassemia is an inherited blood disorders characterized by deficiencies in the rate of production of specific globin chains in Hgb.

14. Transfusions are the foundation of medical management in children with thalassemia with the goal of maintaining the Hgb level above _____ g/dl.

15. In children and adolescents, HIV is most likely to be transmitted:
    a. Perinatal from the mother.
    b. Risky sexual behaviors
    c. To adolescents engaged in IV drug use.
    d. Via all of the above.

16. The American Academy of Pediatrics recommends that all children infected with HIV receive the routine childhood immunizations, but the nurse recognizes that children with HIV who are receiving intravenous immunoglobulin (IVIG) prophylaxis may not respond to the:
    a. Varicella vaccine.
    b. Poliovirus vaccine.
    c. Measles–mumps–rubella vaccine.
    d. Pneumococcal vaccine.

17. _____ _____ _____ is the most common opportunistic infection of children infected with HIV; it occurs most frequently between 3 and 6 months of age.

18. Which of the following is not a clinical manifestation of HIV in children?
    a. Oral candidiasis
    b. Chronic diarrhea
    c. Failure to thrive
    d. Frequent URIs

19. Diagnosis of severe combined immunodeficiency disease (SCID) is primarily based on:
    a. Failure to thrive.
    b. Delayed development.
    c. Feeding problems.
    d. Susceptibility to infections.

20. In Wiskott-Aldrich syndrome, the most notable effect of the disease at birth is:
    a. Bloody diarrhea.
    b. Infection.
    c. Eczema.
    d. Malignancy.

1. The nurse is providing care to the parents of a newly diagnosed infant 8-month-old with sickle-cell anemia Which of the following health teaching strategies would the nurse incorporate into the plan of care? Use an X for the health teachings listed below which are Indicated (appropriate or necessary), Contraindicated (could be harmful), or Non-Essential (makes no difference or not necessary).

Health Teaching	Indicated	Contraindicated	Non-Essential
The child needs to be taken to a physician/provider when seriously ill, not for a common cold.			
Offer genetic counseling. Sickle-cell anemia is an autosomal recessive disease, when both parents carry trait, there is 25% chance with each pregnancy child will have the disease.			
Infant needs to be well hydrated, observe for signs of dehydration (↓ number of wet diapers).			
Prophylactic penicillin			
Factor VIII will be given IV during a crisis.			
Encourage routine vaccine administration			

2. Identify the emergency measures (with rationales) that are used when a child with hemophilia starts to bleed.

44 The Child with Cancer

I. LEARNING KEY TERMS

MATCHING: Match each term with its corresponding definition or description.

1. _____ An abundance of white blood cells in the periphery which can lead to capillary obstruction, microinfarction, and organ dysfunction.

2. _____ A chemical agent which may cause cellular damage to tissues if even minute amounts of the drug infiltrate surrounding tissue.

3. _____ A condition of hyperactive coagulation which may leave the child susceptible to hemorrhage.

4. _____ Where hematopoietic cells previously stored from the patient are given back to the patient by IV infusion.

5. _____ Rapid release of intracellular contents often with possible life-threatening metabolic abnormalities.

6. _____ Can be used for curative purposes and for palliation to relieve symptoms by shrinking the size of the tumor.

7. _____ Loss of hair.

8. _____ A procedure that is done to administer intrathecal drugs.

9. _____ Where hematopoietic cells are obtained from a family member or volunteer donor.

a. Disseminated intravascular coagulation

b. Alopecia

c. Allogeneic

d. Vesicant

e. Hyperleukocytosis

f. Tumor lysis syndrome

g. Radiation

h. Autologous

i. Lumbar puncture

Match each cancer with its corresponding definition or description.

10. _____ This malignancy primarily involves the lymph nodes and usually metastasizes to non-nodal or extra lymphatic sites like the spleen.

11. _____ This is the most common extracranial solid tumor often known as the "silent tumor."

12. _____ Originate from undifferentiated mesenchymal cells in muscles, tendons, bursae, and fascia or in fibrous, connective, lymphatic, or vascular tissue.

13. _____ The most common bone tumor in adolescents and young adults.

14. _____ Immature cells that cannot functioneffectively.

15. _____ This malignancy often presents with painless swelling or a mass in the abdomen.

16. _____ Most common solid tumor in childhood.

17. _____ The second most common malignant bone tumor arising from the marrow spaces.

18. _____ Most common intraocular malignancy with 2-years-old as the average age of diagnosis.

19. _____ Risk factors include infection with EBV, inherited or acquired immunodeficiency, DNA repair syndromes (e.g., ataxia-telangiectasia), and previous cancer.

a. Leukemias

b. Rhabdomyosarcoma

c. Ewing sarcoma

d. Nephroblastoma

e. Neuroblastoma

f. Hodgkin disease

g. Non-Hodgkin disease

h. Central nervous system tumors

i. Osteosarcoma

j. Retinoblastoma

II. REVIEWING KEY CONCEPTS

1. Nursing care of the child with myelosuppression from leukemia or chemotherapeutic agents should include which therapeutic intervention?
   a. Restrict oral intake of fluids.
   b. Institute strict isolation procedures.
   c. Give immunizations appropriate for age.
   d. Good handwashing.

2. The incidence of childhood cancer is more pronounced in children between the ages of ___ and ___ and in adolescents between the ages of ___ and ___.

3. List the eight cardinal symptoms of childhood cancer.

4. A 3-year-old will be receiving his first dose of cisplatin as part of his treatment protocol. The nurse caring for this patient knows anaphylaxis is a potential complication. The nurse is aware the safe minimum time of observation for the possible development of anaphylaxis after administration would be:
   a. 30 minutes.
   b. 45 minutes.
   c. 60 minutes.
   d. 90 minutes.

5. After chemotherapy is begun for a child with acute leukemia, prophylaxis to prevent acute tumor lysis syndrome includes which therapeutic intervention?
   a. Aggressive hydration
   b. Oxygenation
   c. Use of corticosteroids
   d. Aggressive pain management

6. T F The hallmark metabolic disturbances that occur in tumor lysis syndrome include hyperuricemia, hyperkalemia, hyperphosphatemia, and hypocalcemia.

7. Space-occupying lesions located in the chest may cause _____ and lead to _____ compromise and _____ failure.

8. _____ is a common manifestation of spinal cord compression with a(n) _____ as the gold standard diagnostic test.

9. List potential issues a child with an absolute neutrophil count of <500/mm^3 may experience.

10. T F Prophylaxis treatment for *Pneumocystis* pneumonia is typically done with trimethoprim-sulfamethoxazole (Bactrim) routinely given to most children during treatment.

11. The administration of _____ is often used to possibly decrease the side effects caused by low blood counts.

12. Anemia may be a side effect of chemotherapy treatment. Children with profound anemia should:
    a. Be allowed to regulate their physical activity with adult supervision.
    b. Be restricted in their physical activity.
    c. Receive blood transfusions of packed cells until their hemoglobin reaches 12 gm/dL.
    d. Be placed on strict bed rest with no physical activity until their hemoglobin level reaches 10 gm/dL.

13. In teaching parents how to minimize or prevent bleeding episodes when the child is myelosuppressed, the nurse includes what information?
    a. Rectal temperatures are necessary to monitor for infection
    b. Platelet transfusions are given to maintain a count greater than 45,000/mm³
    c. Subcutaneous injections are preferred to intravenous ones.
    d. Meticulous mouthcare is essential to prevent mucositis

14. Children with a platelet count < _____ should avoid activities that may cause injury or bleeding such as riding a bike, skateboarding, or playing at the playground

15. What treatment has been found to be beneficial in decreasing the nausea and vomiting associated with chemotherapy for children?

16. Identify interventions for mouth care in infants and toddlers who may have developed mucosal ulcers as a side effect of chemotherapy.

17. T   F   Viscous lidocaine is an acceptable medication to use in decreasing the pain from mucosal ulcers in young children.

18. What neurologic syndrome may develop 5–8 weeks after central nervous system (CNS) radiation? How long does it typically last?

19. Identify three strategies to possibly decrease the side effect of hemorrhagic cystitis.

20. Postoperative positioning for a child who has had a medulloblastoma brain tumor (infratentorial) removed should be which?
    a. Trendelenburg.
    b. Head of bed elevated 90 degrees.
    c. Flat on operative side with pillows behind the head.
    d. Flat on either side with pillows behind the back.

21. T F The child receiving chemotherapy for cancer should receive all immunizations as scheduled, including live, attenuated vaccines.

22. Discuss the three main consequences of bone marrow infiltration.

23. Which of the following is the gold standard test for a definitive diagnosis in children with leukemia?
    a. MRI
    b. CT scan
    c. Peripheral blood smear
    d. Bone marrow aspiration

24. All children diagnosed with leukemia are at risk for _____ and therefore they receive _____.

25. Hodgkin disease is characterized by which of the following clinical manifestations?
    a. Painless enlargement of lymph nodes
    b. Firm, nontender irregular mass in the thoracic cavity
    c. Painless swelling in the abdomen
    d. A whitish glow in the pupil

26. T F The sibling of a child receiving chemotherapy for cancer can and should receive all immunizations as scheduled, including live, attenuated vaccines.

27. A 16-year-old girl presents to clinic with complaints of awakening with a headache and occasional vomiting not related to eating for the last month. What is most likely responsible for these clinical manifestations?
    a. A supratentorial tumor
    b. An infratentorial tumor
    c. A neuroblastoma
    d. A nephroblastoma

28. The nurse is providing postoperative care for a child following surgical removal of an infratentorial tumor. The nurse notes the child's pupils are now unequal and sluggish to react. Which of the following is the priority intervention at this time?
    a. Recheck the pupils in an hour.
    b. Reposition the patient to facilitate venous drainage.
    c. Notify the provider immediately.
    d. This is an expected finding after this type of surgical procedure.

29. Which vital sign is important to monitor after neurosurgery and why?

30. List nursing care involved in caring for the child who has undergone brain tumor surgery.

31. The signs and symptoms of neuroblastoma depend on the _____ and _____ _____ _____ _____.

32. Why is the prognosis of neuroblastomas so poor?

33. Describe the clinical manifestations of an abdominal neuroblastoma and a nephroblastoma (Wilms tumor).

34. Describe characteristics of phantom limb pain which may develop in children after amputation of their affected limb.

35. When does the discovery of Wilms tumor usually happen?

36. Why is it important not to palpate the abdomen in a child with a Wilms tumor?

37. A 22-month-old child presents to clinic for a well-child checkup. The mother states to the provider, "I have noticed this 'white glow' in her left eye for the last 3 months and am not sure what it is." Based on this clinical manifestation the most likely disease process would be:
    a. Glioma tumor.
    b. Retinoblastoma.
    c. Optic nerve tumor.
    d. Rhabdomyosarcoma.

III. CLINICAL JUDGMENT AND NEXT-GENERATION NCLEX® EXAMINATION-STYLE QUESTIONS

1. Which of the following are reasons to do a lumbar puncture on a child newly diagnosed with leukemia? Select all that apply.

   a. Rule out meningitis.

   b. Assess the central nervous system (CNS) for infiltration.

   c. Give intrathecal chemotherapy.

   d. Determine the presence of increased intracranial pressure.

   e. Stage the leukemia.

2. The nurse is discussing with the family and child undergoing removal of a brain tumor about the possibilities of residual disabilities that could occur postoperatively. Which of the following could be potential disabilities? Select all that apply.

   a. Ataxia

   b. Anorexia

   c. Sensory deficits

   d. Dysphagia

   e. Dysuria

   f. Intellectual deficits

The Child with Genitourinary Dysfunction

I. LEARNING KEY TERMS

MATCHING: Match each term with its corresponding description.

1. _____ Procedure of separating colloids and crystalline substances by circulating a blood filtrate outside the body and exerting hydrostatic pressure across a semipermeable membrane with simultaneous infusion of a replacement solution.

2. _____ Presence of bacteria in the urine.

3. _____ Fluid accumulation in the abdominal cavity.

4. _____ Accumulation of body fluid in the interstitial spaces and body cavities.

5. _____ Meatal opening located on dorsal surface of penis.

6. _____ A reduction in the serum albumin level.

7. _____ Inflammation of the bladder.

8. _____ Procedure in which colloids and crystalline substances are separated by using the abdominal cavity as a semipermeable membrane through which water and solute of small molecular size move by osmosis and diffusion based on concentrations on either side of the membrane.

9. _____ One of the most frequent causes of acute kidney injury clinical features of acquired hemolytic anemia, thrombocytopenia, renal injury, and CNS symptoms.

10. _____ Inflammation of the urethra.

11. _____ Procedure in which colloids and crystalline substance are separated by circulating the blood outside the body through artificial membranes, which permits a similar passage of water and solutes.

12. _____ Opening of urethral meatus on ventral surface of penis.

13. _____ Inflammation of the upper urinary tract and kidneys.

14. _____ Failure of one or both testes to descend normally through inguinal canal.

15. _____ A condition in which there is an abnormal retrograde flow of urine from the bladder into the ureters.

16. _____ Fluid in the scrotum.

17. _____ Febrile urinary tract infection coexisting with systemic signs of bacterial illness; blood culture reveals the presence of urinary pathogen.

a. Bacteriuria

b. Cystitis

c. Urethritis

d. Pyelonephritis

e. Urosepsis

f. Hypospadias

g. Vesicoureteral reflux

h. Hypoalbuminemia

i. Edema

j. Ascites

k. Hemolytic uremic syndrome

l. Epispadias

m. Hydrocele

n. Cryptorchidism

o. Hemodialysis

p. Peritoneal dialysis

q. Hemofiltration

II. REVIEWING KEY CONCEPTS

1. _____-_____ is the most influential factor influencing the occurrence of UTIs.

2. _____ male infants younger than 3 months of age have been reported to have a higher incidence of urinary tract infection than other males or females.

3. Which of the following is not a clinical manifestation of a urinary tract infection in infancy?
   a. Fever
   b. Poor feeding
   c. Frequent urination
   d. Anemia

4. For the child with nephrosis, one aim of the therapy is to reduce:
   a. Excretion of urinary protein.
   b. Excretion of fluids.
   c. Serum albumin levels.
   d. Urinary output.

5. Acute glomerulonephritis is most likely to be suspected when the child presents with the clinical manifestations of:
   a. Normal blood pressure, generalized edema, and oliguria.
   b. Edema, hematuria, and oliguria.
   c. Fatigue, elevated serum lipid levels, and elevated serum protein levels.
   d. Temperature elevation, circulatory congestion, and normal creatinine serum levels.

6. The nurse caring for the child with acute glomerulonephritis would expect to:
   a. Enforce complete bed rest.
   b. Weigh the child daily.
   c. Perform peritoneal dialysis.
   d. Ensure a diet low in protein.

7. The nurse caring for a child with minimal change nephrotic syndrome can expect to administer a _____ as the first-line drug therapy.

8. Clinical manifestations of nephrotic syndrome include:
   a. Hypercholesterolemia, hypoalbuminemia, edema, and proteinuria.
   b. Hematuria, hypertension, periorbital edema, and flank pain.
   c. Oliguria, hypocholesterolemia, and hyperalbuminemia.
   d. Hematuria, generalized edema, hypertension, and proteinuria.

9. When teaching the family of a child with nephrotic syndrome about prednisone therapy, the nurse includes the information that:
   a. Corticosteroid therapy begins after BUN and serum creatinine elevation.
   b. Prednisone is administered orally in a dosage of 4 mg/kg of body weight.
   c. Steroid therapy will occur over several weeks and restarted if a relapse occurs.
   d. The drug is discontinued as soon as the urine is free from protein.

10. Renal injury, acquired hemolytic anemia, central nervous system symptoms, and thrombocytopenia are characteristic clinical manifestations of the disorder known as:
    a. Minimal-change nephrotic syndrome.
    b. Wilms tumor.
    c. Hemolytic-uremic syndrome.
    d. Vesicoureteral reflux.

11. A febrile 8-month-old is being evaluated for a urinary tract infection (UTI). A urinalysis and urine culture have been ordered by the provider. Which of the following is the best way to obtain the urine specimen?
    a. Carefully cleanse the perineum from front to back and apply a self-adhesive urine collection bag to the child's perineum.
    b. Obtain the urine sample by using an indwelling foley catheter.
    c. Place sterile cotton balls inside the child's diaper.
    d. Obtain the urine sample by doing a bladder catheterization.

12. The primary manifestation of acute kidney injury is:
    a. Edema.
    b. Oliguria.
    c. Metabolic acidosis.
    d. Weight gain and proteinuria.

13. The most immediate threat to the life of the child with acute kidney injury is:
    a. Hyperkalemia.
    b. Anemia.
    c. Hypertensive crisis.
    d. Cardiac failure from hypovolemia.

14. A hospitalized child with minimal change nephrotic syndrome is receiving high doses of prednisone. Which of the following interventions would be appropriate to include in the plan of care for this child?
    a. To stimulate their appetite.
    b. To detect evidence of edema.
    c. To minimize risk of infection.
    d. To promote adherence to the antibiotic regimen.

15. The parent of a child hospitalized with acute glomerulonephritis asks the nurse why blood pressure readings are being taken so often. What knowledge should influence the nurse's reply?
    a. Hypotension leading to sudden shock can develop at any time.
    b. Acute hypertension is a concern that requires monitoring.
    c. The antibiotic therapy contributes to increased blood pressure values.
    d. Blood pressure fluctuations indicate that the condition has become chronic.

239

16. A 4-year-old child is admitted with acute glomerulonephritis. Which of the following would the nurse expect the urinalysis during the acute phase to show?
    a. Bacteriuria and hematuria.
    b. Hematuria and proteinuria.
    c. Hypoalbuminemia and increased specific gravity.
    d. Proteinuria and decreased specific gravity.

17. The manifestation of chronic kidney disease that is a major consequence especially in preadolescents is:
    a. Anemia.
    b. Growth restriction.
    c. Bone demineralization.
    d. Septicemia.

18. Which of the following is included in dietary regulation of the child with chronic kidney disease?
    a. Restricting protein intake below the recommended daily allowance.
    b. Dietary protein intake is limited only to the reference daily intake (Recommended Dietary Allowance [RDA]) for the child's age.
    c. Restricting potassium when creatinine clearance falls below 50 mL/min.
    d. Giving vitamin A, E, and K supplements.

19. Methods of dialysis for management of renal failure are _____, _____, and _____.

20. Which of the following major complications is associated with a child with chronic renal failure?
    a. Hypokalemia
    b. Metabolic alkalosis
    c. Water and sodium retention
    d. Excessive excretion of blood urea nitrogen

21. _____ dialysis is usually recommended for small children.

III. CLINICAL JUDGMENT AND NEXT-GENERATION NCLEX® EXAMINATION-STYLE QUESTIONS

1. Which of the following signs and symptoms are indicative of a urinary tract disorder in children under 2 years of age? Select all that apply.

    a. Vomiting

    b. Hypothermia

    c. Jaundice

    d. Pallor

    e. Poor feeding

    f. Foul-smelling urine

2. Which of the following signs and symptoms are indicative of a urinary tract disorder in children greater than 2 years of age? Select all that apply.

   a. Fatigue

   b. Enuresis, incontinence

   c. Abdominal or back pain

   d. Excessive thirst

   c. Hypotension

   f. Muscle cramps

46 The Child with Cerebral Dysfunction

I. LEARNING KEY TERMS

MATCHING: Match each term with its corresponding definition or description.

1. _____ Remaining in a deep sleep, responsive only to vigorous and repeated stimulation.

2. _____ Rigid flexion with the arms held tightly to the body; flexed elbows, wrists, and fingers; plantar flexed feet; legs extended and internally rotated; and possibly the presence of fine tremors or intense stiffness.

3. _____ Brief malfunctions of the brain's electrical system resulting from cortical neuronal discharges; most frequently observed neurologic dysfunction in children; clinical manifestations determined by the site of origin and may include unconsciousness or altered consciousness, involuntary movements, and changes in perception, behaviors, sensations, and posture.

4. _____ A sign of dysfunction at the level of the midbrain or lesions to the brainstem. It is characterized by rigid extension and pronation of the arms and legs, flexed wrists and fingers, a clenched jaw, an extended neck, and possibly an arched back.

5. _____ The most common head injury in which there is a transient disturbance of brain function often traumatically induced that involves a complex pathophysiologic process.

6. _____ Determined by observations of the child's responses to the environment; the earliest indicator of improvement or deterioration in neurologic status.

7. _____ Limited spontaneous movement, sluggish speech, falling asleep quickly.

8. _____ An imbalance in the production and absorption of the cerebral spinal fluid in the ventricular system.

9. _____ No motor or verbal response to noxious (painful) stimuli.

10. _____ An individual who is awake, alert, and oriented to time, place, and person; demonstrating behavior appropriate for age.

11. _____ Depressed cerebral function; the inability to respond to sensory stimuli and to have subjective experiences.

12. _____ Arousable with stimulation.

13. _____ Impaired decision making.

a. Full consciousness

b. Obtundation

c. Unconsciousness

d. Coma

e. Level of consciousness

f. Flexion posturing

g. Extension posturing

h. Confusion

i. Lethargy

j. Stupor

k. Seizure

l. Hydrocephalus

m. Concussion

II. REVIEWING KEY CONCEPTS

1. The nurse is assessing an unconscious child who fell from a second-floor window. The nurse notices the child suddenly has a fixed and dilated pupil. How should the nurse interpret this finding?
   a. This is expected eye damage from the fall.
   b. This is a neurosurgical emergency.
   c. Expected, recheck the pupils in 15 minutes.
   d. This indicated edema of the eye.

2. The sign which can be used to indicate increased intracranial pressure in the infant is:
   a. Projectile vomiting.
   b. Headache.
   c. Bulging fontanel.
   d. Sunken fontanel.

3. The earliest indicator of improvement or deterioration in neurologic status is:
   a. Motor activity.
   b. Level of consciousness.
   c. Reflexes.
   d. Vital signs.

4. Which of the following would be most important when caring for a child during a seizure:
   a. Intervene to halt the seizure.
   b. Restrain the child.
   c. Protect the child from injury.
   d. Place a solid object between the teeth.

5. Which of the following nursing observations would usually indicate pain in a comatose child?
   a. Increased flaccidity
   b. Increased oxygen saturation
   c. Decreased blood pressure
   d. Increased agitation

6. The activity that has been shown to increase intracranial pressure is:
   a. Using earplugs to eliminate noise.
   b. Gentle range-of-motion exercises.
   c. Suctioning.
   d. Osmotherapy and sedation.

7. Which of the following would be important to incorporate in the plan of care for a child who is experiencing a seizure?
   a. Describe and record the seizure activity observed.
   b. Suction the child during a seizure to prevent aspiration.
   c. Attempt to place a tongue blade between the teeth to prevent biting of the tongue.
   d. Attempt to restrain the child during the seizure to prevent injury.

8. Epidural hemorrhage is less common in children under 2 years of age than in adults because:
   a. The middle meningeal artery is embedded in the bone surface of the skull until approximately 2 years of age.
   b. Fractures are less likely to lacerate the middle meningeal artery in children less than 2 years of age.
   c. Separation of the dura from bleeding is more likely to occur in children than in adults.
   d. There is an increased tendency for the skull to fracture in children less than 2 years of age.

9. What finding is a clinical manifestation of increased intracranial pressure (ICP) in children?
   a. Low-pitched cry
   b. Sun setting eyes
   c. Diplopia, blurred vision
   d. Increased heart rate

10. The epidemiology of bacterial meningitis has changed in recent years because of the:
    a. Diphtheria, pertussis, and tetanus vaccine.
    b. Rubella vaccine.
    c. *Haemophilus influenzae* type B vaccine.
    d. Hepatitis B vaccine.

11. The most common mode of transmission for bacterial meningitis is:
    a. Vascular dissemination of an infection elsewhere.
    b. Direct implantation from an invasive procedure.
    c. Direct extension from an infection in the mastoid sinuses.
    d. Direct extension from an infection in the nasal sinuses.

12. _____ _____ occurs in epidemic form and is the only type readily transmitted by droplet infection from nasopharyngeal secretions; it occurs predominantly in school-age children and adolescents.

13. The nurse is caring for a 10-year-old child who has an acute head injury with increased intracranial pressure, a pediatric Glasgow Coma Scale score of 8, and is unconscious. Which of the following is the priority intervention?
    a. Elevate HOB slightly, maintain head in midline position
    b. Perform range of motion exercises every 4 hours
    c. Perform chest percussion every 4 hours
    d. Provide minimal environmental stimuli

14. Which of the following medications is considered first-line drug therapy for a child in status epilepticus?
    a. Intravenous (IV) Levetiracetam (Keppra)
    b. Intravenous (IV) Phenytoin (Dilantin)
    c. Intravenous (IV) Phenobarbital (Luminal)
    d. Intravenous (IV) Lorazepam (Ativan)

15. The nurse is planning care for a 4-year-old child admitted with bacterial meningitis. Which of the following would be the most appropriate intervention to include in the plan of care?
    a. Keep environmental stimuli to a minimum.
    b. Encourage active range of motion by the child every 2–4 hours and prn.
    c. Administer pain medication cautiously as it could dull the sensorium.
    d. Measure head circumference to assess developing complications.

16. Which of the following orders would the nurse question when caring for a 6-month-old immediate post-operative ventriculoperitoneal (VP) shunt placement?
    a. Position the child's head on the unoperated side to prevent pressure on the shunt valve.
    b. Do not pump the shunt.
    c. Elevate the head of the bed 45 degrees.
    d. Measure head circumference daily at the point of largest measurement.

17. The nurse is discussing long-term care with the parents of a child who has a ventriculoperitoneal shunt. Which of the following issues should be addressed?
    a. Most childhood activities must be restricted.
    b. Cognitive impairment is to be expected with hydrocephalus.
    c. Wearing head protection is essential until the child reaches adulthood.
    d. Shunt malfunction or infection requires immediate treatment.

18. Which of the following antiepileptic medications requires monitoring of vitamin D and folic acid?
    a. Topiramate (Topamax)
    b. Valproic acid (Depakene)
    c. Keppra (Levetiracetam)
    d. Phenobarbital (Luminal)

19. When a child has a febrile seizure, it is important for the parents to know that the child will:
    a. Probably not develop epilepsy.
    b. Most likely develop epilepsy.
    c. Most likely develop neurologic damage.
    d. Usually need tepid sponge baths to control fever.

20. A 6-year-old child is seen in the urgent care unit for a history of seizures at home. He begins to have seizures in the urgent care unit that last more than five minutes. Intravenous (IV) access has not been successful. The nurse caring for this child is knowledgeable that which medications may be given to stop the child's seizures?
    a. IM phenytoin
    b. PO Lamical
    c. Intranasal midazolam
    d. IV romazicon

21. A 3-year-old is admitted with a diagnosis of bacterial meningitis. A lumbar puncture is performed. Which of the following CSF findings would be indicative of a bacterial infection?
    a. Increased WBC, elevated protein, decreased glucose.
    b. Decreased WBC, elevated protein, decreased glucose.
    c. Decreased WBC, decreased protein, decreased glucose.
    d. Increased WBC, decreased protein, decreased glucose.

22. A 12-month-old with a history of hydrocephalus and ventriculoperitoneal shunt (VP) placement is brought to the ED by his mother who states that he refuses to eat, is afebrile but extremely fussy, and does not play with any of his toys. The diagnostic evaluation for this child will most likely include:
    a. Urinary catheterization.
    b. Upper GI series.
    c. Skull radiographs.
    d. Head CT or MRI.

III. CLINICAL JUDGMENT AND NEXT-GENERATION NCLEX® EXAMINATION-STYLE QUESTIONS

1. Which of the following would require immediate follow-up in children with a history of headaches? Select all that apply.

    a. The headache progresses in frequency and severity over a brief period.

    b. It occurs in the evening.

    c. It is accompanied by unexplained vomiting.

    d. It is worse at night.

    e. It is characterized by persistent, occipital, or frontal pain.

2. An otherwise healthy 18-month-old child is in the well-child clinic for a follow-up visit after a febrile seizure last approximately two minutes. The parents have some additional questions. Choose the most likely options for the information missing from the statements below by selecting from the list of options provided.

A febrile seizure is a seizure associated with a febrile illness in the absence of a CNS infection, infants and children must have a temperature of at least _____ option 1 _____°C and are between the ages of _____ option 2 _____ to _____ option 2 _____ months. If a febrile seizure lasts greater than _____ option 3 _____ minutes, medical attention should be sought immediately.

Options for 1	Options for 2	Options for 3
37.5 °C	2–24 months	3
38 °C	3–30 months	5
39°C	4 to 48 months	10
40°C	6 to 60 months	15

47 The Child with Endocrine Dysfunction

I. LEARNING KEY TERMS

MATCHING: Match each term with its corresponding definition or description.

1. _____ Protruding eyeballs.

2. _____ Ketone bodies in the urine.

3. _____ Insatiable thirst.

4. _____ Elevation of the blood glucose; usually caused by illness, growth, or emotional upset.

5. _____ Occurs when serum glucose level exceeds the renal threshold (180 mg/dL) and glucose "spills" into the urine.

6. _____ Low blood sugar reaction; usually caused by bursts of physical activity without additional food or delayed, omitted, or incompletely consumed meals.

7. _____ The condition produced by the presence of ketone bodies in the blood; strong acids lower serum pH.

8. _____ Excessive urination.

9. _____ Hyperventilation that is characteristic of metabolic acidosis.

10. _____ Carpal spasm elicited by pressure applied to nerves of the upper arm.

11. _____ Early maturation and development of the gonads with secretion of sex hormones, development of secondary sex characteristics, and sometimes production of mature sperm and ova.

12. _____ Carpopedal spasm, muscle twitching, cramps, seizures, and sometimes stridor; indicative of disorders of the parathyroid function.

13. _____ Excess growth hormone after epiphyseal closure; characterized by facial features such as overgrowth of the head, lips, nose, tongue, jaw, and paranasal and mastoid sinuses.

14. _____ Facial muscle spasm elicited by tapping the facial nerve in the region of the parotid gland.

a. Acromegaly

b. Central precocious puberty

c. Polyuria

d. Polydipsia

e. Exophthalmos

f. Chvostek sign

g. Trousseau sign

h. Tetany

i. Glycosuria

j. Ketonuria

k. Ketoacidosis

l. Kussmaul respirations

m. Hypoglycemia

n. Hyperglycemia

II. REVIEWING KEY CONCEPTS

1. In a child with hypopituitarism, the growth hormone levels are usually:
   a. elevated after 20 minutes of strenuous exercise.
   b. elevated 45–90 minutes after the onset of sleep.
   c. below normal after being stimulated pharmacologically.
   d. below normal at birth.

2. The best time to administer a growth hormone replacement injection is:
   a. midmorning.
   b. at the afternoon nap.
   c. at bedtime.
   d. before breakfast.

3. _____ _____ delay refers to individuals (usually boys) with delayed linear growth, generally beginning as a toddler, and skeletal and sexual maturation that is behind that of age-mates; these children usually achieve normal adult height.

4. Explain the difference between acromegaly and pituitary hyperfunction that would not be considered acromegaly.

5. Recent data suggest that precocious puberty evaluation for a pathologic cause should be performed for Caucasian females younger than _____ years of age or for African American girls younger than _____ years of age; manifestations of sexual development before the age of _____ years in boys would suggest precocious puberty.

6. Parents of the child with precocious puberty need to know that:
   a. dress and activities should be aligned with the child's sexual development.
   b. heterosexual interest will usually be advanced.
   c. the child's mental age is congruent with the chronologic age.
   d. overt manifestations of affection represent sexual advances.

7. The most common cause of thyroid disease in children and adolescents is:
   a. Hashimoto disease (lymphocytic thyroiditis).
   b. Graves disease.
   c. Goiter.
   d. Thyrotoxicosis.

8. A common cause of secondary hyperparathyroidism is:
   a. Maternal hyperparathyroidism.
   b. Chronic renal disease.
   c. Adenoma.
   d. Renal rickets.

9. Pheochromocytoma is a tumor characterized by:
   a. Secretion of insulin.
   b. Secretion of catecholamines
   c. Adrenal crisis.
   d. Myxedema.

10. The parents of a child who has Addison disease should be instructed to:
    a. Use extra hydrocortisone only for crises.
    b. Discontinue the child's cortisone if side effects develop.
    c. Decrease the cortisone dose during times of stress.
    d. Report signs of acute adrenal insufficiency to the physician.

11. Which of the following tests, which yields immediate results, is particularly useful in diagnosing congenital adrenal hyperplasia?
    a. Chromosome typing
    b. Pelvic ultrasound
    c. Pelvic X-ray
    d. Testosterone level

12. Definitive treatment for pheochromocytoma consists of:
    a. Surgical removal of the thyroid.
    b. Administration of potassium.
    c. Surgical removal of the tumor.
    d. Administration of beta blockers.

13. The primary pathologic defect in children with type 1 DM is:
    a. Insulin resistance in which the body fails to use insulin properly.
    b. Destruction of pancreatic βcells resulting in absolute insulin deficiency.

14. The pathologic defect described in the previous question is the basis for the lifelong need for _____ administration in type 1 DM.

15. A child is receiving propylthiouracil for the treatment of hyperthyroidism (Graves disease). The parents and child should be taught to recognize and report which signs or symptoms immediately?
    a. Fatigue, pallor
    b. Nausea, weight loss
    c. Fever, sore throat
    d. Upper respiratory tract infection

16. Glycosylated hemoglobin is an acceptable method to:
    a. Diagnose diabetes mellitus.
    b. Assess the control of diabetes.
    c. Assess oxygen saturation of the hemoglobin.
    d. Determine blood glucose levels most accurately.

17. What time would it be best to administer regular insulin before meals to allow sufficient time for absorption and subsequently a greater reduction in the postprandial rise in blood glucose?
    a. 15 minutes before meals
    b. 30 minutes before meals
    c. 60 minutes before meals
    d. immediately before eating.

18. Exercise for the child with diabetes mellitus:
    a. Is restricted to noncontact sports.
    b. May require a decreased intake of carbohydrate.
    c. May necessitate an increased insulin dose.
    d. May require an increased intake of carbohydrate.

19. Describe what occurs when the glucose concentration in the glomerular filtrate exceeds the renal threshold (180 mg/dl).

20. The nurse is caring for a child with type 1 diabetes. The child is currently nauseated, sweaty, and shaky. Which of the following would be the most appropriate intervention to implement for this child?
    a. Obtain a glucose reading.
    b. Check the child's temperature.
    c. Administer a dose of ondansetron.
    d. Provide the child with a cup of orange juice.

21. The nurse is discussing the various sites used for insulin injections with a newly diagnosed diabetic child and their family. Which of the following sites usually has the fastest rate of absorption?
    a. Arm
    b. Leg
    c. Buttock
    d. Abdomen

22. What is the recommended testing of urine for ketones when an illness is present or when the blood glucose level is greater than 240 mg/dl when illness is not present.
    a. Every hour
    b. Every 2 hours
    c. Every 3 hours
    d. Daily

III. CLINICAL JUDGMENT AND NEXT-GENERATION NCLEX® EXAMINATION-STYLE QUESTIONS

1. The nurse is teaching a 15-year-old adolescent about the management of type 1 DM. The management of type 1 DM for the prevention of complications is based on which of the following. Select all that apply.

    a. A daily insulin regimen.

    b. A periodic insulin regimen.

    c. Blood glucose self-monitoring.

    d. A regular exercise regimen.

    e. A balanced diet.

    f. Limited physical exercise.

2. The nurse is planning to admit an 8-year-old female child with hypoparathyroidism to the pediatric medical unit. Which of the following clinical manifestations would the nurse expect to observe in this child? Select all that apply.

a. Positive Chvostek

b. Muscle cramps

c. Emotional lability

d. Physical restlessness

e. Brittle hair

f. Short stature

48 The Child with Musculoskeletal or Articular Dysfunction

I. LEARNING KEY TERMS

MATCHING: Match each term with its corresponding definition or description.

1. _____ Produced by compression of porous bone; appears as a raised or bulging projection at the fracture site; occurs in the most porous portion of the bone; more common in young children.

2. _____ Occurs when the bone is bent but not broken; a child's flexible bone can be bent 45 degrees or more before breaking.

3. _____ Occurs when a bone is angulated beyond the limits of bending, one side bending and the other side breaking.

4. _____ Used when significant pull must be applied, often applied directly to skeletal structure by a pin or wires.

5. _____ Fractures in which small fragments of bone break off from the fractured shaft and lie in the surrounding tissue.

6. _____ A fracture in which bone fragments cause damage to other organs or tissues such as the lung or liver.

7. _____ Fracture that divides the bone fragments.

8. _____ Applied directly to skin surface and indirectly to skeletal structures.

9. _____ Fracture with an open wound through which the bone is protruding or has protruded.

10. _____ Applied to the body part by the hands placed distal to the fracture site.

11. _____ Helps bones realign and fuse properly.

12. _____ Black and blue discoloration; the escape of blood into the tissues.

13. _____ A fracture that does not produce a break in the skin.

14. _____ When fragments of the bone remain attached.

15. _____ This fracture occurs as slanting but straight between a horizontal and a perpendicular direction.

16. _____ This fracture is slanting and circular, with twisting around the bone shaft.

17. _____ This fracture occurs crosswise at right angles to the long axis of the bone.

18. _____ The process of separating opposing bone to encourage regeneration of new bone in the created space.

19. _____ Partial dislocation.

a. Ecchymosis

b. Simple or closed fracture

c. Compound or open fracture

d. Complicated fracture

e. Comminuted fracture

f. Plastic deformation

g. Buckle or torus fracture

h. Greenstick fracture

i. Complete fracture

j. Traction

k. Manual traction

l. Skin traction

m. Skeletal traction

n. Distraction

o. Incomplete fracture

p. Transverse fracture

q. Oblique fracture

r. Spiral fracture

s. Subluxation

II. REVIEWING KEY CONCEPTS

1. An appropriate nursing intervention for the care of a child with an extremity in a new hip spica plaster cast is:
   a. Keeping the cast covered with a sheet.
   b. Using the fingertips when handling the cast to prevent pressure areas.
   c. Using heated fans or dryers to circulate air and speed the cast-drying process.
   d. Expose the plaster cast to air until dry.

2. Bone healing is characteristically more rapid in children because:
   a. Children have less constant muscle contraction associated with the fracture.
   b. Children's fractures are less severe than adults'.
   c. Children have an active growth plate that helps speed repair with deformity less likely to occur.
   d. Children have thickened periosteum and more generous blood supply.

3. When caring for a 7-year-old child with a suspected fracture which of the following would be an appropriate intervention to implement?
   a. Apply heat to the injured area.
   b. Elevate the injured limb if possible.
   c. Palpate the affected limb.
   d. Immobilize the limb including the joint below the fracture site.

MATCHING: Match each type of traction with its corresponding description.

4. _____ A type of running traction in which the pull is only in one direction; skin traction is applied to the legs, which are flexed at a 90-degree angle at the hips. The child's trunk (with the buttocks raised slightly off the bed) provides counter traction.

5. _____ Uses a system of wires, rings, and telescoping rods that permits limb lengthening to occur.

6. _____ Device is spring loaded, so making burr holes and shaving hair are not required; used for cervical traction.

7. _____ Uses skin traction on the lower leg and a padded sling under the knee.

8. _____ A type of skin traction with the leg in an extended position; used primarily for short-term immobilization.

9. _____ Skeletal traction in which the lower leg is supported by a boot cast or a calf sling.

10. _____ Used with or without skin or skeletal traction; suspends the leg in a flexed position to relax the hip and hamstring muscles.

11. _____ Consists of a steel halo attached to the head by four screws inserted into the outer skull; several rigid bars connect the halo to a vest that is worn around the chest, thus providing greater mobility of the rest of the body while avoiding cervical spinal motion altogether.

12. _____ May be accomplished with the use of a halo brace or halo vest.

a. Gardner-Wells tongs
b. Buck extension
c. Russell traction
d. 90-degree–90-degree traction
e. Balanced suspension traction
f. Halo vest or brace
g. Cervical traction
h. Bryant traction
i. Ilizarov external fixator (IEF)

13. The nurse is caring for a 12-year-old who is immobilized because of a broken femur. Which of the following is a major musculoskeletal consequence of immobilization the nurse should be aware of?
    a. Increased joint mobility will occur.
    b. Will see an increase in muscle size and strength.
    c. Circulatory stasis may develop.
    d. Muscle hypertrophy can occur.

14. Which of the following is the most common dislocation seen in children?
    a. Elbow dislocation
    b. Knee dislocation
    c. Shoulder dislocation
    d. Phalanges dislocation

15. Stress fractures occur most commonly in the _____ _____, particularly the _____ and are more common in those who participate in _____ and _____.

16. The nurse is teaching the parents of a 1-month-old infant with developmental dysplasia of the hip (DDH) about preventing skin breakdown under the Pavlik harness. Which statement by the parent would indicate a correct understanding of the teaching?
    a. "I will apply a lotion for sensitive skin under the straps after my baby has been given a bath to prevent skin irritation."
    b. "I should gently massage the skin under the straps once or twice a day to stimulate circulation."
    c. "I should remove the harness a few times throughout the day and provide passive ROM to all extremities."
    d. "I will place a diaper over the harness for added hip support."

17. What is the most common management of the newborn with hip dysplasia?
    a. Hip spica cast
    b. Pavlik harness
    c. Buck extension traction
    d. Denise-Brown splint

18. Which of the following statements by the parents indicates a need for further teaching with regard to the treatment of congenital clubfoot?
    a. "We'll expose the cast to air to help it dry."
    b. "We'll watch for any swelling of the foot while the cast is on."
    c. "We're happy this is the only cast our baby will need."
    d. "Our baby may need surgery of their foot too."

19. The nurse has been teaching the parents of a child diagnosed with osteogenesis imperfecta (OI) about the use of bisphosphonates for this condition. What statement by the parents indicate a need for further education?
    a. "This medication will help to increase bone mineral density."

    b. "My child's risk for fractures will hopefully be decreased as by taking this medication."
    c. "This drug is commonly used to treat osteogenesis imperfecta."
    d. "This medication will cure my child of this disorder."

20. The nurse is teaching general infant care to parents of an infant diagnosed with osteogenesis imperfecta (OI). Which of the following would be most important to include in the teaching session?
    a. "Vitamin D therapy is beneficial for OI."
    b. "Physical therapy should be avoided as it may cause damage to bones."
    c. "Lift the infant by the buttocks, not the ankles, when changing diapers."
    d. "Braces have not been found to be helpful with ambulation."

21. The nurse is caring for a child with newly applied cast and is assessing for compartment syndrome. Which of the following is considered a late sign of ischemia?
    a. Pallor
    b. Paresthesia
    c. Pain
    d. Petaling

22. The nurse is caring for a 7-year-old with a possible diagnosis of Legg-Calvé-Perthes disease. Which of the following would be an appropriate intervention when planning care for this child?
    a. Strict bed rest and no activities.
    b. Prepare the child for surgical intervention most likely within the first 24 hours of admission.
    c. Promoting hemodynamic stabilization.
    d. Use of physical therapy or range-of-motion exercises to help restore hip motion.

23. A lateral inward curve of the cervical or lumbar curvature is termed _____. An abnormally increased convex angulation in the curvature of the thoracic spine is termed _____.

24. Diagnostic evaluation is important for early recognition of scoliosis. Which of the following is the correct procedure to exam a child for scoliosis.
    a. Standing and walking fully clothed to look for uneven hanging of clothing.
    b. From the front to evaluate bone maturity.
    c. From the left and right side while the child is completely undressed.
    d. From behind while the child is bending forward and is wearing shorts or undergarments.

25. Nursing implementation directed toward nonsurgical management in an adolescent with scoliosis primarily includes:
    a. Promoting self-esteem and positive body image.
    b. Promoting immobilization of the legs.
    c. Promoting adequate nutrition.
    d. Preventing infection.

26. A preadolescent has been diagnosed with scoliosis. The planned therapy is to use a thoracolumbosacral orthotic (TSLO brace). The patient asks how long they will have to wear the brace. The nurse's best response is:
    a. Typically between 6 and 12 months.
    b. Until your growth is complete.
    c. Up until the spinal fusion surgery occurs.
    d. The length of time will be reassessed at age 25.

27. A student athlete was injured during a soccer game. The school nurse observes significant swelling. The player states he thought he "heard a pop," and the pain is "pretty bad," and "my ankle feels like it is coming apart." Based on this description, the school nurse suspects what injury?
    a. Sprain
    b. Strain
    c. Dislocation
    d. Fracture

28. Slipped capital femoral epiphysis is suspected when clinical signs of a _____ or ____ ____ ____ ____ or _____ are reported by the preadolescent or adolescent.

29. A 17-year-old female patient is returning to the pediatric intensive care unit after Luque instrumentation (rods) were placed for scoliosis repair. In addition to the usual immediate postoperative care, what additional intervention will be needed?
    a. Active range of motion to all extremities to decrease risk of neurological injury.
    b. Two-person assist to the bathroom.
    c. Logrolling for position changes.
    d. Elevating the head of the bed to 30–45 degrees to assist with lung deflation.

30. Which of the following nursing interventions is most appropriate when caring for the child with osteomyelitis during the acute phase?
    a. Move and turn the child carefully and gently to minimize discomfort.
    b. Administer po antibiotics with meals.
    c. Implement droplet precautions in children with osteomyelitis.
    d. Provide active range of motion exercises for the affected extremity.

31. A nurse is providing care to an adolescent client diagnosed with a fractured humerus and long arm cast in place. The nurse has completed their assessment. Which assessment finding requires the nurse to contact the health care provider?
    a. Pain rating of 3 out of 10.
    b. Mild itching under the cast.
    c. Capillary refill less than 2 seconds.
    d. Shiny digits.

32. The goal that is most appropriate for the child with juvenile arthritis is for the child to be able to exhibit signs of:
    a. Adequate joint motion and function.
    b. Improved skin integrity.
    c. Weight loss and improved nutritional status.
    d. Adequate respiratory function.

33. A 3-year-old child is admitted to the hospital with osteomyelitis of the right femur. The nurse would expect to start an IV and begin empiric antibiotic therapy after blood is drawn for which lab test?
    a. Hemoglobin and hematocrit
    b. White blood cell count
    c. Culture
    d. C-reactive protein (CRP)

34. A child with juvenile idiopathic arthritis (JIA) has been started on a nonsteroidal anti-inflammatory drug (NSAID). Which of the following nursing considerations should be included in parental education?
    a. Take an apical heart rate before giving the medication.
    b. Administering the medication between meals.
    c. Expect the joint inflammation to be gone in 3–4 days.
    d. Monitor for abdominal discomfort and bloody stools.

1. The nurse is creating a plan of care for a child with a leg cast secondary to a tibia fracture. Which of the following interventions would be appropriate to decrease the risk for ineffective peripheral tissue perfusion related to pressure from cast? Select all that apply.

   a. Assess foot and toes every 4 hours and as necessary for skin temperature and presence of pedal pulses.

   b. Keep leg elevated by a pillow day 1 or as directed by the healthcare provider.

   c. Remind the parents not to allow the child to put anything in the cast.

   d. Assess capillary refill of toes every 4 hours and as necessary.

   e. Educate the child's parents on use of good body mechanics when repositioning the child.

   f. Observe the affected extremity (fingers or toes) for any edema or discoloration every 4 hours and as necessary.

2. The nurse is providing care to a 14-year-old female following a posterior spinal fusion procedure for scoliosis. The instrumentation that is placed along with the spinal fusion procedure itself will result in vigorous pain management for the adolescent during the post-operative period.
   Additionally, what other potential post-operative complications should the nurse be assessing for?
   Choose the most likely options for the information missing from the statements below by selecting from the lists of options provided.
   The nurse is aware the adolescent usually has considerable pain for the first few days after surgery and requires frequent administration of pain medication, preferably _____ option 1 _____ to assist with pain control.
   To prevent damage to the fusion and instrumentation, the adolescent should be _____ option 2 _____ for position changes. The adolescent's _____ option 3 _____ requires special attention and should be evaluated frequently during the post-operative period.

Options for 1	Options for 2	Options for 3
IV NSAIDs (Toradol)	Placed in reverse Trendelenburg position	Pulmonary status
IV opioids (Morphine)	Log rolled	Neurologic status
IV benzodiazepines (Versed)	Ambulating later the first post-operative day	Urine output status

49 The Child with Neuromuscular or Muscular Dysfunction

I. LEARNING KEY TERMS

MATCHING: Match each term with its corresponding definition or description.

1. _____ A visible defect with an external saclike protrusion that contains meninges, spinal fluid, and nerves.

2. _____ Characterized by wide-based gait; rapid repetitive movements, performed poorly; disintegration of movements of the upper extremities when the child reaches for objects.

3. _____ Visible defect with an external saclike protrusion that encases meninges and spinal fluid but no neural elements.

4. _____ Combination of spastic cerebral palsy and dyskinetic cerebral palsy.

5. _____ Type of dyskinetic cerebral palsy characterized by abnormal involuntary movement such as slow, wormlike, writhing movements that usually involve the extremities, trunk, neck, facial muscles, and tongue.

6. _____ Characterized by persistent primitive reflexes, positive Babinski reflex, ankle clonus, exaggerated stretch reflexes, eventual development of contractures.

7. _____ The most common defect of the central nervous system (CNS).

a. Spastic cerebral palsy

b. Athetoid

c. Ataxic

d. Mixed-type cerebral palsy

e. Spina bifida

f. Meningocele

g. Myelomeningocele

II. REVIEWING KEY CONCEPTS

1. The etiology of cerebral palsy (CP) is most commonly related to:
   a. Existing prenatal brain abnormalities.
   b. Maternal obesity.
   c. Post term birth.
   d. Maternal substance abuse.

2. _____ is a congenital malformation in which both cerebral hemispheres are absent.

3. A child is suspected of having CP because they have clinical manifestations of wide-based gait and rapid repetitive movements of the upper extremities when they reach for an object. Based on this information, the clinical classification of CP for this child is most likely:
   a. Dyskinetic (nonspastic).
   b. Ataxic (nonspastic).
   c. Mixed-type (spastic and dyskinesia).
   d. Spastic (pyramidal).

4. Which of the following is the neurosurgical and pharmacologic approach to managing the spasticity associated with CP with intent to improve comfort without as many side effects.
   a. Dantrolene orally.
   b. Botulin A injections.
   c. Valium orally.
   d. Baclofen intrathecally.

5. While performing a physical examination on a 6-month-old infant, the nurse suspects possible CP, because the infant:
   a. Is able to hold on to the nurse's hands while being pulled to a sitting position.
   b. Has no Moro reflex.
   c. Has no tonic neck reflex.
   d. Has an obligatory tonic neck reflex.

6. The goal of therapeutic management for the child with CP is:
   a. Assisting with motor control of voluntary muscle.
   b. Maximizing the capabilities of the child.
   c. Delaying the development of sensory deprivation.
   d. Surgical correction of deformities.

7. The nurse is caring for an infant with a myelomeningocele. The parents ask the nurse why the baby's head is being measured every day. Which of the following would be the best response by the nurse?
   a. We measure all babies' heads to make sure they are growing appropriately.
   b. Babies with myelomeningocele are at risk for hydrocephalus which presents with an increased head circumference.
   c. Many infants with myelomeningocele are at risk for microcephaly which presents with a decreased head circumference.
   d. Because the baby has a hole in her spinal column, she is at risk for meningitis which presents with an increase head circumference.

8. In order to prevent bladder dysfunction in older children with spina bifida, the child and parents are taught:
   a. Clean intermittent catheterization.
   b. Foley catheter care.
   c. Oral fluid challenge.
   d. Bladder irrigations.

9. Which of the following is the most frequent anomaly associated with a meningomyelocele?
   a. Hydrocephalus.
   b. Neurogenic bladder.
   c. Persistence of primitive infantile reflexes.
   d. Sensory impairment.

10. Children with spina bifida are at high risk for the development of _____ _____ and should be screened before any surgical procedure for _____ _____.

11. The nurse is caring for a 1-day-old female infant born with a myelomeningocele. Which of the following interventions would be most appropriate for the infant at this time?
    a. Take vital signs hourly.
    b. Place the infant in the prone position to minimize tension on the sac.
    c. Watch for signs indicating the development of hydrocephalus.
    d. Apply a heat lamp to facilitate drying of the sac.

12. A nurse is caring for an infant with spinal muscle atrophy (SMA) type 1. What will the nurse most likely note when assessing the child?
    a. Spastic upper and lower extremities.
    b. Diaphragmatic breathing with sternal retractions.
    c. Enlarged head (hydrocephalus).
    d. Lusty cry.

13. The nurse is teaching the family members of a child newly diagnosed with muscular dystrophy about signs of the disease process. Which of the following is a characteristic sign of Duchenne Muscular Dystrophy?
    a. Low-grade fevers and increasing fatigue.
    b. Difficulty climbing steps.
    c. Increased muscle strength.
    d. Recurrent respiratory infections.

14. Because Duchenne muscular dystrophy is inherited as an X-linked recessive trait, it is important for the parents of an affected child to:
    a. Seek psychological counseling.
    b. Screen all female offspring for the condition.
    c. Receive genetic counseling.
    d. Undergo voluntary sterilization.

15. A priority nursing consideration for the child in the acute phase of Guillain-Barré syndrome is:
    a. Careful observation for difficulty in swallowing and respiratory involvement.
    b. Prevention of contractures.
    c. Prevention of bowel and bladder complications.
    d. Prevention of sensory impairment.

16. A 16-year-old has arrived in the emergency department with a spinal cord injury from a diving accident. The nurse should be alert to signs of autonomic dysreflexia. Which of the following is a clinical manifestation of this disorder?
    a. Decrease in systemic blood pressure.
    b. Tachycardia.
    c. Piloerection.
    d. Abdominal discomfort.

17. An adolescent whose leg was crushed when they fell off a horse is admitted to the emergency department. The adolescent is up to date on all immunizations, receiving the last tetanus toxoid booster 8 years ago. Which of the following is necessary for therapeutic management of this adolescent to prevent tetanus?
    a. Tetanus toxoid booster is needed because of the type of injury.
    b. Human tetanus immunoglobulin is indicated for immediate prophylaxis.
    c. Concurrent administration of both tetanus immunoglobulin and tetanus antitoxin is needed.
    d. No additional tetanus prophylaxis is indicated. The tetanus toxoid booster is protective for 10 years.

18. Infant botulism usually presents with symptoms of:
    a. Diarrhea and vomiting.
    b. Constipation and generalized weakness.
    c. High fever and seizure activity.
    d. Failure to thrive.

19. It is recommended that infants of what age should not receive honey due to the presence of spores in honey?
    a. Infants older than 12 months of age.
    b. Infants older than 24 months of age.
    c. Infants younger than 12 months of age.
    d. Infants younger than 18 months of age.

III. CLINICAL JUDGMENT AND NEXT-GENERATION NCLEX® EXAMINATION-STYLE QUESTIONS

1. An infant had surgical correction of small myelomeningocele and is 5 days postop. The nurse includes which of the following in the discharge plan for the parents. Select all that apply.

   a. Monitor the operative site for redness or leaking.

   b. Breastfeed or feed the infant a commercial formula as tolerated.

   c. Perform passive range of motion when appropriate.

   d. Place the newborn prone to sleep or side-lying if permitted by provider.

   e. Pick up or hold the newborn as little as possible.

2. A 12-year-old male has been diagnosed with Guillain–Barré syndrome and it is progressing in a classic manner. Place the following sequence of events in the order they typically occur.

Clinical Manifestation	Order in which they occur (earliest to latest)
A. The child is having difficulty producing facial expressions.	
B. The child states that it is difficult to move their legs.	
C. The child reports numbness and tingling in his toes.	
D. The child states that it is difficult to move their arms.	

Chapter **49** **The Child with Neuromuscular or Muscular Dysfunction**

50 The Child with Integumentary Dysfunction

I. LEARNING KEY TERMS

MATCHING: Match each term with its corresponding definition or description.

1. _____ An inflammatory reaction of the skin that evokes a hypersensitivity response or direct irritation.

2. _____ Commonly known as a pimple.

3. _____ Inflammation of skin and subcutaneous tissues with intense redness, swelling, and firm infiltration.

4. _____ Epidermis becomes wrinkled (in days or less), and large bullae appear. _____.

5. _____ Begins as a reddish macule that becomes vesicular, forms heavy honey-colored crusts.

6. _____ Well-circumscribed, gray, or brown, elevated, firm papules with a roughened, finely papillomatous texture, warts.

7. _____ A plant oil which is very potent.

8. _____ More extensive lesion with widespread inflammation and "pointing" at several follicular orifices.

9. _____ Larger lesion with more redness and swelling, also known as a boil.

10. _____ Usually a bacterial infection, organisms such as staph and strep.

11. _____ Formation of ice crystals in tissues caused by excessive heat loss.

12. _____ Redness and swelling of extremities, usually hands when exposed to intermittent temperatures, characterized by intense vasodilation.

13. _____ Hypersensitivity reaction, usually a result of an allergic response to drugs or infection, often see the development of wheals.

14. _____ Cause is unknown; often associated with ingestion of some drugs; develop an erythematous papular rash.

15. _____ Often see round, thick, dry, reddish patches covered with coarse, silvery scales over trunk and extremities.

16. _____ An inherited disorder with characteristic café-au-lait spots.

a. Pyoderma

b. Impetigo

c. Furuncle

d. Verruca

e. Cellulitis

f. Contact dermatitis

g. Scalded skin syndrome

h. Carbuncle

i. Urushiol

j. Folliculitis

k. Chilblain

l. Frostbite

m. Neurofibromatosis

n. Erythema multiforme (Stevens–Johnson Syndrome)

o. Psoriasis

p. Urticaria

II. REVIEWING KEY CONCEPTS

1. Which of the following is the most important function related to the prevention of cross contamination of bacterial skin infections from one patient to another patient?
   a. Antibiotic therapy.
   b. Hand hygiene.
   c. Donning protective eyewear.
   d. Appropriate isolation protocol for the patient.

2. Of the following interventions which would be most appropriate for a child diagnosed with a MRSA infection?
   a. Seal non-washable items in plastic bags for 14 days if unable to dry clean or vacuum.
   b. Treat children and infants older than 2 months of age with permethrin 5% cream.
   c. Application of mupirocin to the nares of patients and families twice daily for 5–10 days to prevent reinfection.
   d. Wearing of a protective cap at night to decrease transmission of the organism.

3. T F Fungal infections can be acquired by animal-to-human transmission; thus, all household pets should be examined for this disorder.

4. T F The major goal in the treatment of cellulitis is to prevent further exposure of the skin to the offending substance.

5. T F When it is known a child has touched a plant with urushiol, the area is immediately flushed as soon as possible with warm running water to neutralize the urushiol not yet bonded to the skin.

6. Of the following medication administration routes, which route is most likely to cause an allergic drug reaction?
   a. Intravenous route
   b. Oral route
   c. Topical route
   d. Intramuscular route

7. A child has just been stung by a bee at recess on the school playground. The child is not allergic to bee stings. Which of the following would be an appropriate intervention for this child to relieve the discomfort from the sting?
   a. Warm compress
   b. Antibiotic cream
   c. Cool compress
   d. Corticosteroid cream

8. Parents of a 10-year-old male call the pediatric clinic as their son is on a camping trip and was apparently bitten by a black widow spider inside the cabin. What action would be most appropriate for the nurse to provide these parents?
   a. Apply a cool compress after running the extremity under cool water.
   b. Carefully scrape off the stinger.
   c. Apply a thin layer of corticosteroid cream and administer an antihistamine (Benadryl).
   d. Have the child to taken to the nearest emergency department.

9. T F Lice can jump and fly.

10. Treatment for Lyme disease depends on the age of the child. For children less than 8 years of age, _____ is prescribed, for children greater than 8 years of age _____ is prescribed. Regardless of age, treatment usually lasts _____ to _____ days to assist in decreasing second stage clinical manifestations.

11. In teaching parents about tick removal, which of the following points would be most important to emphasize?
    a. Apply petroleum jelly to assist with the tick withdrawal.
    b. Apply clear nail polish to smother the tick to make withdrawal easier.
    c. Spray a product containing DEET on the tick as this will enable the removal of the tick.
    d. Use tweezers to remove the tick by pulling it straight out.

12. An infant is being evaluated in clinic for diaper dermatitis. The parent states they are changing the diaper frequently to keep the infant dry, but it does not seem to be helping. Which of the following interventions would be most appropriate to suggest to this parent?
    a. Remove the waste material from the infant's buttocks and reapply the skin barrier cream.
    b. Apply talcum powder after applying the skin barrier cream.
    c. Be certain to cleanse the area thoroughly after each void or stool with commercial wipes.
    d. Use a hair dry on the "cool" setting to assist in drying the buttocks and then reapply the skin barrier cream.

13. Seborrheic dermatitis is a chronic, recurrent, inflammatory reaction of the skin and occurs most commonly where?
    a. The eyelids (blepharitis).
    b. The scalp (cradle cap).
    c. The external ear canal (otitis externa).
    d. The nasolabial folds.

14. The clinic nurse completed health teaching to a 14-year-old patient being treated for acne vulgaris. Which statement indicates understanding of the teaching points?
    a. "I will clean my face daily with a facial scrub pad."
    b. "I will squeeze the whitehead to keep the pores open."
    c. "I will use a gentle cleanser once maybe twice daily."
    d. "I will use an antibacterial soap to cleanse my face daily."

15. T F Ultraviolent A waves are shorter and responsible for tanning, burning, and most of the harmful effects attributed to sunlight, especially skin cancer whereas ultraviolet B waves are longer and cause minimum burning, but play a considerable role in photosensitive and photoallergic reactions.

16. Which of the following statements is appropriate preventative health teaching for parents regarding application of sunscreen during infancy?
    a. Sunscreen does not need to be applied until the infant turns 1-year-of-age.
    b. Sunscreen should be applied liberally before going outside into the sun for an extended period of time.
    c. Sunscreen is not recommended in infants under 6 month-of-age.
    d. Dress the infant in clothing with a tight weave such as polyester fabric to offer good protection from the sun.

17. T F Fires and burns are the 3rd unintentional injury resulting in death in children 5 to 9-years-of-age.

18. This phase of burn care management which extends from the completion of adequate resuscitation through burn coverage is known as?
    a. The acute phase.
    b. The subacute phase.
    c. The management phase.
    d. The rehabilitative phase.

19. A child with major leg burns from a firepit is being assessed after the burning process was stopped. Which of the following would be the most appropriate intervention for this child?
    a. Remove the burned clothing to prevent further damage from smoldering fabric.
    b. Cover the burned area(s) with a wet clean gauze to eliminate air contact and contamination.
    c. Use of neutralizing agents on the skin of a chemical burn to decrease further injury.
    d. Applying cool water over the burned area for at least 15–20 minutes before transporting.

20. Which of the following diets would be most appropriate and encouraged for a 12-year-old with 14%TBSA of their body burned?
    a. High protein, high fat.
    b. High fat, high caloric.
    c. High protein, high caloric.
    d. No special diet is needed.

21. Infection during the acute phase of burn management is a concern in a 7-year-old who experienced a severe scalding burn. Which of the following indicate symptoms of sepsis in this child?
    a. Hypothermia progressing to hyperthermia.
    b. Tachycardia and tachypnea.
    c. An increasing red blood cell count.
    d. Hyperactive bowel sounds.

22. When is the optimal time to administer pain medication in a child needing cleansing and debriding of their burns?
    a. Administered immediately before the procedure.
    b. When the patient asks for the pain medication.
    c. Administered so the peak effect of the drug coincides with the procedure.
    d. Administered immediately before and after the procedure.

III. FILL IN THE BLANK—Use the appropriate burn terms to complete the following sentences.

1. _____ involve the epidermis and varying degrees of the dermal layer. These wounds are painful, moist, red, and blistered.

2. _____ exclude any burn involving the face, hands, feet, perineum, or crossing joints.

3. _____ are full thickness burns that involve underlying structures such as muscle, fascia, and bone.

4. The severity of the burn injury is assessed based on the percentage of _____.

5. In _____ the injury involves the epidermal layer only. There is often a latent period followed by erythema.

6. _____ are serious injuries that involve the entire epidermis and dermis and extend into subcutaneous tissue in which nerve endings, sweat glands, and hair follicles are destroyed.

7. _____ are extensive in nature and involve >20% of the child's TBSA.

8. _____ is particularly useful as a temporary skin covering of surgically excised deep partial- and full-thickness burns and extensive burns.

9. This type of graft is used in areas where cosmetic results are most visible and known as a _____.

10. _____ are available for the management of partial-thickness burns.

11. This type of skin graft is particularly effective in children with partial-thickness scald burns of the hands and face because they allow relatively pain-free movement, which can reduce contracture formation and is known as a _____.

12. _____ are effective in early wound closure and this technique offering an improved rate of survival in patients with extensive burns.

IV. CLINICAL JUDGMENT AND NEXT-GENERATION NCLEX® EXAMINATION-STYLE QUESTIONS

1. The nurse is providing health teaching to the parents of a 10-month-old infant just diagnosed with atopic dermatitis (eczema). Which of the following would be appropriate health teaching goals to include in the plan of care for this infant?

   Use an X for the health teaching to the parents who are concerned about this disease process listed below that is Indicated (appropriate or necessary), Contraindicated (could be harmful), or Non-Essential (makes no difference or not necessary) regarding goals in effectively managing atopic dermatitis.

Health Teaching	Indicated	Contraindicated	Non-Essential
The infant's skin should be thoroughly dried before applying an acceptable emollient preparation			
Fingernails and toenails are cut short, kept clean, and filed frequently to prevent sharp edges			
An anti-seborrheic shampoo containing sulfur and salicylic acid may be used			
Skinfolds and diaper areas need frequent cleansing with plain water			
Colloid baths and cool wet compresses can be uses as they are soothing to the skin and provide antiseptic protection			
Occasional flare-ups may require the use of topical steroids to diminish inflammation			
Bathing may need to be done four to five times per day to prevent skin drying depending on the child's status			
Nonsedating antihistamines such as loratadine (Claritin) or fexofenadine (Allegra) may be prescribed for daytime pruritus relief. As pruritus increases at night, a mildly sedating antihistamine may be prescribed by the provider			

2. The nurse is caring for a 16-year-old female who experienced an allergic reaction to Levetiracetam (Keppra) for a seizure disorder and now presents with probable erythema multiforme (Stevens–Johnson syndrome). What clinical manifestations does the nurse expect to assess in this adolescent? Select all that apply.

    a. Café-au-lait spots.

    b. Erythematous papular rash.

    c. Silvery scales over trunk and extremities.

    d. Red, inflamed, moist, partially denuded, marginated areas.

    e. Lesions usually absent in the scalp region.

    f. Lesions may extend to mucous membranes, especially oral, ocular, and urethral areas.

    g. Wheals that spread irregularly and fade within a few hours.

3. There has been an outbreak of pediculus capitis (head lice) in the local elementary school. A parent's child calls the outpatient pediatric clinic for guidance as their child was sent home with an active case of head lice. Which of the following would be most appropriate for the therapeutic treatment of lice? Select all that apply.

    a. There will need to be manual removal of the nits with a metal nit comb daily.

    b. The house will need sprayed with an insecticide treatment which will be prescribed by the provider.

    c. Permethrin 1% cream rinse (Nix) is the drug of choice followed by a second treatment in 7–10 days.

    d. It will be necessary to machine wash all washable clothing, towels, and bed linens in water greater than 130 °F and dry them in a hot dryer for at least 20 minutes.

    e. Malathion is the recommended drug of choice followed by a second treatment 14–21 days after the initial treatment.

    f. Seal non-washable items in plastic bags for 14 days if unable to dry clean or vacuum.

    g. It is imperative to soak all combs, brushes, and hair accessories in lice-killing products for 1 hour or in boiling water for 10 minutes.

Answer Key

CHAPTER 1

I. Learning Key Terms

1. c 2. g 3. d 4. i 5. f
6. a 7. j 8. b 9. e 10. h

1. Maternity nursing
2. *Healthy People 2020*
3. Sustainable Development Goals
4. Integrative health care
5. Telehealth
6. 60
7. Health literacy
8. Social determinants of health
9. Standards of practice
10. "Do Not Use" list
11. Sentinel event
12. Failure to rescue
13. Standard of care
14. Interprofessional education
15. TeamSTEPPS

II. Reviewing Key Concepts

1. See Maternal Mortality section that identifies many physical and psychosocial factors; consider access to care, reproductive services for adolescents, the incidence of STIs, obesity.
2. See Ethical Issues in Perinatal Nursing and Women's Health Care section that identifies the impact of technology on fertility and pregnancy.
3. a, c; Conventional Western modalities are included, patient autonomy and decision making is encouraged, and the whole patient and not just the disease process is the primary consideration.
4. c; Although the other options are important, the inability to pay, which relates to inadequate or no health care insurance, is the most significant barrier.
5. c
6. d; Obesity is associated with an increased risk for hypertension and diabetes.

III. Clinical Judgment and Next-Generation NCLEX® Examination-style Questions

1. c, e, f, g, h; Social determinants of health play a significant role in maternal and infant outcomes, women during childbearing cycles should have their health across the lifespan considered as part of a "reproductive life plan," income disparities increase morbidity and mortality and should be part of a holistic assessment.
2. Answer should reflect factors associated with IMR, such as the high cost of care management for high-risk pregnancies and compromised infants as compared with the cost and effectiveness of early, ongoing, comprehensive prenatal care.
3. See Social Media section; explain how you could use social media to improve the health care you provide to pregnant women and their families. Identify the precautions you would take to ensure privacy and confidentiality.
4. See Limited Access to Care section; address solutions to the identified barriers—be creative and innovative.
5. See Community-Based Care, Efforts to Reduce Health Disparities, and High-Technology Care sections. You should include information pertaining to monitoring of high risk patients, cost containment, and reduction of disparities in your answer.
6. See Health Literacy section; include therapeutic communication techniques, culturally sensitive approaches, and preparation of bilingual written materials in answer.
7. See Reducing Medical Errors section and access the Patient Fact Sheet identified when formulating your answer.
8. See International Concerns section; discuss both female genital mutilation and human trafficking, consider exploring these issues in greater depth, and investigate media reports regarding these issues.

CHAPTER 2

I. Learning Key Terms

1. b 2. e 3. d 4. c 5. f 6. g
7. a 8. b 9. d 10. c 11. a

12. Culture
13. Cultural relativism
14. Acculturation
15. Assimilation
16. Ethnocentrism
17. Cultural competence
18. Future oriented
19. Past oriented
20. Present oriented
21. Personal space
22. Family
23. Nuclear
24. Extended
25. Single-parent
26. Married-blended
27. Multigenerational
28. Non-biologic-parent
29. Cohabiting-parent
30. Genogram
31. Ecomap
32. Vulnerable populations

II. Reviewing Key Concepts

1. See the Childbearing Beliefs and Practices section for a discussion of communication, personal space, time orientation, and family roles including how the nurse should consider each area when communicating with and caring for patients in a culturally sensitive manner.
2. See Care of the Woman at Home and Guidelines for Nursing Practice sections to formulate your answer. Consider changes in the length of hospital stays, portability of technology, the influence of insurance reimbursement, and the need to reduce health care costs in your answer; describe the need for nurses to broaden their scope of practice.
3. See Introduction to Family, Culture, and Home Care section and the Community Activity to formulate your answer.
4. See separate sections for each of the identified vulnerable populations listed to formulate your answer.
5. See Communication and Technology Applications section; include warm lines, advice lines, and telephonic nursing assessment, consultation, and education.
6. b; Providing explanations, especially when performing tasks that require close contact, can help to avoid misunderstandings; touching the patient, making eye contact, and taking away the right to make decisions can be interpreted by patients in some cultures as invading their personal space.
7. a, b, d, and e; Set meals without regard to a patient's cultural background is not culturally competent.

III. Clinical Judgment and Next-Generation NCLEX® Examination-style Questions

1. See Family Organization and structure section for content needed to answer this question.
2. See Childbearing Beliefs and Practices section and Box 2.2 for the content required to answer this question.
3. See Care of the Woman at Home section and Fig. 2.7 for the content required to answer each part of this question.
4. See Perinatal Services and Homeless Women sections for the content required to answer each part of this question.
5. See Perinatal Services and Immigrant, Refugee, and Migrant Women sections and Box 2.4 for the content required to answer each part of this question.
6. See Communication and Technology Applications section; include questions guided by expected postpartum physical and emotional changes; ask her how she is feeling and managing, condition of her newborn (eating, sleeping, eliminating), the response of other family members to newborn, sources of happiness and stress, adequacy of help and support being received, and need for additional support or referrals.
7. See Care of the Woman at Home, Preparing for the Home Visit, and The First Home Care Visit sections to answer each component of this exercise, including the approach you would take to prepare, your actions during the visit, safety precautions and infection control measures you would follow, how you would end the visit, and the interventions you would follow after the visit, including documentation of assessments, actions, and responses.
8. See Care of the Woman at Home, Perinatal Services, and Patient Referral sections for a and b and Care Management section for c.
9. See Care of the Woman at Home section; include the following in your answer:
   - Ability to observe firsthand, the home environment and family dynamics; natural; adequacy of resources; safety.
   - Teaching can be tailored to the woman, her family, and her home.
   - Services are less expensive than the hospital.
   - Can offer measures for prevention, early detection, and treatment.
   - Services may lead to long-term positive effects on parenting and child health.
   - Use research findings and recommendations of professional organizations to validate the proposal.
   - Investigate insurance reimbursement for home care.
10.

Nursing Action	Indicated	Not Indicated
Chooses a female interpreter from the woman's country of origin.	X	
Uses a quiet location free from interruptions.	X	
Emphasizes that this is an introductory session, and the client can ask questions at a later time.		X
Asks questions while looking at the interpreter.		X
Gathers culturally appropriate reading materials to use during the interaction.	X	
Speaks loudly to enhance understanding		X

CHAPTER 3

I. Learning Key Terms

1. Mons pubis
2. Labia majora
3. Labia minora
4. Prepuce
5. Frenulum
6. Fourchette
7. Clitoris
8. Vaginal vestibule
9. Urethra
10. Perineum

11. Vagina; rugae, Skene, Bartholin, hymen
12. Fornices
13. Uterus; cul-de-sac of Douglas
14. Corpus
15. Isthmus
16. Fundus
17. Endometrium
18. Myometrium
19. Cervix
20. Endocervical; internal os, external os
21. Squamo-columnar junction; transformation
22. Uterine (fallopian) tubes
23. Ovaries; ovulation, estrogen, progesterone, androgen
24. Bony pelvis
25. Breasts
26. Tail of Spence
27. Nipple
28. Areola
29. Montgomery tubercles (glands)
30. Menarche
31. Puberty
32. Climacteric
33. Menopause
34. Perimenopause
35. Menstruation; endometrial, hypothalamic-pituitary, ovarian; 28 days; day 1; 5 days, 3 to 6 days
36. Endometrial; menstrual, proliferative, secretory, ischemic
37. Hypothalamic-pituitary
38. Ovarian; follicular (pre-ovulatory), luteal (postovulatory)
39. Gonadotropin-releasing hormone (GnRH); follicle-stimulating hormone (FSH), luteinizing hormone (LH)
40. Follicle-stimulating hormone (FSH)
41. Luteinizing hormone (LH)
42. Estrogen; spinnbarkeit
43. Progesterone; basal body
44. Mittelschmerz
45. Prostaglandins
46. Preconception counseling and care (Preconception health promotion)
47. Obesity
48. Anorexia nervosa
49. Bulimia nervosa
50. Female genital mutilation (FGM), infibulation, female circumcision
51. Intimate partner violence (IPV), wife battering, spousal abuse, domestic, family
52. Increasing tension, battery, calm, remorse, honeymoon

II. Reviewing Key Concepts

1. Guidelines for each component of the procedure are outlined in Box 3.13: Papanicolaou Test. See Table 3.1 for frequency recommendations.
2. See Barriers to Entering the Health Care System section for a full description of each category of issues listed.
3. See Risky Sexual Practices section and Box 3.8.
4. See Intimate Partner Violence section and Box 3.11.

5. See Nutrition Problems and Eating Disorders section and Box 3.6 to formulate your answer.
6. See separate section for each of the substances listed in the Substance Use and Abuse section.
7. b, e, and f; IPV can occur in any family; battering frequently begins or escalates during pregnancy; women may stay even if the battering is bad because of fear and financial dependence, and shelters often have long waiting lists.
8. c; Self-examination should not be used for self-diagnosis but rather to detect early changes and seek guidance of a health care provider if changes are noted.
9. b; Warming the speculum or using a prewarmed speculum can help increase comfort and relaxation during a pelvic examination.
10. c; Women should not use vaginal medications or douche for 24 to 48 hours before the test; OCPs can continue; the best time for the test is midcycle.
11. a; All women should be screened because abuse can happen to any woman; abuse often escalates during pregnancy; the most commonly injured sites are the head, neck, chest, abdomen, breasts, and upper extremities. If abuse is suspected the nurse needs to assess further to encourage disclosure and then assist the woman to take action and formulate a plan.
12. b, d, and f; Endometrial biopsies are not recommended on a routine basis for most women, but women at risk for endometrial cancer should have one done at menopause; mammograms should be done annually for women over 50 years of age and bone mineral density beginning at age 65 (see Table 3.1).
13. a; All women, not just specific groups, should participate in preconception care 1 year before planning to get pregnant.
14. c and e; Smoking is associated with preterm birth, not post-term pregnancies; smoking can reduce the age for menopause.
15. c; It is essential to first determine what she drinks and how much; once that is established, then intervention regarding alcohol use that is individualized for her can occur.
16. a, b, d, and e; Asking "why" questions revictimizes and blames the victim; the nurse should not talk negatively about the abuser nor talk directly to him about suspicions of abuse.

III. Clinical Judgment and Next-Generation NCLEX® Examination-style Questions

1. See specific sections for each factor and Boxes 3.10 and 3.11.
2. a. See Female Reproductive System—External Structures section; the hymen can be perforated with strenuous exercise, insertion of tampons, masturbation, and during GYN examination, as well as during vaginal intercourse.
   b. See Box 3.13; explain what will occur and each guideline to follow for preparation and why each is important for the accuracy of the test; tell her to

avoid douching, vaginal medications, and intercourse for 24 hours before the examination; she should not be menstruating.

   c. See Ovarian Cycle section; midcycle spotting and pain (mittelschmerz), breast swelling and tenderness, elevated basal body temperature, cervical mucus changes (spinnbarkeit), and other changes in behavior and emotions individual to each woman (premenstrual signs).

3. See Box 3.12 Nurse's Role in Assisting With Pelvic Examination and Box 3.13 Papaniculaou Test.

4. a. See History section and Box 3.10 Health History and Review of Systems for a list and description of components.

   b. Use components of health history as a guide; write questions that are open ended, clear, concise, address only one issue, and progress from general to specific.

   c. See History section.

5. Self-examination techniques involve cognitive, psychomotor, and effective learning; use a variety of methodologies including discussion (when, how often, why, expected and reportable findings, who to call, what will be done if abnormal findings are experienced); explore feelings regarding self-examination; provide literature with illustrations; demonstrate and have patient redemonstrate using practice models and then self as appropriate. See Vulvar Self-Examination section.

6. See Cultural Considerations and Communication Variations in the History and Physical section.
   - Approach the woman in a respectful and calm manner.
   - Consider modifications in the examination to maintain her modesty.
   - Modify plan of care to individually meet her needs.
   - Take time to learn about the woman's cultural beliefs and practices regarding well-woman assessment and care.

7. See Intimate Partner Violence section including Legal Tip, Boxes 3.10 and 3.11, and Figs. 3.10 and 3.11 for content required to answer all parts of the question.

8. See Box 3.12, Nurse's Role in Assisting With Pelvic Examination and Box 3.13 Papanicolaou Test for the content required to answer each part of this question.

9. See Preconception Counseling and Care section and Box 3.2; this nurse should:
   - Define preconception counseling and care and what it entails and stress the importance of both partners participating.
   - Identify the impact of a woman's health status and lifestyle habits on the developing fetus during the first trimester.
   - Describe how preconception counseling can help a couple choose the best time to begin a pregnancy.

10. See Nutrition Problems and Eating Disorders and Lack of Exercise sections:

   - Start with 24-hour to 3-day dietary recall; based on analysis of woman's current nutritional habits, suggest the use of MyPlate, emphasize complex carbohydrates and foods high in iron and calcium, reduce fat intake, and ensure adequate fluid intake, avoiding those high in sugar, alcohol, or caffeine; use weight changes and activity patterns to determine the adequacy of caloric intake.
   - Aerobic exercise: Discuss weight-bearing versus non–weight-bearing exercises as well as frequency and duration of exercise sessions for maximum benefit.

11. See Pregnancy section and Box 3.3 Major Goals of Prenatal Care to answer this question.

12. Identify the following: "complaining of fatigue, insomnia, headaches, and feeling anxious", "never can seem to find time for herself or to socialize with her friends", "drinking more wine to help her sleep", "started to smoke again to help her relax", "lost some weight", "diminished appetite". See Stress, Sleep Disorders, Alcohol Consumption, Cigarette Smoking, Nutrition Problems, and Eating Disorders sections and Box 3.7 Stress Symptoms content. She is showing signs of stress which can have negative health outcomes, the nurse should assess for how much alcohol she is drinking, follow up regarding tobacco use education and intention to quit, assess her eating habits to assess for appropriate nutrition intake and healthy eating habits. The nurse should further assess each risk factor and abnormal finding.

13. See Cigarette Smoking section and Box 3.4 Interventions for Smoking Cessation: The Five A's.
   - Discuss the impact of smoking on pregnancy using statistics, illustrations, research, and case studies to convince her that smoking does have harmful effects on her, her pregnancy, and on the baby before and after it is born.
   - Help her change her behavior by referring her to smoking cessation programs; use the motivation of pregnancy to at least limit smoking, if she cannot stop completely.

14. See Intimate Partner Violence including Legal Tip and Battering During Pregnancy sections and Boxes 3.10 and 3.11 for content to answer all parts of this question.

CHAPTER 4

I. Learning Key Terms
1. Amenorrhea
2. Hypogonadotropic amenorrhea
3. Female athlete triad
4. Dysmenorrhea
5. Primary dysmenorrhea
6. Secondary dysmenorrhea
7. Premenstrual syndrome (PMS)

8. Premenstrual dysphoric disorder (PMDD)
9. Cyclic perimenstrual pain and discomfort (CPDD)
10. Endometriosis
11. Oligomenorrhea
12. Hypomenorrhea
13. Menorrhagia
14. Metrorrhagia
15. Abnormal uterine bleeding (AUB)
16. Fibroids (uterine leiomyomas or myomas)
17. Sexually transmitted infections (STIs)
18. Condom (male, female)
19. Chlamydia
20. Gonorrhea
21. Syphilis; chancre; symmetric maculopapular rash, lymphadenopathy; Condylomata lata
22. Pelvic inflammatory disease (PID)
23. Human papillomavirus (HPV)
24. Herpes simplex virus (HSV)
25. Hepatitis A virus (HAV)
26. Hepatitis B virus (HBV)
27. Hepatitis C virus (HCV)
28. Human immunodeficiency virus (HIV); Acquired immunodeficiency syndrome (AIDS)
29. Bacterial vaginosis
30. Vulvovaginal candidiasis
31. Trichomoniasis
32. Group B streptococcus (GBS)

II. Reviewing Key Concepts

1. b   2. d   3. a   4. f   5. e   6. c
7. Box 4.3 Assessing Sexually Transmitted Infection and Human Immunodeficiency Virus Risk Behaviors: The Five Ps cites many common risk behaviors according to sexual, drug use–related, and blood-related risks.
8. See Box 4.6 Standard Precautions for a full description of Standard Precautions.
9. See Human Immunodeficiency Virus section and Box 4.3 for a description of risk behaviors.
10. See Zika Virus section.
11. See Malignant Conditions of the Breast and Clinical Manifestations and Diagnosis sections and Box 4.7 Risk Factors for Breast Cancer for the content required to answer each part of this question.
12. See Care Management for Women with Breast Cancer and Malignant Conditions of the Breast and Screening and Diagnosis sections for a description of each approach.
13. b; The 13-year-old reflects several of the risk factors associated with this menstrual disorder, namely: presently in a growth period, she is underweight, and in a competitive sport where she participates in strenuous exercise.
14. c; Choices a, b, and d interfere with prostaglandin synthesis, whereas acetaminophen does not have the same anti-prostaglandin properties as NSAIDs; prostaglandins are a recognized factor in the etiology of dysmenorrhea.

15. b; Caffeine should be avoided; other substances listed can be helpful in relieving the discomforts of PMS.
16. b, d, e, and f; Exercise increases endorphins, dilates blood vessels, and helps to reduce ischemia; peaches and watermelon have a natural diuretic effect.
17. c, d, e, and f; Women taking danazol often experience masculinizing changes; amenorrhea is an outcome of taking this medication; ovulation may not be fully suppressed; therefore, birth control is essential because this medication is teratogenic.
18. a; Dysmenorrhea is painful menstruation; dysuria is painful urination; dyspnea is difficulty breathing.
19. a; Because these infections are often asymptomatic, they can go undetected and untreated causing more damage including an ascent of the pathogen into the uterus and pelvis, resulting in PID and infertility; many effective treatment measures are available, including for chlamydia.
20. b; Choice a is indicative of candidiasis; choice c is indicative of HSV-2; choice d is indicative of trichomoniasis.
21. b; Flagyl is used to treat bacterial vaginosis and trichomoniasis; ampicillin is effective in the treatment of chlamydia or gonorrhea; acyclovir is used to treat herpes.
22. b; Choices a, c, and d are not used to treat GBS infection; acyclovir is used orally to treat herpes; there are no lesions with GBS.
23. d; Recurrent infections commonly involve only local symptoms that are less severe; stress reduction, healthy lifestyle practices and acyclovir can reduce recurrence rate; nonantiviral ointments, especially those containing cortisone should be avoided—use lidocaine ointment or an antiseptic spray instead.
24. c, e, and f; Breast cancer is more common among Caucasian women; most breast cancers are not related to genetic factors; one in eight women could develop breast cancer in her lifetime.
25. b; The right arm should be used as much as possible to maintain mobility and prevent lymphedema; loose nonrestrictive clothing should be worn; tingling and numbness are expected findings for as long as a few months after surgery.
26. a; Pain is a common finding; it usually begins a week before the onset of menses; leakage from the nipples is not associated with this disorder; surgery is unlikely and is only attempted in a few selected cases; common, benign condition
27. d; Fibroadenomas are generally small, unilateral, firm, non-tender, moveable lumps located in the upper outer quadrant; borders are discrete and well defined; discharge is not associated with this disorder.
28. c; Tamoxifen is an antiestrogenic drug; the woman may experience hot flashes because estrogen activity is blocked; nonhormonal or barrier form of contraception should be used because tamoxifen may-be teratogenic.

III. Clinical Judgment and Next-Generation NCLEX® Examination-style Questions

1. See Hypogonadotropic Amenorrhea section for the content required to answer each part of this question; Nursing Diagnosis: Disturbed body image related to delayed onset of menstruation and development of secondary sexual characteristics.

2. See Primary Dysmenorrhea section.

3. See Premenstrual Syndrome section for the content required to answer each part of this question; Nursing diagnoses could include acute pain, activity intolerance, disturbed sleep pattern, diarrhea, constipation, ineffective role performance; use assessment findings to determine those that would apply to a particular patient including those that are priority; obtain a detailed history and encourage woman to keep a diary of physical and emotional manifestations (what occurs, when, contributing circumstances) from one cycle to another.

4. See Endometriosis section for the content required to answer each part of this question.

5. See Sexually Transmitted Infections section, Box 4.2 Sexually Transmitted Infections, and Box 4.3 Assessing Sexually Transmitted Infection and Human Immunodeficiency Virus Risk Behaviors: The Five Ps for the content required to answer each part of this question.

6. See Human Immunodeficiency Virus sections to formulate your answer; include antiviral therapy recommended, use of elective cesarean birth, and breastfeeding recommendations.

7. See Pelvic Inflammatory Disease section for the content required to answer each part of this question.

8. See Gonorrhea section, and Table 4.2 Sexually Transmitted Infections and Drug Therapies for Women for the content required to answer each part of this question.

9. See Human Papillomavirus section for content required to answer each part of this question.

10. See Herpes Simplex Virus section for content required to answer each part of this question.

11. See Human Immunodeficiency Virus section for content required to answer each part of this question; use Sonya's risky behaviors as a basis for discussing prevention measures, including safer sex practices; discuss impact HIV could have on her health and that of her fetus when pregnant.

12. See Fibrocystic Changes section for content required to answer each part of this question.

13. See Malignant Conditions of the Breast section, Box 4.7, Box 4.8, and Box 4.11 Patient Teaching Box After a Mastectomy Without and With Reconstruction for content required to answer each part of this question.

14. See Malignant Conditions of the Breast section—Screening and Diagnosis to formulate your answer.

15. Identify the following statements: "67-year-old"; "Caucasian"; "High breast tissue density"; "started her period at 11 years of age"; "Current BMI of 32"; "Had her first child at 36"

CHAPTER 5

I. Learning Key Terms

1. Infertility
2. Fecundity
3. Assisted reproductive technology (ART)
4. In vitro fertilization-embryo transfer (IVF-ET)
5. Intracytoplasmic sperm injection
6. Gamete intrafallopian transfer (GIFT)
7. Zygote intrafallopian transfer (ZIFT)
8. Therapeutic donor insemination
9. Gestational carrier (embryo host)
10. Surrogate motherhood
11. Assisted hatching
12. Donor oocyte
13. Donor embryo (embryo adoption)
14. Therapeutic donor insemination
15. Cryopreservation
16. Preimplantation genetic diagnosis
17. Semen analysis
18. Hysterosalpingography
19. Urinary ovulation predictor kit
20. Hysterosalpingo-contrast sonography
21. Contraception
22. Birth control
23. Family planning
24. Contraceptive failure
25. Long-acting reversible contraception (LARC)
26. Coitus interruptus
27. Fertility awareness methods
28. Natural family planning
29. Calendar rhythm method
30. Standard days method
31. Basal body temperature (BBT) method
32. Cervical mucus ovulation-detection method
33. Spinnbarkeit
34. Symptothermal method
35. TwoDay method of family planning
36. Lactation amenorrhea method (LAM)
37. Spermicide
38. Condom
39. Diaphragm
40. Cervical cap
41. Contraceptive sponge
42. Combined oral contraceptive pills (COCs)
43. Transdermal contraceptive system (patch)
44. Vaginal contraceptive ring
45. Single-rod etonogestrel implant (Implanon, Nexplanon)
46. Plan B One-Step; Next Choice
47. Intrauterine device (IUD)
48. Sterilization; female sterilization (bilateral tubal ligation); vasectomy
49. Induced abortion; elective abortion; therapeutic abortion

II. Reviewing Key Concepts

1. See Cervical Mucus Ovulation-Detection Method section and Guidelines box, Cervical Mucus Characteristics.

2. See Abortion section; preserve life and health of the woman, genetic disorder of the fetus, rape/incest, pregnant woman's request.

3. a, c, d, e, and h; Spermicide should be applied to the surface of the diaphragm and the rim; diaphragm should not be removed for at least 6 hours; it should be washed with warm water and mild soap, and then cornstarch should be applied.

4. b; Spinnbarkeit refers to the stretchiness of cervical mucus at ovulation to facilitate passage of sperm; there is an LH surge before ovulation; BBT rises in response to increased progesterone after ovulation; cervical mucus becomes thinner and more abundant with ovulation.

6. a; Although choices b, c, and d are all temporary side effects, the most common is the irregular pattern of vaginal bleeding that occurs; women report that this bleeding is also the most distressing side effect.

7. c; The longer a woman uses Depo-Provera, the more significant the loss of bone mineral density; weight gain not loss can occur.

8. a, d, and e; The string should be checked after menses, before intercourse, at the time of ovulation, and if expulsion is suspected; a missing string or one that becomes longer or shorter should be checked by a health care professional; ParaGard is a copper IUD—it contains no hormone; NSAIDs are safe to use for discomfort.

9. d; Clomiphene citrate is taken orally; therefore, there is no need to teach the patient's husband how to give an IM injection; b refers to nafarelin and c is used as part of treatment with menotropins.

III. Clinical Judgment and Next-Generation NCLEX® Examination-style Questions

1. See Infertility-Care Management, Assessment of Male Infertility, Psychosocial, and Nonmedical Therapy sections, and Box 5.4 for content required to answer each part of this question.

2. See Assisted Reproductive Technology section and Table 5.3 for the content required to answer each part of this question; the answer should discuss such issues as
   - Who should pay? Insurance coverage; wealthy versus poor couples
   - Children: Who are their biological parents? What is their medical history?
   - Availability to married couples only
   - Ownership of ovum, sperm, embryos
   - Attempt to create the "perfect" child

3. See Contraceptive section including Care Management, Table 5.4 and Box 5.6 for content required to answer each part of this question; Potential Nursing Diagnosis: Anxiety-related to lack of knowledge regarding contraception.

4. See Oral Contraceptives section, Box 5.8, and Table 5.4 for content required to answer each part of this question.

5. See Intrauterine Devices section and Box 5.9 Signs of Potential Complications: Intrauterine Devices, which uses the acronym of PAINS to identify signs of problems; be sure to include in your answer:
   - Teach how and when to check strings.

- Stress importance of appropriate genital hygiene and sexual practices.
- Inform when IUD needs to be replaced.

6. See Sterilization section for content required to answer each part of this question.

7. See Symptothermal Method, Basal Body Temperature, and Home Predictor Test Kits for Ovulation sections, and Cervical Mucus Characteristics Guidelines box, for content required to answer each part of this question.

8. See Abortion section – Care Management, Surgical (Aspiration) Abortion, Safety Alert, and Nursing Considerations and for content required to answer each part of this question.

9. See Medical Abortion section for a description of the drugs used.

10. See Emergency Contraception section for content required to answer each part of this question; be sure to include each of the following in your answer:
    - Explore the possibility of pregnancy and options related to continuing pregnancy if it occurs.
    - Explore options for emergency contraception to prevent pregnancy: methods available, how each works, timing, side effects, how administered.
    - Emphasize the importance of follow-up to check for effectiveness of the method used and occurrence of infection.
    - Discuss methods of contraception and infection prevention measures to prevent recurrence of this situation.

11.

Health Teaching	Effective	Not Effective
"I can stop using barrier methods with my sexual partners."		X
"With oral contraceptives, my menstrual periods should be shorter with decreased blood loss."	X	
"I will need to take the oral pills at the same time each day."	X	
"If I try the calendar rhythm method, I will need track my body temperature daily."		X
"I can tell I am ovulating if my cervical mucus is thick and white."		X
"If I miss more than two pills, I will need to use a barrier method for birth control."	X	

269

Contraception methods, other than barrier methods, do not provide protection from STIs; therefore, condoms are still recommended to prevent transmission; basal body temperature method requires her to take her temperature every day, the calendar rhythm method is based on the number of days in the cycle; cervical mucus will be thin, clear, and watery right before ovulation, not thick and white.

CHAPTER 6

I. Learning Key Terms

1. Conception
2. Gametes; sperm, ovum (egg)
3. Gametogenesis; spermatogenesis, oogenesis
4. Fertilization; ampulla (outer third); zonal reaction; diploid (46)
5. Zygote; morula; blastocyst; trophoblast
6. Implantation; chorionic villi; decidua; decidua basalis; decidua capsularis
7. Embryo
8. Fetus
9. Amniotic membranes; chorion; amnion
10. Amniotic fluid
11. Umbilical cord; arteries, vein
12. Wharton's jelly
13. Placenta; hormones, oxygen, nutrients, waste products, carbon dioxide
14. Viability
15. Pulmonary surfactants; lecithin-sphingomyelin (L/S)
16. Ductus arteriosus
17. Ductus venosus
18. Foramen ovale
19. Hematopoiesis; the yolk sac
20. Meconium
21. Dizygotic; fraternal
22. Monozygotic; identical

1. j   2. b   3. m   4. h   5. k   6. c
7. l   8. i   9. q   10. a   11. r   12. f
13. o   14. g   15. s   16. d   17. n   18. p
19. t   20. e

1. Genetic testing
2. Direct or molecular testing
3. Linkage analysis
4. Biochemical testing
5. Cytogenetic testing
6. Predictive testing; pre-symptomatic; pre-dispositional
7. Carrier screening
8. Pharmacogenomics
9. Gene therapy (transfer)
10. Homologous
11. Homozygous; heterozygous
12. Genotype
13. Phenotype
14. Karyotype
15. Multifactorial
16. Unifactorial

17. Autosomal dominance
18. Autosomal recessive
19. Inborn errors of metabolism

II. Reviewing Key Concepts

1. See Yolk Sac, Amniotic Fluid, Umbilical Cord, and Placenta sections for each of these structures' functions.
2. See Primary Germ Layers section, and Fig. 6.7, for identification of tissues and organs that develop from the ectoderm, mesoderm, and endoderm.
3. See Fig. 6.3, a risk factors questionnaire: Ask questions that would elicit information regarding health status of family members; abnormal reproductive outcomes; history of maternal disorders, drug exposures, and illnesses; advanced maternal and paternal age; and ethnic origin.
4. See Genetics—Estimation of Risk section.
5. See Human Genome Project and Implications for Clinical Practice - Ethical, Legal, Social Implications sections: consider the impact of being able to determine vulnerability to certain disorders and the impact this can have on an individual physically, socially, economically, and emotionally.
6. a; Autosomal dominant inheritance is unrelated to exposure to teratogens; each pregnancy has the same potential for expression of the disorder; there is no reduction if one child is already affected; if the gene is inherited, the disorder is always expressed.
7. b; There is a 25% chance females will be carriers; if males inherit the X chromosome with the defective gene, the disorder will be expressed and they can transmit the gene to female offspring; females are affected if they receive the defective gene from both parents.
8. d; Cystic fibrosis, as an inborn error of metabolism, follows an autosomal recessive pattern of inheritance; two defective genes (one from each parent) are required for the disorder to be expressed; she does not have the disorder and the father does not have the defective gene; therefore, none of their children will have the disorder, but there will be a 50% chance they will be carriers of the defective gene.

III. Clinical Judgment and Next-Generation NCLEX® Examination-style Questions

1. a. See Table 6.1 to formulate your answer; use of illustrations and life-size models would facilitate learning.
   b. See Pulmonary Surfactants section; discuss how the respiratory system develops including the critical factor, surfactant production; describe how surfactant helps the newborn breathe.
   c. See Musculoskeletal section; explain that the woman's perception of fetal movement occurs at about 16 to 20 weeks of gestation.
   d. Discuss sensory capability of the fetus using Sensory Awareness section; fetus can hear sounds such as parents' voices, respond to light and touch, and perceive temperature and taste.

e. See Reproductive System section; discuss the function of X and Y chromosomes; sex of her fetus will become recognizable around 12 weeks of gestation.

f. See Multifetal Pregnancy—Twins section; discuss monozygotic (identical) and dizygotic (fraternal) twinning and how each occurs; emphasize that fraternal twinning tends to occur in some families.

2. See Genetic Counseling, Clinical Genetics, and Autosomal Recessive Inheritance sections.

a. Tay-Sachs is an autosomal recessive disorder that follows a unifactorial pattern of inheritance; Mr. G. needs to be tested because he must also be a carrier to produce a child with the disorder; emphasize the nurse's role in terms of emotional support, facilitation of the decision-making process, and interpretation of diagnostic test results and how they can influence future childbearing decisions.

b. See Estimation of Risk section: There is a 25% chance the child will be unaffected, a 25% chance that the child will express the disorder, and a 50% chance that the child will be a carrier; this pattern is the same for every pregnancy; there is no reduction in risk from one pregnancy to another. See Fig. 6.2.

c. Discuss the nature of this disorder, the extent of risk, and consequences if the child inherits the disorder; options available include amniocentesis, continuing or not continuing the pregnancy if the child is affected, and use of reproductive technology or adoption; be sensitive to cultural and religious beliefs; encourage the expression of feelings; refer for further counseling or support groups as appropriate.

3. c, e, f, and h; The sex of a baby is determined at conception; the heart begins to pump blood by the 3rd week and a beat can be heard with ultrasound by the 8th week of gestation; prenatal genetic testing only tests for genetic abnormalities.

CHAPTER 7

I. Learning Key Terms

1. Thoracic (chest) breathing
2. Trimesters
3. Progesterone
4. Estrogen
5. Serum prolactin
6. Oxytocin
7. Supine hypotensive syndrome; vena cava
8. Human chorionic gonadotropin (hCG)
9. Braxton Hicks contractions
10. Uterine souffle
11. Funic souffle
12. Quickening
13. Supine hypotensive syndrome
14. Pruritus gravidarum
15. Pica

16. c	17. p	18. k	19. t	20. s	21. u
22. j	23. n	24. v	25. b	26. g	27. a

28. o	29. i	30. q	31. e	32. m	33. w
34. f	35. h	36. d	37. r	38. l	39. x

II. Reviewing Key Concepts

1. b; Friability refers to cervical fragility resulting in slight bleeding when scraped or touched; Chadwick sign refers to a deep bluish color of the cervix and vagina as a result of increased circulation; Hegar sign refers to softening and compressibility of the lower uterine segment.

2. See Cardiovascular System and Respiratory System sections, and Tables 7.1 Cardiovascular Changes in Pregnancy and 7.3 Respiratory Changes in Pregnancy for content needed to answer the question.

3. See Home Pregnancy Tests section.

4. a. See Blood Components section and Table 7.2 Laboratory Values for Pregnant and Nonpregnant Women.

   b. See Blood Components section and Table 7.2 Laboratory Values for Pregnant and Nonpregnant Women.

   c. See Respiratory System section.

5. a. See Renal System section; slowed passage of more alkaline urine and dilation of the ureters as a result of progesterone increases the risk for UTIs; bladder irritability, nocturia, urinary frequency, and urgency (first and third trimesters after lightening).

   b. See Gastrointestinal section; constipation and hemorrhoids; effect of increased progesterone, which decreases peristalsis and intestinal displacement by enlarging the uterus.

6. c; Although little change occurs in respiratory rate, breathing becomes more thoracic in nature with the upward displacement of the diaphragm; women normally experience a greater awareness of breathing and may even complain of dyspnea at rest as pregnancy progresses; supine hypotension syndrome with a decrease in systolic pressure as much as 30 mm Hg occurs as a result of vena cava and aorta compression by the uterus when the woman is in a supine position; baseline pulse rate increases by 10 to 20 beats per minute; systolic and diastolic pressure may slightly decrease beginning in the second trimester, returning to first trimester levels in the third trimester.

III. Clinical Judgment and Next-Generation NCLEX® Examination-style Questions

1. a. See Cervix section; discuss cervical and vaginal friability and increased vascularity; makes the vagina and cervix softer and more delicate so spotting after intercourse is expected; caution that any bleeding should be reported so it can be evaluated.

   b. See Pregnancy Tests section: emphasize the importance of following directions because each brand of test is slightly different; use first-voided morning specimen for the most concentrated urine and notify health care provider regardless of the test result.

c. See Vagina and Vulva and Urinary System sections: discuss the impact of increased vaginal secretions and impact of stasis of urine that contains nutrients and has a high pH; review prevention measures at this time.

d. See Breasts section; discuss changes in breasts such as enlargement of Montgomery glands and development of lactation structures resulting in larger breasts that are tender during the first trimester; changes in consistency and presence of lumpiness during BSE; changes are bilateral.

e. See Uteroplacental Blood Flow, Blood Pressure, and Renal Function sections; discuss supine hypotensive syndrome and importance of the lateral position when at rest; also emphasize safety when changing position from supine to upright and to do so slowly as pregnancy progresses to reduce effects of orthostatic hypotension and dizziness.

f. See Respiratory System section; discuss the impact of estrogen-stimulated increase in the upper airway vascularity, which increases edema, congestion, and hyperemia of the tissue making nosebleeds more common.

g. See Renal System and Fluid and Electrolyte Balance sections; explain that the swelling of her ankles is a result of the pressure of the enlarging uterus and the dependent position of her legs; elevating her legs and exercising them helps decrease edema; caution her to never take someone else's medications or to self-medicate.

h. See Musculoskeletal section; lordosis occurs as a result of the enlargement of the uterus, which decreases abdominal muscle tone and increases mobility of the pelvic joints, tilting the pelvis forward and resulting in lower back pain, a change in posture, and a shifting forward of the center of gravity.

i. See Changes in Contractility section; the woman is describing false labor contractions because they diminish with activity; these contractions facilitate blood flow and promote oxygen delivery to the fetus; compare these contractions with true labor contractions.

2. See Blood Pressure section for content required to answer each part of this question.

3. Identify the following statements: "She has had elevated blood pressures per her report"; "She has had irregular and painless contractions, but state they have become more frequent"; "Blood pressure 143/94"; "2-hour postprandial blood glucose of 134"; "Platelets 124,000"

CHAPTER 8

I. Learning Key Terms

1. Gravidity
2. Parity
3. Gravida
4. Nulligravida
5. Nullipara
6. Primigravida
7. Primipara
8. Multigravida
9. Multipara
10. Viability
11. Preterm
12. Full term
13. Postterm
14. Presumptive changes
15. Probable changes
16. Positive changes
17. Naegele rule; 3, 7, last menstrual period (LMP), 7, last menstrual period
18. Fundal height
19. Developmental tasks; accepting pregnancy, identifying with the role of mother, reordering personal relationships, establishing a relationship with unborn child, preparing for childbirth
20. Emotional lability
21. Ambivalence
22. Mother-child relationship; biologic fact of pregnancy; "I am going to have a baby"; birth;"I am going to be a mother."
23. Orthostatic (postural) hypotension
24. Ultrasound measurements, fundal height
25. Doula
26. Birth plan

II. Reviewing Key Concepts

1. Nancy (3-1-1-0-1); Alma (4-2-0-1-2); Malak (4-1-1-1-3).
2. Use the Naegele rule: Subtract 3 months and add 7 days and 1 year to the first day of the last menstrual period.
   a. February 12, 2023
   b. October 26, 2022
   c. April 11, 2022
3. See Culturally Sensitive Care section.
   a. Consider the following factors: barriers to care, communication difficulties, concerns regarding modesty and gender of health care provider, fear of invasive procedures, view of pregnancy as a healthy state whereas health care providers imply illness, view pregnancy problems as a normal part of pregnancy.
4. See Initial Visit and Follow-Up Visits sections and Table 8.2 Routine Tests in the Prenatal Period.
5. a. See Table 8.4 Signs of Potential Complications During
   b. • Discuss the signs, possible causes, when and to whom to report.
      • Present the signs verbally and in written form.
      • Provide time to answer questions and discuss concerns; make follow-up phone calls.
      • Gather full information of signs that are reported; use information as a basis for action.
      • Document all assessments, actions, and responses.

6. See Fundal Height section; consider woman's position, type of measuring tape used, measurement method (Fig. 8.6), and conditions of the examination such as an empty bladder and relaxed or contracted uterus.

7. See Preparation for Breastfeeding section.

8. See Partner Adaptation—Accepting the Pregnancy section for a discussion of each phase.

9. a, b, and f; Choices c and e are probable signs and choice d is a positive sign, diagnostic of pregnancy.

10. a; Use Naegele's rule by subtracting 3 months and adding 7 days and 1 year to the first day of the last menstrual period (September 10, 2021).

11. d; Supine hypotension related to compression of aorta and vena cava is being experienced; the first action is to remove the cause of the problem by turning the woman on her side; this should alleviate the symptoms being experienced, including nausea; assessment of vital signs can occur after the woman's position is changed.

12. a and e; Intake of at least 2 to 3 liters per day is recommended; she does not have to abstain from intercourse, but she should empty her bladder before and after intercourse and drink a large glass of water.

13. d; Continuous support is critical and involves praise, encouragement, reassurance, comfort measures, physical contact, and explanations; the doula does not get involved in clinical tasks; she is not a substitute for the father but rather encourages his participation as a partner with her in supporting the laboring woman.

14. a, c, and e; hCG indicates a positive pregnancy test and is a probable sign of pregnancy along with other changes that can be observed by the examiner; breast tenderness and amenorrhea are presumptive signs; fetal heart sounds are a positive sign of pregnancy.

15. d; Gravida (total number of pregnancies including the present one is 5); para (term birth of daughter at 39 weeks = 1; preterm stillbirth at 32 weeks and triplets at 30 weeks = 2; spontaneous abortion at 8 weeks = 1; total number of living children = 4).

III. Clinical Judgment and Next-Generation NCLEX® Examination-style Questions

1. See Initial Prenatal Visit and Follow-Up Visits sections sections.
   a. • Establish a therapeutic relationship with the pregnant woman and her family.
      • Plan time for purposeful communication to gather baseline data related to the woman's subjective appraisal of her health status and to gather objective information based on observation of the woman's effect, posture, body language, skin color, and other physical and emotional signs.
      • Update information and compare to baseline information during follow-up interviews.
   b. Be sure questions reflect principles of effective questioning; consider the need to ask follow-up questions to clarify and gather further information when a problem is identified.
   c. Focus on updating baseline information and asking questions related to anticipated events and changes for the woman's gestational age at the time of the visit.

2. See Adolescents section; the answer should emphasize the following:
   • Establishing a therapeutic, trusting relationship so the woman will feel comfortable continuing with prenatal care
   • Teaching the woman about the importance of prenatal care for her health and that of her baby
   • Involving her boyfriend in the care process so he will encourage her participation in prenatal care
   • Following guidelines for health history interview, physical examination, and laboratory testing; ensure privacy and comfort during the examination and teach her about how her body is changing and will continue to change with pregnancy
   • Evaluating the couple's reaction (e.g., same or different) to pregnancy and the need for community agency support

3. a. Reliability depends on the accuracy of date used and the regularity of her menstrual cycles; birth can normally occur 2 weeks before or after the date or from week 38 to 42.
   b. See Kegel Exercises section.
   c. See Sexuality section and Patient Teaching Sexuality in Pregnancy; emphasize that intercourse is safe as long as the pregnancy is progressing normally and it is comfortable for the woman; sexual expression should be in tune with the woman's changing needs and emotions; inform that spotting can normally occur related to the fragility of the vaginal mucosa and cervix and that changes in positions and activities may be helpful as pregnancy progresses.
   d. See Table 8.3 Discomforts Related to Pregnancy; fully assess what she is experiencing; then discuss why it happens, how long it will likely last, and relief measures that are safe and effective (also see Coping With Nutritional-Related Discomforts of Pregnancy section of Chapter 9).

4. See Physical Activity section and Patient Teaching Box: Exercise Tips for Pregnant Women; assess her usual pattern of exercise and activity and consider their safety during pregnancy; discuss precautions and guidelines for safe, effective exercise; emphasize that moderate physical activity benefits her and her baby and will prepare her for the work of labor and birth; caution her to take note of the effects of exercise in terms of temperature, heart rate, and feeling of well-being.

5. a. Risk for urinary tract infection related to lack of knowledge regarding changes of the renal system

273

during pregnancy (see Prevention of Urinary Tract Infections section):

- Woman will drink at least 2–3 liters of fluids per day; woman will empty the bladder at the first urge.

b. Acute pain in lower back related to neuromuscular changes associated with pregnancy at 23 weeks of gestation (see Table 8.3 Discomforts Related to Pregnancy):

- Woman will experience lessening of lower back pain following implementation of suggested relief measures.
- Explain basis for lower back pain and relief the measures, including back massage, pelvic rock, and posture changes; encourage woman to change her footwear for better stability and safety.

c. Anxiety related to lack of knowledge concerning the process of labor and birth and appropriate measures to cope with the pain and discomfort (see Maternal Adaptation and Partner Adaptation sections):

- Couple will enroll in a childbirth education program in the seventh month of pregnancy.
- Explain the childbirth process and describe the many nonpharmacologic and pharmacologic measures to relieve pain; discuss the role of coach and the possibility of hiring a doula; make a referral to a childbirth education program and assist with the preparation of a birth plan; discuss childbirth options and prebirth preparations.

6. a. See Fundal Height section; purpose of fundal height: indirect assessment of how her fetus is growing.

b. See Clothing section; consider safety and comfort in terms of the low-heeled shoe and nonrestrictive clothing.

c. See Table 8.3 Discomforts Related to Pregnancy: Constipation and Flatulence with bloating and belching sections.

d. See Table 8.3 Discomforts Related to Pregnancy: Pruritus (noninflammatory) section for the basis of discomfort and relief measures.

e. See Travel section; tell her that she may travel if her pregnancy is progressing normally; emphasize the importance of staying hydrated, wearing a seat belt, doing breathing and lower extremities exercises, ambulating every hour for 15 minutes, and voiding every 2 hours.

7. See Emergency Treatment: Supine Hypotension for content required to answer each part of this question.

8. a. See Preparation for Breastfeeding section; Assess nipples for eversion; if they are not, the woman can be taught to use a nipple shell to help her nipples protrude; no special exercises are recommended because they could stimulate preterm labor in a susceptible woman as a result of secretion of oxytocin; keep nipples and areola clean and dry.

b. Ankle edema: see Table 8.3 Discomforts Related to Pregnancy: Ankle edema (nonpitting) to lower extremities; discuss the basis of the edema and encourage the use of lower extremities exercises and elevation of legs periodically during the day; emphasize importance of fluid intake.

c. Leg cramps: see Table 8.3 (Discomforts Related to Pregnancy: Leg cramps and Fig. 8.9; discuss basis of leg cramps, and then demonstrate relief measures such as pressing weight onto foot when standing or dorsiflexing the foot while lying in bed; avoid pointing the toes; ensure adequate intake of calcium.

9. a. Anxiety related to perceived risk for preterm labor and birth; the woman will identify signs suggestive of preterm labor and the action to take if they occur.

b. See Table 8.4 Signs of Potential Complications During Pregnancy.

10. See Sibling Adaptation section and Patient Teaching Box: Sibling Preparation During Pregnancy, which provide tips for sibling preparation; emphasize importance of considering each child's developmental level; prepare children for prenatal events, time during hospitalization, and the homecoming of the new baby; refer to sibling classes and encourage sibling visitation after birth; suggest books and videos that parents could use to prepare their children for birth; provide opportunities to spend time with newborns/infants if possible.

11. a. Deficient knowledge related to pregnant spouse's mood changes; Tom will explain the basis for wife's mood swings and strategies that he can use to cope with these changes and support his spouse.

b. See Maternal Adaptation section and Table 8.3 Discomforts Related to Pregnancy: Psychosocial responses: mood swings, mixed feelings, increased anxiety section; discuss the basis for the mood swings and experiences during the first trimester including ambivalence; identify measures he can use to support her.

12. See Creating a Birth Plan and Birth Setting Choices sections, the answer should include:

- Descriptions of each option along with the criteria for use and the advantages and disadvantages.
- Onsite visits and interaction with health care providers responsible for care at each site should be encouraged.
- Speak to couples who gave birth in these settings to get their impressions.
- Emphasize that the decision is theirs and that they should choose what is comfortable for them; a decision should be made on the basis of a full understanding of each option.
- Assist couple with the creation of a birth plan to facilitate their control over the childbirth process and a more positive birthing experience.

13. See Doula section for the content required to answer each part of this question.

14. See Home Birth section for content required to answer each part of this question.
15. a and d; Ambivalence is a common response when preparing for a new role and mood swings or emotional lability is commonly related to hormonal changes; a woman's partner or the father of the baby is usually the greatest source of support; attachment begins with the pregnancy and intensifies during the second trimester; fatigue is common throughout pregnancy, and not a concrete sign of depression; not accepting the pregnancy does not mean that she will reject the child once it is born.

CHAPTER 9

I. Learning Key Terms

1. Low birth weight (LBW)
2. Folate (folic acid); neural tube defects, 0.4 mg (400 mcg)
3. Dietary reference intake (DRI)
4. BMI; underweight (low); normal; overweight (high); obese
5. Lacto-vegetarian
6. Physiologic anemia
7. Lactose intolerance
8. Pica
9. Food cravings
10. MyPlate
11. Nausea and vomiting of pregnancy ("morning sickness")
12. Hyperemesis gravidarum
13. Constipation
14. Pyrosis

II. Reviewing Key Concepts

1. See separate sections for each nutrient in Nutrient Needs During Pregnancy section and Table 9.1 to complete this activity.
2. See Box 9.2 to identify the five risk indicators.
3. See Pattern of Weight Gain sections.
4. See Vegetarian Diets section. These diets tend to be low in vitamins B12 and B6, iron, calcium, zinc, and perhaps calories; supplements may be needed. Food needs to be combined to ensure that all essential amino acids are provided.
5. See Table 9.4 Physical Assessment of Nutritional Status for several signs of good and inadequate nutrition.
6. See Weight Management and Pattern of Weight Gain sections to determine weight gain patterns based on each woman's BMI; keep in mind that each woman should gain 1 to 2.5 kg in the first trimester; weight gain per week is recommended for the second and third trimester.
   a. June: BMI 21.3 (normal); total 11.5 to 16 kg; 0.4 kg/week
   b. Alisa: BMI 29 (overweight); total 7 to 11.5 kg; 0.3 kg/week

c. Siobhan: BMI 15.8 (underweight); total 12.5 to 18 kg; 0.5 kg/week
7. b, d, e, and f; Bran, tea, coffee, milk, oxalate-containing vegetables (spinach, Swiss chard), and egg yolks all decrease iron absorption; tomatoes and strawberries contain vitamin C, which enhances iron absorption; meats contain heme iron, which also enhances absorption.
9. b; BMI indicates the woman is at a normal weight; recommended weight gain of approximately 0.45 kg/week during the second and third trimesters.
10. c; Small, frequent meals are better tolerated than large meals that distend the stomach; hunger can worsen nausea; therefore, meals should not be skipped; avoid large amounts of fluid early in the day; a bedtime snack is recommended.
11. b, d, and e; Legumes are a good source for folic acid along with whole grains and fortified cereals, oranges, asparagus, liver, and green leafy vegetables; choices a, c, and f are not good sources of folic acid though they do supply other important nutrients for pregnancy (see Box 9.1).

III. Clinical Judgment and Next-Generation NCLEX® Examination-style Questions

1. a. Concern regarding amount of recommended weight gain during pregnancy:
   - See Weight Management, Pattern of Weight Gain, and Low Pre-pregnancy Weight and Inadequate Weight Gain sections and Table 9.2 Tissues Contributing to Maternal Weight Gain at 40 Weeks of Gestation to identify components of maternal weight gain.
   - Discuss impact of maternal weight gain on fetal growth and development; association between inadequate maternal weight gain and low birth weight and infant mortality.
   - Discuss weight gain total and pattern recommended for a woman with a BMI of 18 (underweight).
   b. See Weight Management and Nutrient Needs During Pregnancy sections.
   - Place emphasis on quality of food that meets nutritional requirements, not on the quantity of food.
   - Discuss expected weight gain total and pattern for a woman with a normal BMI of 21.4.
   c. See Water-Soluble and Fat-Soluble Vitamins sections. Discuss vitamin supplementation during pregnancy: determine what and how much she takes; compare to recommendations for pregnancy; discuss potential problems with toxicity, especially with overuse of fat-soluble vitamins.
   d. See Nutrients section and Table 9.1 Recommendations for Daily Intakes of Selected Nutrients During Pregnancy and Lactation. Discuss factors that increase nutritional needs

275

during pregnancy: growth and development of uterine-placental-fetal unit, expansion of maternal blood volume and RBCs, mammary changes, increased basal metabolic rate (BMR).

e. See Energy Needs, Weight Management, Patterns of Weight Gain, and Obesity and Excessive Weight Gain sections. Discuss weight reduction diets during pregnancy:

- BMI indicates overweight status; discuss appropriate weight gain.
- Discuss hazards of inadequate caloric intake during pregnancy in terms of growth and development of fetus and pregnancy-related structures.
- Discuss quality of foods and development of good nutritional habits to be used during the postpartum period as part of a sensible weight loss program.
- Discuss importance of exercise and activity during pregnancy.

f. See Fluids section. Discuss importance of and types of fluid to meet demands of pregnancy-related changes, regulate temperature, and prevent constipation and urinary tract infections (UTIs); consider possible association between dehydration and preterm labor and oligohydramnios.

g. See Calcium and Usual Maternal Diet sections and Box 9.4, Calcium Sources for Women Who Do Not Drink Milk. Discuss basis for problem; reduce lactose intake by using lactose-free products, nondairy sources of calcium, and calcium supplements; take lactase supplements.

2. See Iron section, Patient Teaching box Iron Supplementation, and Table 9.1 Recommendations for Daily Intakes of Selected Nutrients During Pregnancy and Lactation for iron sources.
- Discuss importance of iron.
- Emphasize importance of vitamin C for iron absorption; discuss food sources high in iron and vitamin C; discuss foods to avoid when taking iron.
- Discuss ways to take iron supplements to enhance absorption and minimize side effects including GI upset and constipation.

3. See appropriate section for each nutrition-related discomfort in Coping With Nutrition-Related Discomforts of Pregnancy section.
a. See Nausea and Vomiting section and Patient Teaching: Managing Nausea and Vomiting During Pregnancy for several relief measures.
b. See Constipation section; include adequate fluid and roughage/fiber intake, exercise and activity, regular time for elimination.
c. See Pyrosis section; small frequent meals, drink fluids between not with meals, avoid spicy foods, remain upright after eating.

4.

Health Teaching	Indicated	Not Indicated
Counsel her to begin a lifestyle change for weight reduction		X
Recommend a total weight gain goal of 4 kg during pregnancy		X
Set a weight gain goal of 0.2 kg per week during the second and third trimesters	X	
Limit her third trimester calorie increase to no more than 600 kcal more than prepregnant needs		X
Her recommended total weight gain is 11 to 20 pounds during pregnancy	X	
Recommend a low calorie, low-carbohydrate, high-protein diet during the second and trimesters		X

A BMI of 33 indicates that this woman is obese; she should not consider a weight loss regimen until healing is complete in the postpartum period; increase in calories should reflect energy expenditure of the pregnancy during the third trimester; it is not recommended for her to go on a diet to try and lose weight during pregnancy.

CHAPTER 10

I. Learning Key Terms

1. High risk
2. Daily fetal movement count (DFMC) or kick count; fetal alarm signal (FAS)
3. Ultrasound (ultrasonography); transvaginal, abdominal
4. Doppler blood flow analysis
5. Biophysical profile (BPP); ultrasound; fetal breathing movements, fetal movements, fetal tone, amniotic fluid volume, nonstress test.
6. Magnetic resonance imaging (MRI)
7. Amniocentesis
8. Percutaneous umbilical blood sampling (PUBS)
9. Chorionic villus sampling (CVS)
10. Maternal serum alpha-fetoprotein (MSAFP)
11. Multiple marker screens
12. Coombs (indirect)
13. Nonstress test
14. Vibroacoustic stimulation test (fetal acoustic stimulation test)

15. Contraction stress test; nipple-stimulated contraction stress, oxytocin-stimulated contraction stress

II. Reviewing Key Concepts

1. See Box 10.1 Categories of High-Risk Factors and Assessment of Risk Factors section, which describe several risk factors in each category listed.

2. See Nurses' Role in Assessment and Management of High Risk Pregnancy section; answer should emphasize education, support measures, and assisting with or performing the test and follow-up care for each test discussed in the chapter.

3. See Box 10.2, which lists risk factors for each pregnancy-related problem identified.

4. d; An amniocentesis with analysis of amniotic fluid for the L/S ratio and presence of phosphatidylglycerol (Pg) is used to determine pulmonary maturity; choice b refers to a contraction stress test; choice c refers to serial measurements of fetal growth using ultrasound.

5. c; Food/fluid is not restricted before the test; the test will evaluate the response of the fetal heart rate (FHR) to fetal movement—acceleration is expected; external not internal monitoring is used.

6. b; The multiple marker test is used to screen the older pregnant woman for the possibility that her fetus has Down syndrome; serum levels of alpha fetoprotein (AFP), unconjugated estriol, and hCG are measured; maternal serum alpha-fetoprotein alone is the screening test for open neural tube defects such as spina bifida; a glucose test is used to screen for gestational diabetes; Coombs testing would be used to check for Rh antibodies.

7. c; A suspicious result is recorded when late decelerations occur with less than 50% of the contractions; a negative test result is recorded when no late decelerations occur during at least three uterine contractions within a 10-minute period; a positive test is recorded when there are persistent late decelerations with more than 50% of the contractions; unsatisfactory is the result recorded when there is a failure to achieve adequate uterine contractions.

8. a; A supine position with hips elevated enhances the view of the uterus; a lithotomy position may also be used; a full bladder is not required for the vaginal ultrasound but would be needed for most abdominal ultrasounds; during the test the woman may experience some pressure but medication for pain relief before the test is not required; contact gel is used with the abdominal ultrasound; water-soluble lubricant may be used to ease insertion of the vaginal probe.

III. Clinical Judgment and Next-Generation NCLEX® Examination-style Questions

1. See Ultrasonography section:
   a. This woman was tested to determine location of gestational sac because PID could have resulted in narrowing of fallopian tube, thereby increasing risk for ectopic pregnancy; in addition, a determination of gestational age and estimation of date of birth would be done related to irregular cycles and unknown date of last menstrual period (LMP).
   b. Explain purpose of test, how it will be performed, and how it will feel; assist her into a lithotomy position or supine position with hips elevated on a pillow; point out structures on monitor as test is performed.

2. See Ultrasonography section; instruct woman to come for test with full bladder if appropriate; explain purpose of test and method of examination; assist her into a supine position with head and shoulders elevated on pillow and hip slightly tipped to right or left side; observe for supine hypotension during test and orthostatic hypotension when rising to upright position after test; indicate how the fetus is being measured and point out fetus and its movements.

3. See Biophysical Profile section and Tables 10.2 Scoring the Biophysical Profile and 10.3 Biophysical Profile Management for identification of variables tested and scoring. 1. Noninvasive ultrasound; 2. A quiet sleep; 3. 8 to 10

4. See Amniocentesis including Safety Alert section and The Nurse's Role in Assessment and Management of High Risk Pregnancy section.
   a. Explain procedure, witness informed consent, assess maternal vital signs and health status and FHR before the test; ensure that ultrasound is performed to locate placenta and fetus before the test.
   b. Explain what is happening and what she will be feeling; help her relax; encourage her to ask questions and voice concerns and feelings; assess her reactions.
   c. Monitor maternal vital signs, status, and FHR; tell her when test results should be available and whom to call; administer RhoGAM because she is Rh negative; teach her to assess herself for signs of infection, bleeding, rupture of membranes, and uterine contractions; make a follow-up phone call to check her status.

5. See Nonstress Test section.
   a. Test measures response of FHR to fetal activity to determine adequacy of placental perfusion and fetal oxygenation.
   b. Tell her that she can eat before and during the test; schedule test at a time of day that fetus is usually active; assist woman into a semirecumbent or seated position.
   c. Attach tocotransducer to fundus and Doppler transducer at site of point of maximum intensity (PMI); instruct woman to indicate when fetus moves; assess change, if any, in FHR following the movement.
   d. See Figs. 10.9 and 10.10, and Box 10.11 for the criteria to determine the test result.

6. See Contraction Stress Test section.
   a. The test is a way of determining how her fetus will react to the stress of uterine contractions as they would occur during labor; uterine contractions

decrease perfusion through the placenta leading to fetal hypoxia; late decelerations during this test could be interpreted as an early warning of fetal compromise.

b. Assess woman's vital signs, general health status, and contraindications for the test; attach external electronic fetal monitor and assess FHR and uterine activity; assist woman into a lateral, semirecumbent, or seated position; determine whether an informed consent is required because contractions will be stimulated.

c. See Nipple-Stimulated Contraction Stress Test section.

d. See Oxytocin-Stimulated Contraction Stress Test section.

e. See Table 10.5 for criteria used to interpret the test results and to document as **negative:** no late decelerations are noted; as **positive:** late decelerations with more than half of the contractions; **equivocal-suspicious: intermittent** late decelerations or significant variable decelerations; **equivocal:** late decelerations with excessive uterine contractions or tone; or **unsatisfactory:** recording is inadequate.

CHAPTER 11

I. Learning Key Terms

1. Diabetes mellitus
2. Hyperglycemia
3. Euglycemia
4. Hypoglycemia
5. Polyuria
6. Polydipsia
7. Polyphagia
8. Glycosuria
9. Ketoacidosis
10. Type 1 diabetes mellitus
11. Type 2 diabetes mellitus
12. Pregestational
13. Gestational
14. Glycosylated hemoglobin A$_{1c}$
15. Macrosomia
16. Hydramnios (polyhydramnios)
17. Hyperinsulinism
18. Cardiac decompensation; 25, 30
19. Functional classification of heart disease; asymptomatic without limitation of physical activity; symptomatic with slight limitation of activity; symptomatic with marked limitation of activity; symptomatic with inability to carry on any physical activity without discomfort
20. Peripartum cardiomyopathy
21. Rheumatic heart disease
22. Mitral valve stenosis; Aortic stenosis
23. Myocardial infarction
24. Infective endocarditis
25. Mitral valve prolapse
26. Anemia; iron
27. Sickle cell hemoglobinopathy (anemia)
28. Thalassemia (Mediterranean or Cooley anemia)
29. Asthma
30. Cystic fibrosis
31. Pruritus gravidarum
32. Polymorphic eruption of pregnancy or pruritic urticarial papules and plaques of pregnancy (PUPPP)
33. Intrahepatic cholestasis of pregnancy
34. Epilepsy
35. Multiple sclerosis
36. Bell palsy
37. Systemic lupus erythematosus (SLE)

II. Reviewing Key Concepts

1. See Diabetes Mellitus sections for a list of all major complications.
2. See Screening for Gestational Diabetes Mellitus section.
3. See Thyroid Disorders sections for a description of hyperthyroidism and hypothyroidism; consider effects of these disorders on reproductive development, sexuality, fertility in terms of ability to conceive and to sustain a pregnancy to viability, and potential fetal/newborn complications related to maternal treatment of her thyroid disorder.
4. See Cardiovascular Disorders section; maternal arrhythmias, preterm labor and birth, IUGR, maternal mortality, and fetal death.
5. See Substance Abuse—Screening section and Box 11.4 for a full description of the tool and why it is used.
6. d; The woman is exhibiting signs of DKA; insulin is the required treatment, with the dosage dependent on blood glucose level; intravenous fluids may also be required; choice a is the treatment for hypoglycemia; choices b and c, although they may increase the woman's comfort, are not priorities.
7. c; A 2-hour postprandial blood glucose should be less than 120 mg/dL; choices a, b, and d fall within the expected normal ranges.
8. a, b, and c; A suggested intake of 33% to 40% carbohydrates, 20% protein, and 40% fat is recommended daily.
9. d; Washing hands is important but gloves are not necessary for self-injection; vial should be gently rotated, not shaken; regular insulin should be drawn into the syringe first; because she is obese, a 90-degree angle with skin taut is recommended. See Patient Teaching: Self-Administration of Insulin and Box 11.1 Helpful Hints for Using Insulin
10. b, e, and f; Other signs of cardiac compensation include moist, productive, frequent cough, and crackles at bases of lungs; pulse becomes rapid, weak, irregular. See Box 11.3 Signs of Potential Complications: Cardiac Decompensation
11. a; This woman is exhibiting signs of cardiac decompensation; further information regarding her cardiac status is required to determine what further action would be needed.

12. c; Furosemide is a diuretic; propranolol is a beta blocker that is used to manage hypertension and tachycardia; ibuprofen is an NSAID and is not used during pregnancy or as an anticoagulant.

13. b; Bed rest is not required for a woman with a class II designation; she will need to avoid heavy exertion and stop activities that cause fatigue and dyspnea; actions in a, c, and d are all appropriate and recommended for class II.

III. Clinical Judgment and Next-Generation NCLEX® Examination-style Questions

1. See Preconception Counseling section.
   - Discuss purpose in terms of planning pregnancy for the optimum time when glucose control is established within normal ranges, because this will decrease incidence of congenital anomalies; diagnose any vascular problems; emphasize the importance of her health before the pregnancy, helping to ensure a positive outcome.
   - Discuss how her diabetic management will need to be altered during pregnancy; include her husband, because his help and support during the pregnancy are important.

2. Identify the following statements: "She has had type 1 diabetes since she was 15 years old"; "Recently, she has been experiencing some nausea and is eating less as a result"; "took her usual dose of regular and NPH insulin"; "eating a very light breakfast of tea and a piece of toast"; "experience nervousness and weakness"; "felt dizzy and became diaphoretic and pale"; "Heart rate 108"; "Blood glucose 67"

3. See Pregestational Diabetes subsections for the content required to answer each part of this question.

4. See Gestational Diabetes Mellitus section, Fig. 11.1 Changing Insulin Needs During Pregnancy for the content required to answer each part of this question.

5. See Cardiovascular Disorders section, Patient Teaching box: The Pregnant Woman at Risk for Cardiac Decompensation, and Box 11.3 Signs of Potential Complications: Cardiac Decompensation for the content required to answer each part of this question.

6. See Antepartum section.
   a. Discuss importance of taking an anticoagulant to prevent thrombus formation; inform heparin does not cross the placenta.
   b. Information to ensure safe use of heparin:
      - Safe administration; teach subcutaneous injection technique to Allison and family.
      - Stress importance of routine blood tests to assess clotting ability; discuss alternative sources for folic acid.
      - Review side effects, including unusual bleeding and bruising and measures to prevent injury (soft toothbrush, no razors to shave legs).

7. See Epilepsy section including the Safety Alert; inform her that effects of pregnancy on epilepsy are unpredictable; convulsions may injure her or her fetus and lead to miscarriage, preterm labor, or separation of the placenta; medications that will be given in the lowest therapeutic dose must be taken to prevent convulsions; folic acid supplementation is important because anticonvulsants can deplete folic acid stores.

8. See Substance Abuse section and Boxes 11.4 Screening With the 4Ps Plus and 11.5 CRAFFT Substance Abuse Screen for Adolescents and Young Adults for description of principles to follow; emphasize:
   - Family focus including childcare and education and support for parenting
   - Empowerment building
   - A community-based interdisciplinary approach with multiplicity of services, including those related to sexual and physical abuse and lack of social support
   - Continuum of care
   - Pregnancy as a window of opportunity related to motivation for change

CHAPTER 12

I. Learning Key Terms

1. Hypertension
2. Gestational hypertension
3. Preeclampsia
4. Preeclampsia with Severe Features
5. Eclampsia
6. Chronic hypertension
7. Generalized vasospasm
8. HELLP syndrome; hemolysis, elevated liver enzymes, low platelets
9. Proteinuria
10. 48 hours
11. Hyperemesis gravidarum
12. Miscarriage (spontaneous abortion)
13. Missed miscarriage
14. Recurrent (habitual) miscarriage
15. Cervical insufficiency
16. Cerclage
17. Ectopic pregnancy
18. Molar pregnancy (Hydatidiform mole)
19. Complete hydatidiform mole
20. Partial hydatidiform mole
21. Complete placenta previa
22. Marginal placenta previa
23. Premature separation of the placenta (abruptio placentae, placental abruption)
24. Vasa previa; velamentous insertion of the cord; succenturiate placenta
25. Battledore
26. Disseminated intravascular coagulation (DIC)
27. Asymptomatic bacteriuria
28. Cystitis
29. Pyelonephritis
30. Appendicitis
31. Cholelithiasis
32. Cholecystitis

II. Reviewing Key Concepts

1. See Table 12.2 Diagnostic Criteria for Preeclamsia and Preeclampsia With Severe Features.
2. See Nursing Care Management—Physical Examination section.
   a. Hyperreflexia and ankle clonus: see Table 12.4 Assessing Deep Tendon Reflexes which grades deep tendon reflex (DTR) responses and Fig. 12.5 for illustrations depicting performance of DTRs and ankle clonus.
   b. Proteinuria: describe dipstick and 24-hour urine collection methods to determine level of protein in urine.
   c. Pitting edema: see Figs. 12.3 and 12.4, which illustrate assessment of pitting edema and classifications.

3. e   4. c   5. b   6. a   7. d
8. c   9. g   10. d   11. a   12. h
13. b   14. f   15. e

16. c; The woman should be seated or in a lateral position, she should rest for 5 to 10 minutes, the ideal cuff will have a bladder length that is 80% and a width that is 40% of the arm circumference.
17. a; With severe preeclampsia, the DTRs would be more than 3+ with possible ankle clonus; the BP would be more than 160/110; thrombocytopenia with a platelet level less than 150,000 mm³.
18. b, d, and f; The loading dose should be an IV of 4 to 6 g diluted in 100 mL of intravenous fluid; maternal assessment should occur every 15 to 30 minutes and FHR and UC continuously; respirations should be less than 12.
19. b; Magnesium sulfate is a CNS depressant given to prevent seizures.
20. b; Labetalol is a beta blocker used for hypertension; oral hygiene is important when NPO and after vomiting episodes to maintain the integrity of oral mucosa; taking fluids between, not with, meals reduces nausea, thereby increasing tolerance for oral nutrition.
21. a; The woman is experiencing a threatened abortion; therefore, a conservative approach is attempted first; b reflects management of an inevitable and complete or incomplete abortion; blood tests for HCG and progesterone levels would be done; cerclage or suturing of the cervix is done for recurrent, spontaneous abortion associated with premature dilation of the cervix.
22. c; Choices a, b, and d are appropriate nursing diagnoses, but deficient fluid is the most immediate concern, placing the woman's well-being at greatest risk.
23. b; Methotrexate destroys rapidly growing tissue, in this case the fetus and placenta, to avoid rupture of the tube and need for surgery; follow-up with blood tests is needed for 2 to 8 weeks; alcohol and vitamins containing folic acid increase the risk for side effects with this medication or exacerbating the ectopic rupture.

24. c; The clinical manifestations of placenta previa are described; dark red bleeding with pain is characteristic of abruptio placentae; massive bleeding from many sites is associated with DIC; bleeding is not a sign of preterm labor.
25. a; Hemorrhage is a major potential postpartum complication because the implantation site of the placenta is in the lower uterine segment, which has a limited capacity to contract after birth; infection is another major complication, but it is not the immediate focus of care; b and d are also important but not to the same degree as hemorrhage, which is life threatening.

III. Clinical Judgment and Next-Generation NCLEX® Examination-style Questions

1. See Preeclampsia section, Boxes 12.1 and 12.2, Tables 12.1, 12.2, 12.3, and 12.5, and Patient Teaching boxes for the content required to answer each part of this question.
2. See Preeclampsia and Eclampsia sections, Emergency Treatment box: Eclampsia, Boxes 12.2 and 12.3, Tables 12.1, 12.2, 12.3, and 12.5 for the content required to answer each part of this question.
3. See Hyperemesis Gravidarum section and Patient Teaching box: Diet for Hyperemesis for content required to answer each part of this question.
4. See Ectopic Pregnancy section and Box 12.4 for content required to answer each part of this question.
5. See Miscarriage sections and Table 12.6 for content required to answer both parts of this question.
6. See Miscarriage sections, Patient Teaching box: Care After Miscarriage, and Table 12.6 for content required to answer each part of this question; be sure to determine what she means by a lot of bleeding, and whether she is experiencing any other signs and symptoms related to miscarriage such as pain and cramping; determine the gestational age of her pregnancy and whether there is anyone to bring her to the hospital if inevitable abortion is suspected; priority nursing diagnosis at this time: Deficient fluid volume related to blood loss secondary to incomplete abortion; acknowledge her loss and provide time for her to express her feelings; inform her about how she may feel (mood swings, depression); refer her for grief counseling, support groups, clergy; make follow-up phone calls.
7. See Molar Pregnancy section for content required to answer this question.
8. See Placenta Previa and Premature Separation of the Placenta (Abruptio Placentae [Placental Abruption]) sections and Table 12.7 to compare findings for each disorder in terms of characteristics of bleeding, uterine tone, pain and tenderness, and ultrasound findings regarding location of placenta and fetal presentation/position; priority nursing diagnoses: consider diagnoses related to major physical problems such as deficient fluid volume related to blood

loss, ineffective tissue perfusion (placenta), and risk for fetal injury; major psychosocial nursing diagnoses could include fear/anxiety, interrupted family processes, and anticipatory grieving; comparison of care management approaches: consider home care versus hospital care for woman with placenta previa; hospital care is the safest approach for woman experiencing abruptio placentae; discuss active versus expectant management for each disorder; postpartum complications include increased risk for hemorrhage and infection as well as the emotional impact of a major pregnancy-related complication.

9. See Trauma During Pregnancy section, Table 12.8, Emergency Treatment boxes: Cardiopulmonary Resuscitation for the Pregnant Woman and Relief of Foreign Body Airway Obstruction, and Fig. 12.19 for the content required to answer each part of this question.

10. b, d, e, and g; Magnesium sulfate is administered intravenously in the hospital with severe preeclampsia; she should monitor her blood pressure and report any increases to her health care provider immediately, fluid intake should be six to eight 8-ounce glasses a day along with roughage to prevent constipation; gentle exercise improves circulation and helps preserve muscle tone and a sense of well-being; modified bed rest with diversional activities is recommended for mild preeclampsia. She should be monitoring for signs of worsening preeclampsia, such as headaches that are not relieved with medication, right upper quadrant pain or epigastric pain. Her provider may place her on 81 mg of aspirin daily, but she should not take 325 mg q 6 hours.

CHAPTER 13

I. Learning Key Terms

1. Passenger (fetus, placenta), passageway (birth canal), powers (contractions), position of the mother, psychologic response
2. Fontanels
3. Molding
4. Presentation; cephalic presentation, breech presentation, shoulder presentation
5. Presenting part; occiput, sacrum, scapula
6. Lie; longitudinal (vertical), transverse (horizontal, oblique)
7. Attitude (posture); flexion
8. Biparietal; suboccipitobregmatic
9. Position
10. Engagement
11. Station
12. Bony pelvis, soft tissue
13. Effacement
14. Dilation
15. Lightening
16. Involuntary uterine contractions

17. Bearing down (pushing; contraction of abdominal muscles and diaphragm)
18. Bloody show
19. Mechanism of labor (cardinal movements); engagement, descent, flexion, internal rotation, extension, external rotation (restitution), expulsion
20. Valsalva maneuver
21. Latent (passive fetal descent); active pushing
22. Labor
23. Ferguson reflex
24. First; Regular uterine contractions; latent (early), active
25. Second; Dilated, birth of the infant
26. Third; placenta
27. Fourth; delivery of the placenta
28. Maternal position, uterine contractions, blood pressure, umbilical cord blood flow
29. Endogenous endorphins

II. Reviewing Key Concepts

1. See separate sections for each of the five factors in Factors Affecting Labor section; consider the factors of passenger, passage, powers, position of mother, psychologic response.
2. a, c, d, and e; Station is 1 cm above the ischial spines (−1); 7 cm more to reach full dilation of 10 cm.
3. c, d, e, and f; Systolic blood pressure increases with uterine contractions in the first stage, whereas both systolic and diastolic blood pressures increase during contractions in the second stage; WBC increases.
4. a, d, and e; Quickening refers to the woman's first perception of fetal movement at 16 to 18 weeks of gestation; urinary frequency, lightening, weight loss of 0.5 to 1 kg occur to signal that the onset of labor is near; backache, stronger Braxton Hicks and bloody show are also noted; shortness of breath is relieved once lightening occurs reducing pressure on the diaphragm.

III. Clinical Judgment and Next-Generation NCLEX® Examination-style Questions

1. • Examination I: ROP (right occiput posterior, cephalic [vertex] presentation, longitudinal lie, flexed attitude), −1 (station at 1 cm above the ischial spines), 50% effaced, 3 cm dilated.
   • Examination II: RMA (right mentum anterior, cephalic [face] presentation, longitudinal lie, extended attitude), 0 (station at the ischial spines, engaged), 25% effaced, 2 cm dilated.
   • Examination III: LST (left sacrum transverse, breech presentation, longitudinal lie, flexed attitude), +1 (station at 1 cm below the ischial spines), 75% effaced, 6 cm dilated.
   • Examination IV: OA (occiput anterior, cephalic [vertex] presentation, longitudinal lie, flexed attitude), +3 (station at 3 cm below the ischial spines near or on the perineum), 100% effaced, 10 cm (fully dilated).

2.

Nurse's Responses	Mother's Statements	Appropriate Nurse's Response for each Question
"Labor starts when your progesterone levels increase to a high enough level to start uterine contractions."	"What gets labor to start?"	"There is no one single cause, there will be changes to your hormones, uterus, and cervix as true labor begins."
"Yes, this is an excellent way to push while having your baby."	"Are there things I should watch for that would tell me my labor is getting closer to starting?"	"You may notice a surge of energy, bloody show, a backache, or feeling less pressure below your ribcage."
"There is no one single cause, there will be changes to your hormones, uterus, and cervix as true labor begins."	"My friend just had a baby and she told me the nurses kept helping her change her position and even encouraged her to walk! Isn't that dangerous for the baby and painful for the mom?"	"Frequent position changes can actually increase your comfort and reduce fatigue. You should work to find positions that are comfortable for you with the help of your nurse."
"Unfortunately, there is no way to tell."	"I have heard that the best way to push is to bear down and hold my breath, is this true?"	"You are actually encouraged to not hold your breath and bear down; this is called the Valsalva maneuver."
"Frequent position changes can actually increase your comfort and reduce fatigue. You should work to find positions that are comfortable for you with the help of your nurse."		
"You may notice a surge of energy, bloody show, a backache, or feeling less pressure below your ribcage."		
"You should try and stay as calm and still as possible during your labor to save your energy for when you need to push."		
"You are actually encouraged to not hold your breath and bear down; this is called the Valsalva maneuver."		

CHAPTER 14

I. Learning Key Terms

1. Uterine ischemia
2. Visceral
3. Somatic
4. Referred
5. Pain threshold
6. Gate-control theory of pain
7. Beta endorphins
8. Cleansing breath
9. Slow-paced breathing
10. Modified-paced breathing
11. Patterned-paced breathing (pant-blow breathing)
12. Hyperventilation
13. Effleurage
14. Counterpressure
15. Water therapy (hydrotherapy)
16. Transcutaneous electrical nerve stimulation (TENS)
17. Acupressure
18. Acupuncture
19. Aromatherapy
20. Intradermal water block

II. Reviewing Key Concepts

1. See Pain During Labor and Birth and Factors Influencing the Pain Response sections for content required to answer each part of this question.
2. See Gate-control Theory of Pain section.

3. b 4. f 5. h 6. a 7. g 8. j

9. m 10. d 11. i 12. l 13. c 14. e

15. k 16. n

17. See individual sections for each regional anesthetic listed.
18. See Systemic Analgesics section including Safety Alert and Medication Guide for Analgesics for content required to answer each part of this question.
19. See Administration of Medications sections; onset of action is faster and more reliable and predictable when administered intravenously.
20. d; Woman can and should change her position while in the bath, using lateral and hand-and-knees positioning when indicated; as long as amniotic fluid is clear or only slightly meconium tinged, a whirlpool

can continue; there is no limit to the time she can spend in the water—she can stay as long as she wishes. The temperature should be maintained between 36° C/96.8° F and 37.5° C/99.5° F.

21. a; Promethazine is a phenothiazine, butorphanol is an opioid agonist-antagonist analgesic; fentanyl is an opioid agonist analgesic.

22. c; Metoclopramide is used to prevent or treat nausea and vomiting, it does not provide analgesia nor cause respiratory depression; it can increase the effectiveness of opioid analgesics.

23. d; As a pure opioid agonist, meperidine will not cause abstinence syndrome; adverse effects of normeperidine, an active metabolite of meperidine, cannot be reversed with naloxone; this medication is a potent opioid agonist analgesic; while it can cause respiratory depression, that is more likely to occur with morphine.

24. c; Administration of Narcan is given to reverse effects of sedation as the client is experiencing potential symptoms and/or in this case delivery is imminent and the provider wants to counteract possible fetal effects as a result of maternal narcotic administration. The nurse should continue to monitor maternal condition for possible side effects of the medication.

25. a, b, and c; Choices d, e, and f are not associated with opioid abstinence syndrome.

26. b; Changing the woman to a lateral position will enhance cardiac output and raise the blood pressure because compression of the abdominal aorta and vena cava is removed; administering oxygen and notifying the health care provider would follow along with increasing intravenous fluid administration; administration of a vasopressor, if ordered by the physician, would follow if the other measures are not sufficient to restore the blood pressure.

III. Clinical Judgment and Next-Generation NCLEX® Examination-style Questions

1. See Pain During Labor and Birth sections and Factors Influencing Pain Response sections; describe why pain occurs and its very real basis including the types of pain and their origin; discuss how women experience the pain and factors that influence the experience; identify measures they can use to help their partners reduce and cope with the pain.

2. See Pain During Labor and Birth, Nonpharmacologic Pain Management, and Pharmacologic Pain Management sections and Box 14.1 for content required to answer each part of this question; include the following points in your answer:
   • Basis of pain and its potentially adverse effects on the maternal-fetal unit and the progress of labor
   • The variety of nonpharmacologic and pharmacologic measures that are safe and effective to use during labor and can have beneficial effects on the maternal-fetal unit and can enhance the progress of labor
   • To emphasize that the mother and fetus will be thoroughly assessed before, during, and after use of any measure to ensure safety

3. See Water Therapy (Hydrotherapy) section for content required to answer each part of this question.
   • Describe the beneficial effects of water therapy and how it can facilitate the labor process thereby decreasing the possibility of cesarean birth; use research findings to substantiate these claims.
   • Describe the successful experiences of other agencies that have implemented water therapy; state how it has affected the number of births.
   • Use favorable reports of women who have used water therapy; consider how this could affect other women preparing for childbirth.

4. See Emergency Treatment box: Maternal Hypotension With Decreased Placental Perfusion for content required to answer each part of this question.

5. See Epidural Anesthesia or Analgesia (Block) sections including Nursing Alerts, Figs. 14.10 and 14.11, and Box 14.7 for content required to answer each part of this question.

6.

Nursing Actions	Indicated	Not Indicated
Assist the woman into a modified left lateral recumbent position or upright position with back curved for administration of the block.	X	
Alternate her position from side to side every hour.	X	
Assess the woman for headaches because they commonly occur in the postpartum period if an epidural is used for labor.		X
Assist the woman to urinate every 2 hours during labor to prevent bladder distention.	X	
Prepare the woman for use of forceps- or vacuum-assisted birth because she will be unable to bear down.		X
Assess blood pressure frequently because severe hypotension can occur.	X	

Spinal headache is rare because the dura is not punctured; using a combined anesthetic-analgesic and reducing dosage can allow a woman to push when the time is right.

CHAPTER 15

I. Learning Key Terms

1. Intermittent auscultation
2. Ultrasound stethoscope (Doppler ultrasound)
3. Electronic fetal monitoring; external, internal
4. Ultrasound transducer
5. Tocotransducer
6. Spiral electrode
7. Intrauterine pressure catheter (IUPC)
8. Hypoxemia
9. Intrauterine resuscitation
10. Fetal stimulation
11. Oligohydramnios
12. Anhydramnios
13. Amnioinfusion
14. Tocolytic therapy

II. Reviewing Key Concepts

1. i 2. j 3. m 4. h 5. g 6. k

7. f 8. c 9. b 10. d 11. e 12. a

13. 13. l
14. See Fetal Response section for a description of each factor that reduces fetal oxygen supply.
15. See Uterine Activity and Fetal Compromise section, Box 15.1, and Table 15.1 for content required to answer each part of this question.
16. See Categorizing Fetal Heart Rate Tracings and Nursing Management of Abnormal Patterns sections and Figs. 15.6, 15.7, 15.8, 15.9, 15.10; include a description of baseline rate, baseline variability, presence of periodic or episodic changes in FHR, uterine activity pattern, efficiency of equipment.
17. See Monitoring Techniques sections and Boxes 15.7 and 15.9 for content required to answer each part of this question; be sure to include advantages and disadvantages for each method in answer.
18. See Legal Tip: Fetal Monitoring Standards section; evaluate FHR pattern at frequency that reflects professional standards, agency policy, and condition of maternal-fetal unit; correctly interpret FHR pattern as reassuring or nonreassuring; take appropriate action; evaluate response to actions taken; notify primary health care provider in a timely fashion; know the chain of command if a dispute about interpretation occurs; document assessment findings, actions, and responses.
19. d; The average resting pressure should be 10 mm Hg; a, b, and c are all findings within the expected ranges.
20. a, c, d, and e; The tocotransducer is always placed over the fundus but the ultrasound transducer, which requires the use of gel, should be repositioned when the fetus moves or as needed; woman's position should be changed even though it may mean repositioning the transducers.

21. b; See Nursing Management of Abnormal Patterns section and Box 15.8.
22. b and d; The baseline rate should be 110 to 160 beats/min; late deceleration pattern of any magnitude is nonreassuring (abnormal), especially if it is repetitive.
23. c; The FHR increases as the maternal core body temperature rises; therefore, tachycardia would be the pattern exhibited; it is often a clue of intrauterine infection because maternal fever is often the first sign; diminished variability reflects hypoxia and variable decelerations are characteristic of cord compression; early decelerations are characteristic of head compression and are not considered an abnormal pattern.

III. Clinical Judgment and Next-Generation NCLEX® Examination-style Questions

1. See Monitoring Techniques and External Monitoring sections and Box 15.9 for content required to answer each part of this question; include the following points in your answer:
   - Discuss how fetus responds to labor and how the monitor will assess these responses.
   - Explain the advantages of monitoring.
   - Show her a monitor strip and explain what it reveals; tell her how to use the strip to help her with breathing techniques.
2. See Fetal Heart Rate Patterns section, Boxes 15.5 and 15.8, and Figs. 15.6, 15.13, and 15.14 for content required to answer each part of this question; the pattern described is a late deceleration pattern with baseline variability change.
3. See Fetal Heart Rate Patterns section, Boxes 15.6 and 15.8, and Figs. 15.15 and 15.16 for content required to answer each part of this question; discuss variable deceleration patterns associated with cord compression.
4. See Intermittent Auscultation section and Box 15.2 for the content required to answer this question.
5.

Nursing Actions	Indicated	Not Indicated
Change the woman's position to her left side.		X
Document the finding on the woman's chart.	X	
Notify the physician.		X
Perform a vaginal examination to check for cord prolapse.		X
Reassure her that this finding is not a cause for concern.	X	
Administer oxygen via nonrebreather.		X

The pattern described is an early deceleration pattern, which is considered to be benign, reassuring, and requiring no action other than documentation of the finding; it is associated with fetal head compression; changing a woman's position, notifying the physician, and administering oxygen would be appropriate if nonreassuring signs such as late or variable decelerations were occurring; prolapse of cord is associated with variable decelerations as a result of cord compression.

CHAPTER 16

I. Learning Key Terms

1. Regular uterine contractions, effacement, dilation
2. 3; 4, 7
3. Baby's birth
4. Birth of the baby, placenta is expelled, fundus, discoid, globular ovoid, gush of dark blood, umbilical cord, fetal membranes
5. 1 to 2
6. e   7. f   8. h   9. g   10. b   11. k
12. a   13. n   14. i   15. l   16. d   17. m
18. c   19. j
20. Uterine contractions
21. Increment
22. Acme
23. Decrement
24. Frequency
25. Intensity
26. Duration
27. Resting tone
28. Interval
29. Bearing-down effort

II. Reviewing Key Concepts

1. See First Stage of Labor sections and Boxes 16.2 and 16.3 for content required to answer each part of this question.
2. See Box 16.9 and Ambulation and Positioning section for content required to answer each part of this question.
3. See appropriate sections that discuss general systems Assessment, vital signs, Leopold maneuvers, assessment of FHR and pattern, assessment of uterine contractions, and vaginal examination; see Boxes 16.3, 16.5, and 16.6 and Tables 16.1 and 16.2 for content required to answer this question.
4. See Laboratory and Diagnostic Tests section for content required to answer this question.
5. See Second Stage of Labor section for content required to answer this question.
6. See Ambulation and Positioning section for content required to answer this question; include squatting, side-lying, semirecumbent, standing, and hands-and-knees positions in your answer.
7. See Fourth Stage of Labor section for content required to answer this question; discuss how breastfeeding will have positive physiologic effects for the mother and enhance attachment and success of breastfeeding.
8. See Second Stage of Labor section; Table 16.4/Box 16.11 for content required to answer this question.
9. a; Although b, c, and d are all important questions, the first question should gather information regarding whether or not the woman is in labor.
10. c; pH of amniotic fluid is alkaline at 6.5 or higher, ferning is noted when examining fluid with a microscope, and the fluid is relatively odorless; a strong odor is strongly suggestive of infection.
11. b and d; The only indicators of true labor are cervical change. Other statements are subjective based on maternal perception.
12. c; O or occiput indicates a vertex presentation with the neck fully flexed and the occiput in the transverse section (T) of the woman's pelvis; the station is 2 cm below the ischial spines (+2); the woman is entering the active phase of labor as indicated by 4 cm of dilation; the lie is longitudinal (vertical) because the head (cephalic/vertex) is presenting.
13. b; Research has indicated that enemas are not needed during labor; according to research findings a, c, and d have all been found to be beneficial and safe during pregnancy.

III. Clinical Judgment and Next-Generation NCLEX® Examination-style Questions

1. See First Stage of Labor—Assessment section and Patient Teaching box: How to Distinguish True Labor From False Labor for content required to answer each part of this question.
   a. Determine the status of her labor; if there is any doubt about the information being given or her status, the patient should be advised to come in for evaluation.
   b. Questions should be clear, concise, open ended, and directed toward distinguishing her labor status and determining the basis for action.
   c. Discuss assessment measures, comfort, distraction, emotional support, and who and when to call; it is important that the nurse make follow-up calls to determine how the woman is progressing.
2. a. and b.: See Table 16.4 to determine phase; Denise (active); Teresa (active); Danielle (latent).
   c. See Box 16.11, Tables 16.3 and 16.4, Supportive Care During Labor and Birth sections for care measures required by each woman according to her phase of labor.
   d. See Box 16.10 and Partner Support section for several suggested measures the nurse can use to support the support person of the laboring woman.
3. See Box 16.5, and Leopold Maneuvers and Assessment of Fetal Heart Rate and Pattern sections for content required to answer this question; realize that presentation and position affect location of PMI and the PMI will change as the fetus progresses through the birth canal.

4. See Vaginal Examination section and Box 16.6 for content required to answer each part of this question; explain to the woman the data obtained from monitoring and the vaginal examination and tell her what she can do to decrease her discomfort; privacy and discussion of the results is critical.

5. See Assessment of Amniotic Membranes and Fluid and Assessment of Fetal Heart Rate and Pattern sections, and Table 16.2 (prolapse of the cord could have occurred, compressing the cord and leading to hypoxia and variable deceleration patterns); vaginal examination (status of cervix, check for cord prolapse); assess fluid, document findings and notify primary health care provider; cleanse perineum as soon as possible once status of fetus, mother, and labor are determined; strict infection control measures after rupture because risk for infection increases.

6. See First Stage of Labor—Care Management section emphasizing supportive care during labor and birth for content required to answer this question.
   - Nursing diagnosis: Anxiety related to lack of knowledge and experience regarding the process of childbirth.
   - Expected outcome: Couple will cooperate with measures to enhance progress of labor as their anxiety level decreases.
   - Nursing measures: Provide explanations, demonstrate and assist with simple breathing and relaxation techniques; make use of phases of labor to tailor health teaching.

7. See Cultural Factors, Culture and Father Participation, and the Non–English Speaking Woman in Labor sections and Box 16.10 for content required to answer each part of this question.

8. See Ambulation and Positioning and Preparing for Birth sections and Box 16.9 for content required to this question. 1. Cesarean birth; 2. Upright; 3. Lateral; 4. Hands-and-knees

9. See Mechanism of Birth: Vertex Presentation, Immediate Assessments and Care of Newborn, and Fourth Stage of Labor sections and Box 16.12, Guidelines for Assistance at the Emergency Birth of a Fetus in the Vertex Presentation, for content required to answer each part of this question.

10. See Maternal Position and Bearing-Down Efforts sections for the criteria to use to determine correctness of the bearing down technique.

11. See Perineal Trauma Related to Childbirth section; compare episiotomies with spontaneous lacerations in terms of tissue affected, long-term sequelae, healing process, discomfort; compare reasons given for performing an episiotomy with what research findings demonstrate to be true.

12. See Siblings During Labor and Birth section: Include research findings regarding effect of sibling participation on family and on the sibling; consider the developmental readiness of the child and use developmental principles to prepare him or her for the experience; offer family and sibling classes to prepare them for participation in the birth process; evaluate parental comfort with this option; arrange for a support person to remain with the child during the entire childbirth process.

13. See Fourth Stage of Labor and Family-Newborn Relationships sections for content required to answer each section of this question.

CHAPTER 17

I. Learning Key Terms
1. Preterm labor
2. Preterm birth
3. Low birth weight (LBW)
4. Fetal fibronectins
5. Cervical length
6. Prelabor rupture of membranes (PROM)
7. Preterm prelabor rupture of membranes (PPROM)
8. Chorioamnionitis
9. Dystocia (dysfunctional labor)
10. Hypertonic uterine dysfunction *or* primary dysfunctional labor
11. Hypotonic uterine dysfunction
12. Pelvic dystocia
13. Soft tissue dystocia
14. Dystocia of fetal origin
15. Cephalopelvic disproportion (CPD) *or* fetopelvic disproportion (FPD)
16. Occipitoposterior
17. Breech
18. Multifetal pregnancy
19. Prolonged latent phase, protracted active-phase dilation, secondary arrest: no change, protracted descent, arrest of descent, failure of descent
20. Precipitous labor
21. External cephalic version (ECV)
22. Trial of labor
23. Induction of labor
24. Bishop score
25. Amniotomy
26. Augmentation of labor
27. Cervical ripening
28. Tachysystole
29. Forceps-assisted birth
30. Vacuum-assisted birth *or* vacuum extraction
31. Cesarean birth
32. Postterm *or* postmature *or* prolonged; postmaturity
33. Shoulder dystocia
34. Prolapse of umbilical cord
35. Amniotic fluid embolus (AFE) *or* anaphylactoid syndrome of pregnancy

II. Reviewing Key Concepts
1. See Spontaneous Versus Indicated Preterm Birth sections and Boxes 17.1 and 17.2 for content required to answer this question.

2. See Activity Restriction section for content required to answer this question.

3. b   4. c   5. e   6. a   7. d   8. f
9. e   10. f   11. c   12. d   13. a   14. g
15. h   16. b

17. See Dysfunctional Labor (Dystocia) sections and specific sections for each factor for content required to answer this question.
18. See Abnormal Uterine Activity section.
   - Purpose: Help woman experiencing hypertonic uterine dysfunction to rest/sleep so active labor can begin usually after a 4- to 6-hour rest period.
   - What: Use shower or warm bath for relaxation, comfort measures, administration of analgesics to inhibit contractions, reduce pain, and encourage rest/sleep and relaxation.
19. See Abnormal Uterine Activity section and Table 17.1 for content required to answer this question.
20. See Oxytocin section and Box 17.4 where several indicators and contraindications are listed.
21. a, d, and f; Weight loss, not gain, occurs and there is a decrease in cardiac output.
22. a; Magnesium sulfate is a central nervous system (CNS) depressant; woman should alternate lateral positions to decrease pressure on cervix, which could stimulate uterine contractions; calcium gluconate would be used if toxicity occurs; infusion should be discontinued if respiratory rate is <12.
23. c; It is inserted into the posterior vaginal fornix; the woman should remain in bed for 2 hours; induction can begin within 30 to 60 minutes of the insert's removal.
24. d; A Bishop score of 9 indicates that the cervix is already sufficiently ripe for successful induction; 10 units of Pitocin is usually mixed in 1000 mL of an electrolyte solution such as Ringer lactate; the Pitocin solution is piggybacked at the proximal port (port nearest the insertion site).
25. a; Frequency of uterine contractions should not be less than every 2 minutes to allow for an adequate rest period between contractions; b, c, and d are all expected findings within the normal range.
26. c; The presentation of this fetus is breech; the soft buttocks are a less efficient dilating wedge than the fetal head; therefore, labor may be slower; the ultrasound transducer should be placed to the left of the umbilicus at a level at or above it; passage of meconium is an expected finding as a result of pressure on the abdomen during descent; knee-chest position is most often used for occipitoposterior positions.
27. d; The dosage is correct at 12 mg × 2 doses; it should be given intramuscularly; dosages should be spaced 24 hours apart; therefore the next dose should be given at 11 A.M. the next day.
28. a; The definitive sign of preterm labor is significant change in the cervix.

III. Clinical Judgment and Next-Generation NCLEX® Examination-style Questions

1. See Preterm Labor and Birth section and Boxes 17.1, 17.2, and 17.3 for content required to answer this question; keep in mind that as many as 50% of women go into preterm labor without identifiable risk factors.
2. See Early Recognition and Diagnosis, Prevention, and Suppression of Uterine Activity sections, Boxes 17.2 and 17.3, Patient Teaching box What to Do If Symptoms of Preterm Labor Occur, and Medication Guides: Tocolytic Therapy for Preterm Labor and Antenatal Glucocorticoid Therapy with Betamethasone or Dexamethasone for content required to answer each part of this question.
3. See Suppression of Uterine Activity and Lifestyle Modifications sections, Medication Guide: Tocolytic Therapy for Preterm Labor, Box 17.3, and Patient Teaching boxes for content required to answer each part of this question.
4. See Malposition section for the content required to answer this question; LOP indicates that the fetus is in a posterior position—the most common type of malpresentation.
5. See Cesarean Birth and Trial of Labor and Vaginal Birth After Cesarean sections, Emergency Treatment box: Immediate Management of the Newborn with Meconium-Stained Amniotic Fluid, and Patient Teaching boxes for the content required to answer each part of this question.
   a. Implement typical preoperative care measures as for any major surgery in a calm and professional manner, explaining the purpose of each measure that must be performed; use a family-centered approach.
   b. Assess for signs of hemorrhage, pain level, respiratory effort, renal function, circulatory status to extremities, signs of postanesthesia recovery, emotional status, and attachment/reaction to newborn.
   c. Measures include assessment of recovery, pain relief, coughing and deep breathing, leg exercises and assistance with ambulation, nutrition and fluid intake (oral, IV); provide opportunities for interaction and care of newborn, assisting her as needed; provide emotional support to help her deal with her disappointment and feelings of failure; help her and her family prepare for discharge, making referrals as needed.
   d. Situational low self-esteem related to inability to reach goal of a vaginal birth secondary to occurrence of fetal distress.
   - Discuss and review why Anne needed a cesarean birth, how she performed during labor, and that she had no control over the fetal distress.
   - Discuss vaginal birth after cesarean (VBAC) and likelihood of it being an option because the reason for her primary cesarean (fetal distress) may not occur again; discuss trial of labor next time to determine her ability to proceed to vaginal birth.
   - Use follow-up phone calls to assess progress in accepting cesarean birth.

6. See Malpresentation section; right sacrum anterior (RSA) indicates a breech presentation; consider that descent may be slower, meconium is often expelled, increasing danger of meconium aspiration, and risk for cord prolapse is increased; depending on progress of labor and maternal characteristics, cesarean or vaginal birth may occur or external cephalic version (ECV) may be attempted.
7. See Induction of Labor section.
   a. See Table 17.3 for factors assessed to determine degree of cervical ripening in preparation for labor process.
   b. Her score should be >9 to ensure a successful induction; cervical ripening will be needed before induction.
   c. See Cervical Ripening Methods section and Medication Guide for guidelines for use and adverse reactions; consider how and where it is inserted, protocol to follow after the insertion, and adverse reactions and what to do if they occur.
   d. See Box 17.8, Procedure: Assisting With Amniotomy; explain what will happen, how it will feel, and why it is being done; assess maternal-fetal unit before and after the procedure; document findings; support woman during procedure telling her what is happening; document procedure and outcomes/reactions appropriately.
   e. Induction protocol:
      1. A   2. NA   3. A   4. A   5. A
      6. NA   7. NA   8. A   9. NA   10. NA
   f. See Box 17.5—focus on factors related to mother, fetus, and labor process.
   g. See Emergency box, Uterine Tachysystole With Oxytocin.
8. See Postterm Pregnancy, Labor, and Birth section and Patient Teaching box Postterm Pregnancy for content required to answer each part of this question.
9. See Obesity section for content required to answer this question.
10. Identify the following statements: "pregnant with twins"; "currently a smoker"; "BMI is 18.9"; "My sister delivered both of her kids early"; "My mom said both me and my sister were also born early"

CHAPTER 18

I. Learning Key Terms

1. Profuse diaphoresis
2. Afterpains/afterbirth pains
3. Prolactin; oxytocin
4. Episiotomy
5. Melasma
6. Hemorrhoid
7. Involution
8. Autolysis
9. Puerperium; fourth trimester
10. Diastasis recti abdominis
11. Lochia
12. Lochia rubra
13. Lochia serosa
14. Lochia alba
15. Engorgement
16. Subinvolution; retained placental fragments, infection
17. Exogenous oxytocin (Pitocin)
18. Dyspareunia
19. Kegel exercises
20. Colostrum
21. Postpartal diuresis
22. Striae gravidarum

II. Reviewing Key Concepts

1. See Urethra and Bladder section of Urinary System for content required to answer each part of this question.
2. See Gastrointestinal System section for content required to answer this question.
3. See Gastrointestinal System section for content required to answer this question.
4. See Blood Components section for content required to answer this question.
5. See Box 18.1 for the information to complete your answer.
6. d; Fundus should be at midline; deviation from midline could indicate a full bladder; bright to dark red uterine discharge refers to lochia rubra; edema and erythema are common shortly after repair of a wound; decreased abdominal muscle tone and enlarged uterus result in abdominal protrusion; separation of the abdominal muscle walls, diastasis rectus abdominis, is common during pregnancy and the postpartum period.
7. b; The woman is describing the normal finding of postpartum diaphoresis, which is the body's attempt to excrete fluid retained during pregnancy; documentation is important but not the first nursing action; infection assessment and physician notification are not needed at this time.
8. d; Afterpains are most likely to occur in the following circumstances: multiparity, overdistention of the uterus (macrosomia, multifetal pregnancy, hydramnios), breastfeeding (endogenous oxytocin secretion), and administration of an oxytocic.

III. Clinical Judgment and Next-Generation NCLEX® Examination-style Questions

1. a. Afterpains: Breastfeeding with newborn sucking causes the posterior pituitary to secrete oxytocin, stimulating the let-down reflex; uterine contractions are also stimulated, leading to afterpains, which will occur for the first few days postpartum.
   b. See Involution section; progress of uterine descent in the abdomen is described.
   c. See Lochia section; discuss characteristics of rubra, serosa, and alba lochia in terms of color, consistency, amount, odor, and duration.
   d. See Musculoskeletal System section for content required to answer question—focus on reason for the occurrence and what can be done to restore abdominal muscle tone safely.

e. See Fluid Loss section; discuss normalcy of these processes designed to rid the body of fluid retained during pregnancy. Be sure to ask questions regarding characteristics of urine, including amount and any pain with urination, to rule out a bladder infection or urinary retention evidenced by frequent voiding of small amounts of urine (overload).

f. See Pituitary Hormones and Ovaries sections; emphasize that breastfeeding is not a reliable method because the return of ovulation is unpredictable and may precede menstruation; discuss appropriate contraceptive methods for a breastfeeding women, taking care to avoid hormonal-based methods until lactation is well established.

g. See Nonbreastfeeding Mothers section for content required to answer this question; discuss the process of natural lactation suppression, why it is used now, and what she can do to enhance her comfort and facilitate the process.

2. 1. 2-3; 2. 4-6; 3. An increase; 4. More common

CHAPTER 19

I. Learning Key Terms

1. Couplet care; mother/baby care, rooming-in
2. Fundal massage
3. Oxytocic
4. Uterine atony
5. Sitz bath
6. Afterpains
7. Splanchnic engorgement, orthostatic hypotension
8. Kegel
9. Engorgement
10. Rubella
11. RhoGAM (Rh immune globulin)
12. Warm line

II. Reviewing Key Concepts

1. See Promoting Breastfeeding section for the content required to answer this question.
2. See Preventing Bladder Distention section for content required to answer this question.
3. See Promoting Ambulation section including safety alert for content required to answer this question; in addition to activity include the use of support hose (if varicosities are present) and importance of remaining well hydrated.
4. See Lactation Suppression section for content required to answer this question.
5. See Preventing Excessive Bleeding section; include each measure in your answer:
   • Maintain uterine tone
   • Prevent bladder distention
6. See Box 19.2 and Promoting Psychosocial Well-being section for the content required to answer the question.
7. c; The woman should be assisted into a supine position with head and shoulders on a pillow, arms at sides, and knees flexed; this will facilitate relaxation of abdominal muscles and allow deep palpation.

8. b; A direct and indirect Coombs must be negative, indicating that antibodies have not been formed, before RhoGAM can be given; it must be given within 72 hours of birth; the newborn needs to be Rh positive; it is often given in the third trimester and then again after birth.
9. d; This is a medical aseptic procedure; therefore, clean, not sterile, equipment is used; the water should be warm at 38° to 40.6°C; it is often used 2 to 3 times a day for 20 minutes each time.
10. d and e; The sitz bath should be used 2 to 3 times per day for 20 minutes each time; topical medications should be used sparingly only 3 to 4 times per day.

III. Clinical Judgment and Next-Generation NCLEX® Examination-style Questions

1. See Promoting Comfort sections; assess characteristics of pain and relief measures already tried and effectiveness; use a combination of pharmacologic and nonpharmacologic measures as indicated by the nature of the pain being experienced; if breastfeeding, administer a systemic analgesic just after a feeding session; make sure medication is not contraindicated for breastfeeding women.
2. See Preventing Excessive Bleeding section for content required to answer each part of this question.
3. See Rubella Vaccination section including Legal Tip for the content required to answer this question.
4. See Preventing Rh Isoimmunization section including Nursing Alert and Medication Guide for content required to answer this question.
5. See Sexual Activity and Contraception section for content required to answer this question.
6. See related sections for content required to answer this question
   a. Nursing diagnosis: Risk for infection of episiotomy related to ineffective perineal hygiene measures.
      Expected outcome: Episiotomy will heal without infection.
      Nursing management: See Prevention of Infection section and Box 19.1 for full identification of measures to enhance healing and prevent infection.
   b. Nursing diagnosis: Constipation related to inactivity and lack of knowledge.
      Expected outcome: Women will have soft formed bowel movement.
      Nursing management: See Promotion of Bowel Function section.
   c. Nursing diagnosis: Acute pain related to episiotomy and hemorrhoids.
      Expected outcome: Women will experience a reduction in pain following implementation of suggested relief measures.
      Nursing management: See Promotion of Comfort section and Box 19.1.
7. See Preventing Bladder Distention section; discuss implications of bladder distention and measures to facilitate emptying of the bladder.

289

8. See Promoting Ambulation section including safety alert for content required to answer this question.
9. See Planning for Discharge, Discharge Teaching, and Follow-up after Discharge sections for the content required to answer each part of this question.
10. See Effects of Cultural Beliefs and Practices section for the content required to answer each part of this question.
11. See Chapter 19 and Table 19.1 for the content required to answer each part of this question.
    a. Position for fundal palpation: supine, head and the shoulder on pillow, arms at sides, knees slightly flexed.
    b. Fundal characteristics to assess: consistency (firm or boggy), height (above, at, below the umbilicus), location (midline or deviated to the right or left).
    c. Position for assessment of perineum: lateral or modified left lateral recumbent position with upper leg flexed on hip.
    d. Episiotomy characteristics to assess: REEDA (redness, edema, ecchymosis, drainage, approximation); presence of hematoma; adequacy of hygiene, including cleanliness, presence of odor, the method used to cleanse perineum and to apply topical preparations.
    e. Characteristics of lochia to assess: stage, amount, odor, clots.
12. See Transfer From the Recovery Area section for a discussion of essential information that should be reported regarding the woman, the baby, and the significant events and findings from her prenatal and childbirth periods.
13. See Preventing Infection section and Box 19.1 for content required to answer each part of this question.
14. b, d, f, and g; Temperature of 38°C during the first 24 hours may be related to deficient fluid and is therefore not a concern; fundus should be firm, not boggy; saturation of the pad in 15 minutes or less would be a concern; usually women have a good appetite after birth; each voiding should be at least 100 mL. Saturated perineal pads in under 15 minutes or less are a sign of excessive blood loss. Sore nipples are most likely a sign of an ineffective latch technique. Fatigue is a common complaint during this time period.

CHAPTER 20

I. Learning Key Terms

1. Attachment; bonding
2. Acquaintance
3. Mutuality
4. Signaling behaviors
5. Executive behaviors
6. Claiming
7. En face
8. Entrainment
9. Biorhythmicity
10. Reciprocity
11. Synchrony
12. Transition to parenthood
13. Eye contact
14. Adaptation
15. Perinatal education
16. Becoming a mother
17. "Pink" period; "blue" period (postpartum blues; baby blues)
18. Engrossment
19. Responsivity

II. Reviewing Key Concepts

1. See Parental Attachment, Bonding, and Acquaintance and Assessment of Attachment Behaviors sections, Tables 20.1, 20.2, and 20.3, and Box 20.1 for content required to answer each part of the question.
2. See Parental Tasks and Responsibilities section for content required to answer this question.
3. See Parent-Infant Contact—Early Contact and Extended Contact section for the content required to answer each part of this question.
4. See Touch section for a description of touch as it progresses from an exploration with fingertips to gentle stroking, patting, and rubbing.
5. Factors influencing parental responses to the birth of their child: see section for each factor in the Diversity in Transitions to Parenthood and Parental Sensory Impairment sections.
6. d; Choice a reflects the first phase of identifying likenesses; choice b reflects the second phase of identifying differences; choice c reflects a negative reaction of claiming the infant in terms of pain and discomfort; choice d reflects the third or final stage of identifying uniqueness.
7. b; Early close contact is recommended to initiate and enhance the attachment process.
8. a; Engrossment refers to a father's absorption, preoccupation, and interest in his infant; b represents the claiming process phase I, identifying likeness; c represents reciprocity; d represents en face or face-to-face position with mutual gazing.
9. a, d, and e; See also Table 20.1 Infant Behaviors Affecting Parental Attachment.

III. Clinical Judgment and Next-Generation NCLEX® Examination-style Questions

1. See Communication Between Parent and Infant section and Tables 20.1 and 20.2 for the content required to answer each part of this question.
2. See Parental Attachment, Bonding, and Acquaintance and Parent-Infant Contact sections for the content to answer this question; be sure to emphasize that the process of attachment is ongoing and the delay in interacting with her newborn will not affect this process.
   • Help her meet her own physical and emotional needs so that she develops readiness to meet her newborn's needs.
   • Help her get to know her baby and interact with and care for him; point out newborn characteristics, including how the baby is responding to her efforts.

- Show her how to communicate with her newborn and how her newborn communicates with her.
- Arrange for follow-up after discharge to assess how attachment is progressing.

3. See Sibling Adaptation section and Box 20.5; caution her that adjustment takes time and is strongly related to the developmental level and experiences of the sibling(s); give mother suggestions regarding what she can do now and what she did previously.

4. See Parental Attachment, Bonding, and Acquaintance and Communication Between Parent and Infant sections and Tables 20.1, 20.2, and 20.3 for content required to answer each part of this question; Nursing diagnosis: Risk for impaired parent-infant attachment related to lack of knowledge and feeling of incompetence regarding infant care.

5. See Parental Tasks and Responsibilities section; foster attachment, acquaintance, and claiming; help parents get acquainted with the infant and reconcile the real child with the fantasy child; discuss the basis of molding, caput succedaneum, and forceps marks and how they will be resolved; be alert for problems with attachment and care so follow-up can be arranged.

6. See Grandparent Adaptation section; observe the interaction between grandparents and parents taking note of signs of effective interaction and conflict; involve grandparents in teaching sessions as appropriate for this family; spend time with grandparents to help them be supportive without "taking over" or being critical; help the new parents recognize the unique role grandparents can play as parenting role models, nurturers, and providers of respite care.

7. See Becoming a Mother and Postpartum Blues sections and Box 20.2 Coping With Postpartum Blues for content required to answer this question; Nursing diagnosis: Ineffective maternal coping related to hormonal changes and increased responsibilities following birth; Expected outcome: Woman will report feeling more contented with her role as mother following use of recommended coping strategies.

8. See Becoming a Father section and Table 20.3 to discuss the transition process to fatherhood and nursing measures that provide the father with support, teaching, demonstrations, and practice and interaction time with the newborn.

9.

Health Teaching	Indicated	Not Indicated
"Postpartum blues usually happen in pregnancies that are high risk or unplanned, so there is no need for you to worry."		X
"Try to become skillful in breastfeeding and caring for your baby as quickly as you can."		X

Health Teaching	Indicated	Not Indicated
"Get as much rest as you can and sleep when the baby sleeps, because fatigue can precipitate the blues or make them worse."	X	
"I will call your doctor before you leave to get you a prescription for an antidepressant to prevent the blues from happening."		X
"The 'baby blues" can cause you to cry for no apparent reason, and may experience anxiety, anger, or insomnia."	X	
"As long as you love your baby, you don't need to worry about depression after delivery."		X

Approximately 50% to 80% of women experience postpartum blues; new parents should be reassured that their skills as parents develop gradually and they should seek help to develop these skills; postpartum blues that are self-limiting and short-lived do not require psychotropic medications; support and care of the postpartum woman and her newborn by her partner and family is the most effective prevention and coping strategy; feelings of fatigue from childbirth and meeting demands of a newborn can accentuate feelings of depression; postpartum depression can happen to any woman, and it is not due to her loving her infant; it is important to stay supportive and educate the woman on the signs and symptoms of the postpartum "baby" blues and postpartum depression so she will know the signs to monitor for.

CHAPTER 21

I. Learning Key Terms

1. Postpartum hemorrhage (PPH); Early (acute, primary) PPH; Late (secondary) PPH
2. Uterine atony
3. Pelvic hematoma; vulvar hematomas
4. Placenta accreta
5. Placenta increta
6. Placenta percreta
7. Inversion
8. Subinvolution
9. Hemorrhagic (hypovolemic) shock
10. Idiopathic (immune) thrombocytopenic purpura; von Willebrand disease
11. Disseminated intravascular coagulation
12. Venous thromboembolism
13. Thrombophlebitis

14. Superficial venous thrombosis
15. Deep vein thrombosis (DVT)
16. Pulmonary embolism
17. Postpartum, puerperal infection
18. Endometritis
19. Mastitis
20. Uterine prolapse
21. Perinatal mood and anxiety disorders
22. Postpartum blues
23. History of psychiatric disorders prior to or during pregnancy
24. Postpartum depression
25. Postpartum psychosis
26. Paternal perinatal depression
27. Detachment
28. Psychotherapy
29. Antidepressants
30. Bipolar disorder
31. Edinburgh Postnatal Depression Screen (EPDS)
32. Method, availability, specificity, and lethality
33. Generalized anxiety disorder
34. Panic disorder

II. Reviewing Key Concepts

1. See Hemorrhagic (Hypovolemic) Shock section and Emergency box: Hemorrhagic Shock; restore circulating blood volume to enhance perfusion of vital organs and treat the cause of the hemorrhage.

2. See Postpartum Hemorrhage and Hemorrhagic (Hypovolemic) Shock sections for content required to answer this question; cite interventions related to improving and monitoring tissue perfusion, treating the cause of the hemorrhage, enhancing healing, supporting the woman and her family, fostering maternal-infant attachment as appropriate, and planning for discharge.

3. See Legal Tip—Standard of Care for Bleeding Emergencies for content required to answer this question.

4. See Postpartum Infection sections and Box 21.2 for a list of prevention measures including good prenatal nutrition to control anemia and intrapartal hemorrhage, perineal hygiene, and adherence to aseptic techniques.

5. See Postpartum Psychiatric Disorders sections to answer this question.

6. See Maternal Death section to answer this question.

7. See Postpartum Psychiatric Disorders sections including the Nursing Alert for the content required to answer each part of this question; identify the possibility of woman harming herself, her baby, or both of them.

8. b; Although a, c, and d are correct actions, the woman's hypertensive status would be a contraindicating the factor for its use; therefore, the order should be questioned as the nurse's first action.

9. d; Hemabate is a powerful prostaglandin that is the third-line medication given to treat excessive uterine blood loss or hemorrhage related to uterine atony; it has no action related to pain, infection, or clotting.

10. a; Puerperal infections are infections of the genital tract after birth; pulse will increase, not decrease, in response to fever; lochia characteristics will change, but this will not be the first sign exhibited; WBC count would already be elevated related to pregnancy and birth.

11. b, c, d, and f; Heparin and warfarin (Coumadin) are safe for use by breastfeeding women; heparin, which is administered intravenously or subcutaneously, is the anticoagulant of choice during the acute stage of DVT; warfarin is administered orally, not parenterally.

12. a; Although the other questions are appropriate, the potential for harming herself or her baby is the most serious and very real concern.

13. c; Hemabate is contraindicated in women with a history of asthma. It can cause bronchoconstriction.

14. d; Tachypnea is a sign and symptom of a pulmonary embolus. All others are not.

15. a, b and c; All are techniques used to manage postpartum hemorrhage.

III. Clinical Judgment and Next-Generation NCLEX® Examination-style Questions

1. See Postpartum Hemorrhage section, Medication Guide: Uterotonic Drugs to Manage Postpartum Hemorrhage, Box 21.1, and Emergency box: Hemorrhagic Shock for the content required to answer each part of this question.

   a. Risk factors for early postpartum hemorrhage: parity (5-1-0-7), vaginal full-term twin birth 1 hour ago; hypotonic uterine dysfunction treated with oxytocin (Pitocin); use of forceps for birth; increased manipulation with the birth of twins.

   b. Nurse's response to excessive blood loss: Most common cause of the excessive blood loss 1 hour after birth would be uterine atony, especially because woman exhibits several risk factors.

   • Assess fundus for consistency, height, and location; massage if boggy.

   • Express clots, if present, once the uterus is firm.

   • Check bladder for distention (distended bladder will reduce uterine contraction); check perineum for swelling and ask woman about experiencing perineal pressure (hematoma formation is possible related to use of forceps for birth).

   c. Guidelines for administering Pitocin IV: Use Medication Guide.

   d. Signs of developing hemorrhagic shock: See Emergency box.

   e. Nursing measures to support the woman and family:

   • Explain progress, including the meaning of findings and need for treatment measures being used, including their purpose and effectiveness.

   • Use a calm, professional, organized approach that incorporates periods of uninterrupted rest.

   • Initiate comfort measures.

   • Provide opportunities for interaction with newborn and updates on the newborn's status.

2. See Postpartum Infection section and Box 21.2 for the content required to answer each part of this question.
4. See Venous Thromboembolic Disorders section for content required to answer each part of this question.
   a. Risk factors: In addition to hypercoagulability of pregnancy continuing into the postpartum period, other risk factors for this woman would be cesarean birth, obesity, age over 35 years, multiparity, smoking habit, and varicosities in both legs.
   b. Signs and symptoms indicative of DVT: see Clinical Manifestations section.
   c. Nursing diagnosis: Anxiety related to unexpected development of a postpartum complication.
   d. Expected care management: see Medical Management and Nursing Interventions sections including Nursing Alert.
   e. Discharge instructions:
      • How to assess leg and to assess for signs of unusual bleeding
      • Proper use of elastic/support stockings
      • How to take anticoagulants safely and the importance of follow-up to assess progress
      • Practices to prevent bleeding while taking an anticoagulant and importance of avoiding pregnancy because warfarin is teratogenic
      • Importance of avoiding aspirin and NSAIDs for pain and food/vitamin supplements that are sources of vitamin K because they can interact with warfarin (Coumadin)
5. See Hematomas section to answer all parts of this section
6. See Postpartum Psychiatric Disorders section and Patient Teaching boxes: Signs of Postpartum Blues, Depression, and Psychosis and Preventing Postpartum Depression for content required to answer each part of this question.

   Identify the following statements: "Tom tries to help Mary with the baby but he has to spend long hours at work to establish his position"; "Mary's prenatal record reveals that she often exhibited anxiety about her well-being and that of her baby"; "she always wants to sleep and just cannot seem to get enough rest"; "Mary is very concerned that she is not being a good mother"; "Sometimes I just do not know what to do to care for my baby the right way, and I am not even breastfeeding my baby"; ". It seems that Tom enjoys spending what little time he has at home with the baby and not with me."; "I even find myself yelling at him for the silliest things."
7. See information under Postpartum Hemorrhage related to interprofessional health care teams.
8. See information under Postpartum Infection and Urinary Tract Infection to answer this question.

CHAPTER 22

I. Learning Key Terms
1. Neutral thermal environment
2. Thermogenesis
3. Nonshivering thermogenesis
4. Convection
5. Radiation
6. Evaporation
7. Conduction
8. Hyperthermia
9. Cold stress
10. Nevus simplex (telangiectatic nevi)
11. Molding
12. Caput succedaneum
13. Cephalhematoma
14. Mongolian spots
15. Acrocyanosis
16. Vernix caseosa
17. Milia
18. Jaundice
19. Meconium
20. Erythema toxicum (neonatorum)
21. Uric acid crystals
22. "Wink" reflex
23. Hydrocele
24. Ecchymosis
25. Murmur
26. Lanugo
27. Subgaleal hemorrhage
28. Desquamation
29. Nevus flammeus (port-wine stain)
30. Infantile hemangioma
31. Pseudomenstruation
32. Prepuce
33. Surfactant
34. Epstein pearls
35. Polydactyly; oligodactyly
36. Syndactyly
37. Sleep-wake states
38. Deep sleep; light sleep; increasing
39. Drowsy, quiet alert, active alert, crying
40. Quiet alert
41. State regulation
42. Habituation
43. Orientation
44. Consolability
45. Temperament
46. Crying

II. Reviewing Key Concepts
1. See Respiratory System section for a description of how a newborn begins to breathe; include chemical, mechanical, thermal, and sensory factors in your answer.
2. j   3. f   4. b   5. i   6. d   7. h
8. a   9. e   10. g   11. c   12. k
13. See Stages of Transition to Extrauterine Life section at beginning of the chapter for identification of each

phase and description of timing/duration and typical newborn behaviors for each phase.

14. a; The rash described is erythema toxicum; it is an inflammatory response that has no clinical significance and requires no treatment because it will disappear spontaneously.

15. b; Physiologic jaundice does not appear until 24 hours after birth; a further investigation would be needed if it appears during the first 24 hours, because that would be consistent with pathologic jaundice; a, c, and d are all expected findings.

16. d; Choices b and c are common newborn reflexes used to assess the integrity of the neuromuscular system; syndactyly refers to webbing of the fingers.

17. c; Telangiectatic nevi (nevus simplex) are also known as stork bite marks and can also appear on the eyelids; milia are plugged sebaceous glands and appear like white pimples; nevus vasculosus or a strawberry mark is a raised, sharply demarcated, bright or dark red swelling; nevus flammeus is a port-wine, flat red to a purple lesion that does not blanch with pressure.

III. Clinical Judgment and Next-Generation NCLEX® Examination-style Questions

1. See Thermogenesis, Hypothermia and Cold Stress section and Figs. 22.2 and 22.3 for the content required to answer each part of this question. Nursing Diagnosis: Risk for imbalanced body temperature—hypothermia related to immature thermoregulation associated with newborn status; Expected outcome: newborn's temperature will stabilize between 36.5° and 37.2° C within 8 to 10 hours of birth.

2. See Integumentary System and Skeletal System sections; discuss each finding in terms of cause, significance for the newborn's health status and adjustment, and how/when it will be resolved; refer to Figs. 22.14 and 22.15 to facilitate parental understanding.

3. See Respiratory System section for the content required to answer this question.

4. See Sensory Behaviors section including vision, hearing, smell, taste, and touch:
   a. Discuss and demonstrate newborn's capability regarding vision, hearing, touch, taste, and smell.
   b. Face-to-face/eye-to-eye contact, objects (bright or black-and-white changing, complex patterns), sound (talking to infant, music, heartbeat simulator), touch (infant massage, cuddling).

5. Discuss the characteristics and cause of Mongolian spots (see Mongolian Spots section and Fig. 22.8).

6. a, b, and c; The newborn at 5 hours old is in the second period of reactivity, during which tachycardia, tachypnea, increased muscle tone, skin color changes, increased mucus production, and passage of meconium are normal findings; and respiratory rate should range between 30 and 60 BPM; expiratory grunting and nasal flaring and retractions of the sternum are signs of respiratory distress. Blue mucus membranes would indicate circumoral cyanosis, which is a sign of hypoxemia. An Axillary temperature of 38.0°C is considered hyperthermia.

7. See Bilirubin Synthesis, Physiologic Jaundice, Pathologic Jaundice, and Jaundice Related to Breastfeeding sections for the content to compare and contrast each type of jaundice listed.

CHAPTER 23

I. Learning Key Terms

1. Apgar score; heart rate, respiratory effort, muscle tone, reflex irritability, color
2. Bulb syringe
3. Thermistor probe
4. Ophthalmia neonatorum (neonatal conjunctivitis); Erythromycin
5. Vitamin K
6. New Ballard score
7. Appropriate for gestational age (AGA)
8. Large for gestational age (LGA)
9. Small for gestational age (SGA)
10. Late preterm
11. Preterm
12. Full-term
13. Postterm
14. Post mature
15. Early term
16. Petechiae
17. Physiologic jaundice
18. Colostrum
19. Transcutaneous bilirubinometry Monitor
20. Phototherapy
21. Hypoglycemia
22. Bradypnea
23. Tachypnea
24. Handwashing (hand hygiene)
25. Fiberoptic blanket
26. Circumcision

II. Reviewing Key Concepts

1. See Protective Environment section; discuss each of the following in your answer:
   a. Environmental modifications
   b. Infection control measures
   c. Safety in terms of security precautions and identification measures

2. See Baseline Measurements of Physical Growth section and Table 23.3 for content required to answer this question.

3. See Discharge Planning and Parent Education, Vital Signs, Elimination, and Sleeping, Positioning, and Holding sections, Safety Alerts, and Patient Teaching box: Home Care: Bathing, Cord Care, Skin Care, and Nail Care for content required to answer each part of this question.

4. See Airway Maintenance and Maintaining an Adequate Oxygen Supply sections for the content required to answer each part of this question.

5. d, e, and f; Thinning of lanugo with bald spots, descent of testes and absence of scarf sign are consistent with full-term status; pulse and weight are not part of the Ballard scale; the popliteal angle for a full-term newborn would be 90 degrees or less.

6. b; Signs of hypoglycemia include cyanosis along with apnea, hypothermia, jitteriness/twitching, irregular respirations, high-pitched cry, difficulty feeding, hunger, lethargy, eye-rolling, and seizures.

7. a; The control panel should be set between 36° and 37° C; the probe should be placed in one of the upper quadrants of the abdomen below the intercostal margin, never over a rib; axillary, not rectal, temperatures should be taken.

8. b; Acetaminophen should be given every 4 hours for a maximum of 5 doses in 24 hours; the site should be checked every 15 to 30 minutes for the first hour and then every hour for the next 4 to 6 hours; diaper wipes should not be used on the site because they contain alcohol, which would delay healing and cause discomfort; the yellow exudate is a protective film that forms in 24 hours, and it should not be removed.

9. b, c, and d; Mother does not have to be hepatitis B positive for the vaccine to be given to her newborn; use a 5/8-inch 25-gauge needle and insert it at a 90-degree angle.

III. Clinical Judgment and Next-Generation NCLEX® Examination-style Questions

1. See Table 23.2 and the Apgar Score section for the content to answer this question.
   a. Baby boy Smith: heart rate: 160 (2); respiratory effort: good, crying (2); muscle tone: flexion, active movement (2); reflex irritability: cry with stimulus (2); color: acrocyanosis (1); score is 9 and is within normal limits; interpretation: score of 7 to 10 indicates that the infant is not having difficulty adjusting to extrauterine life.
   b. Baby girl Doe: heart rate: 102 (2); respiratory effort: slow, irregular, weak cry (1); muscle tone: some flexion (1); reflex irritability: grimace with stimulus (1); color: pale (0); score is 5; interpretation: score of 4–6 indicates a moderate difficulty adjusting to extrauterine life.

2. See Tables 23.1 and 23.2 and Initial Physical Assessment, Apgar Score, Immediate Care After Birth, Protective Environment, and Promoting Parent-Infant Interaction sections for the content to answer each part of this question; be sure to include the following in your answer:
   • Assessment of physical status and stabilization of respiration and airway patency
   • Maintenance of body temperature
   • Immediate interventions in terms of identification, prophylactic medications, infection control measures, security, promotion of bonding/attachment

3. See Discharge Planning and Parent Education, Protective Environment, and Promoting Parent-Infant Interaction sections, Table 23.1, and Patient Teaching box Signs of Illness for the content required to answer each part of this question; by including the parents you have a chance to observe parent-infant interactions and to identify and meet learning needs; foster active involvement in assessment and care of their newborn; encourage discussion of concerns and

asking of questions; a chance to explain and demonstrate newborn characteristics and capabilities.

4. See Airway Maintenance and Maintaining an Adequate Oxygen Supply sections and Patient Teaching box: Suctioning With a Bulb Syringe for the content required to answer each part of this question; Nursing diagnosis: Impaired gas exchange related to upper airway obstruction with mucus.

5. See Discharge Planning and Parent Education section, Patient Teaching box: Care of the Circumcised Newborn at Home, and Patient Teaching box: Home Care: Bathing, Cord Care, Skin Care, and Nail Care for the content required to answer each part of this question; Nursing diagnosis: Risk for infection related to the removal of foreskin and healing umbilical cord site; Expected outcome: cord and circumcision site will heal without infection.

6. See Phototherapy for Hyperbilirubinemia and Promoting Parent-Infant Interaction sections and Chapter 22 for a full discussion of the basis for physiologic (non-pathologic) jaundice for the content required to answer each part of this question. Be sure that your answer includes the importance of telling parents in simple terms that their newborn is exhibiting physiologic jaundice, explaining why it occurs, what impact it will have on their newborn's health, and how it will be resolved; in addition, ensure that they are given time to interact with their newborn during feeding times when the infant is out of the lights and even when under the lights.

7. See Circumcision and Neonatal Responses to Pain sections, Box 23.5 for the content required to answer this question.

8.

Nursing Actions	Indicated	Not Indicated
Maintain skin-to-skin and administer the ointment at 4 hours of life.		X
Explain that it is not recommended because he was born by cesarean.		X
Cleanse eyes if secretions are present.	X	
Squeeze an ointment ribbon of 1 to 2 inches into the lower conjunctival sac.		X
Wipe away excess ointment after 1 minute.	X	
Apply the ointment from inner to the outer canthus.	X	

Administer within 1 to 2 hours; it is recommended for infants who are born by cesarean, squeeze a 1- to 2-cm ribbon of ointment into the lower conjunctival sac.

CHAPTER 24

I. Learning Key Terms

1. Lobes
2. Alveoli
3. Milk ducts
4. Montgomery glands
5. Nipple-erection reflex
6. Myoepithelial cells
7. Areola
8. Lactation (lactogenesis)
9. Prolactin
10. Oxytocin
11. Flat, inverted
12. Breast shell
13. Reverse pressure softening
14. Colostrum
15. Human milk
16. Feeding-readiness cues
17. Let-down; milk ejection
18. Rooting reflex
19. Latch (latch-on)
20. Engorgement
21. Football hold
22. Cradle hold
23. Lactation consultant
24. Mastitis
25. Commercial infant formula
26. Frenotomy
27. Weaning
28. Foremilk
29. Hindmilk
30. Early-onset jaundice (breastfeeding-associated jaundice)
31. Late-onset jaundice (breast milk jaundice)

II. Reviewing Key Concepts

1. See Benefits of Breastfeeding section and Table 24.1; emphasize the importance and benefits of breastfeeding for infants, mothers, and family/society.
2. See Positioning section and Fig. 24.5; describe the positions of football hold, cradle (traditional), modified cradle (across the lap), and side-lying.
3. See Breastfeeding Initiation section for the content required to answer each part of this question.
4. See Latch section and Figs. 24.6 and 24.7 for the content required to answer each part of this question.
5. b; Birthweight is regained in 10 to 14 days; 6 to 8 wet diapers are expected at this time; should be fed every 2 to 3 hours for a total of 8 to 10 times per day.
6. d; Mother should be encouraged to let her newborn begin to suck on her clean finger until the baby begins to calm down then switch to the breast; a, b, and c are all appropriate actions to calm a fussy baby.
7. d; No soap should be used because it could dry the areola and increase the risk for irritation; vitamin E should not be used because it is a fat-soluble vitamin that the infant could ingest when breastfeeding; lanolin or colostrum/milk are the preferred substances to be applied to the area; plastic liners can trap moisture and lead to sore nipples.
8. b; A combination hormonal contraceptive could decrease the milk supply if given before lactation is well established during the first 6 weeks after birth; after 6 weeks, a progestin-only contraceptive could be used because it is the least likely hormonal contraceptive to affect lactation; even complete breastfeeding is not considered to be a reliable method because ovulation can occur unexpectedly even before the first menstrual period; diaphragm used before pregnancy would have to be checked to see whether it fits properly before the woman uses it again.
9. b; Supplements are not required when using prepared formulas; a 2-week-old infant should consume approximately 90 to 150 mL of formula at each feeding; formula should never be heated in the microwave because it could be overheated or unevenly heated.
10. a, c, and d; Nipples should not be washed using soap; plastic liners can keep nipples and areola moist and increase the risk for tissue breakdown; bring baby to breast, not breast to baby.
11. c; Limiting the length of feeding does not protect the nipples and areola; b and d are correct actions but not the most important.

III. Clinical Judgment and Next-Generation NCLEX® Examination-style Questions

1. See Decision-Making About Breastfeeding section, Evidence-Based Practice Box: Infant Feeding Decision-Making.
   a. Decisional conflict regarding feeding method for their newborn related to lack of knowledge and experience with newborn feeding methods.
   b. Couple will choose the feeding method for their newborn that is most comfortable for them.
   c. Both should learn about the pros and cons of feeding methods with an emphasis on the benefits of breastfeeding and how the partner can help with the method.
   d. The prenatal period is a less stressful time, allowing for full consideration of options, how feeding methods would be incorporated into life activities (such as work outside the home), and learning about breastfeeding by attending a prenatal breastfeeding class and reading.
   e. Provide information about feeding methods in a nonjudgmental manner while still emphasizing the importance of breastfeeding as the preferred method, dispel myths, address personal concerns of the couple, and make needed referrals to WIC, lactation consultant, breastfeeding classes, and the La Leche League.

2.

Nurse's Responses	Mother's Statements	Appropriate Nurse's Response for each Question
"This is a normal finding, particularly in the first few days. It happens because baby is latching."	"Every time I breastfeed, I get cramps and my flow seems to get heavier. Is there something wrong with me?"	"This is a normal finding, particularly in the first few days. It happens because baby is latching."
"Unfortunately, breastfeeding is not considered an effective method of contraception. While the lactational amenorrhea method may be effective, let's talk about other effective contraception methods so you know all of your options."	"Everyone keeps talking about this let-down that is supposed to happen. What is it and how will I know I have it?"	"Let-down is when the milk is ejected from the breast. You may feel a warm rush or tingling, and you may experience milk leaking from the opposite breast."
"This is one of the major benefits of breastfeeding, you can trust the process and know that it is working."	"How can I possibly know if my baby is getting enough if I cannot tell how many ounces he gets with each feeding?"	"It is important to keep track of her urine and stool output to tell if she is getting enough milk. A feeding diary can help with this."
"If your cramps get worse during breastfeeding, please let your provider know immediately. This can be a sign of retained placental fragments."	"It is only the first day that I am breastfeeding and my nipples already feel sore. What can I do to relieve this soreness and prevent it from getting worse?"	"Next time she breastfeeds, I would like to observe her latch. Some mild discomfort can be normal in the first few sucks but making sure she has a good latch is critical to preventing sore nipples."
"It is important to keep track of her urine and stool output to tell if she is getting enough milk. A feeding diary can help with this."	"I am so glad I do not have to worry about getting pregnant again as long as I am breastfeeding. I hate using birth control and my friend told me I do not have to as long as I am breastfeeding."	"Unfortunately, breastfeeding is not considered an effective method of contraception. While the lactational amenorrhea method may be effective, let's talk about other effective contraception methods so you know all of your options."
"Let-down is when the milk is ejected from the breast. You may feel a warm rush or tingling, and you may experience milk leaking from the opposite breast."		
"Next time she breastfeeds, I would like to observe her latch. Some mild discomfort can be normal in the first few sucks but making sure she has a good latch is critical to preventing sore nipples."		
"Let-down is typically painful for the first week, but you can tell that it is happening due to increased thirst and uterine cramping."		

3. See Frequency of Feedings and Sleepy Baby sections for the content required to answer each part of this question.
   a. Nursing diagnosis: Imbalanced nutrition less than body requirements related to infrequent feeding of newborn.
   Expected outcome: Mother will awaken the infant every 2 to 3 hours during the day and every 4 hours at night to feed the infant, achieving at least 8 feedings per day.
   b. Nursing approach: Discuss feeding readiness cues to facilitate proper timing of feedings; discuss techniques to wake sleeping baby and signs indicating adequate intake.
4. See Formula-Feeding section and Patient Teaching box: Formula Preparation and Feeding for the content required to answer each part of this question.
   a. Discuss how the mother can facilitate close contact and socialization with the infant during feeding; reassure that properly prepared formula will

297

fully meet her newborn's need for nutrients and fluid.

b. Discuss how to choose a formula type; amount and frequency of feedings; how to prepare formula, safety measures, cues of feeding readiness and satiety, and burping.

5. See Assessment of Effective Breastfeeding section and Box 24.2 to determine what to assess; formulate questions that address the assessment factors; in addition ask questions about such areas as frequency and duration of feedings, breastfeeding techniques used, how she feels about breastfeeding and how well she feels she is doing, family support for breastfeeding; her ability to rest; and nutrient and fluid intake.

CHAPTER 25

I. Learning Key Terms

1. m	2. n	3. o	4. p	5. q	6. i
7. a	8. l	9. r	10. j	11. k	12. h
13. g	14. c	15. e	16. f	17. b	18. s
19. d	20. t	21. u	22. v		

23. TORCH
24. Herpes simplex virus
25. Hand washing
26. Fetal alcohol spectrum disorder (FASD)
27. Hemolytic disease of the newborn
28. Erythroblastosis fetalis; hydrops fetalis
29. RhoGAM
30. Neonatal abstinence syndrome
31. Meconium
32. Inborn errors of metabolism
33. Phenylketonuria (PKU)
34. Galactosemia
35. Congenital hypothyroidism
36. Clavicle
37. Phrenic nerve paralysis
38. Therapeutic hypothermia
39. Retinopathy of prematurity
40. Necrotizing enterocolitis
41. Intermittent gavage feeding
42. Bronchopulmonary dysplasia
43. Respiratory distress syndrome
44. Persistent pulmonary hypertension of the newborn

II. Reviewing Key Concepts

1. See Drug-Exposed Infants and Box 25.2
   CNS—irritability, hyperactivity, tremors, high-pitched cry, seizures, exaggerated Moro reflex
   Gastrointestinal—poor feeding, diarrhea, vomiting
   Respiratory—tachypnea, nasal congestion
   Autonomic—diaphoresis, disrupted sleep patterns, temperature instability

2. See Infants of Diabetic Mothers section. With maternal diabetes there is an increase in maternal insulin production as a result of hyperglycemia; insulin does not cross the placental circulation to the fetus, thus the fetus increases insulin production to manage the added glucose which easily passes from the maternal circulation to the fetus. At birth, the newborn pancreas continues to produce large amounts of insulin and glucose stores are rapidly depleted thus resulting in hypoglycemia.

3. See Infants of Diabetic Mothers section. Encourage woman to seek pregestational care because euglycemia before and during pregnancy is a major factor in preventing complications including congenital anomalies associated with diabetes during pregnancy.

4. See Rh Incompatibility (Isoimmunization) and ABO incompatibility sections. Basically human blood cells contain a variety of antigens, also known as agglutinogens, substances capable of producing an immune response if recognized by the body as foreign. The reciprocal relationship between antigens on RBCs and antibodies in the plasma cause agglutination (clumping). In other words, antibodies in the plasma of one blood group (except the AB group, which contains no antibodies) produce agglutination when mixed with antigens of a different blood group. In the ABO blood group system, the antibodies occur naturally. In the Rh system, the person must be exposed to the Rh antigen before significant antibody formation takes place and causes a sensitivity response known as isoimmunization. If the Rh (D)–negative mother conceives an Rh (D)–positive fetus and the fetus's blood cells enter into the maternal circulation, the antibody formation sequence (anti-Rh) is initiated. Fetal blood cells are destroyed by the maternal antibodies if maternal cells (anti-Rh) come in contact with the fetal circulation thus causing fetal anemia and an increased production of fetal erythrocytes, which are immature red cells. See the discussion on isoimmunization for further discussion of erythroblastosis fetalis. The placenta processes the bilirubin produced by destroyed fetal red cells, but at birth the newborn liver is immature and cannot handle the circulating volume of bilirubin, thus jaundice ensues. In ABO incompatibility the immune response and production of antibodies to fetal cells is less dramatic than the Rh response, thus the fetal red cell destruction is less severe in the majority of cases. See Table 25.6 for ABO group incompatibilities.

5. b, c, d, e, f

6. See Preterm Infants and Late-Preterm Infants sections and Table 25.7
   Respiratory function—immature alveolar development and function leading to respiratory distress; decreased chest wall musculature; decreased diaphragmatic excursion.
   Cardiovascular function—delayed closure of functional fetal shunts such as the ductus arteriosus which increases blood flow to the lungs by mixed oxygenated and deoxygenated blood, thus placing an increased the workload on the heart and lungs; hypoxemia and

high circulating levels of prostaglandins keep the ductus arteriosus from closing in the neonatal period.

Thermoregulation—decreased subcutaneous fat tissue and immature CNS thermoregulatory function contribute to poor thermoregulation with ensuing increased glucose metabolism and often poor glucose stores; nonshivering thermogenesis increases glucose metabolism and oxygen consumption; eventual outcome in a cold preterm infant is a metabolic acidosis, respiratory compromise, and possibly death if no interventions occur.

CNS function—immature CNS regulation; stimulation capable of taxing neonates and causing stress as the neonate is unable to self-regulate and respond to environmental stimuli; pain sensation is enhanced.

Nutritional status—functional immaturity of GI system in relation to the ability to physically consume the amount of caloric intake required to maintain positive nitrogen balance and promote growth; increased susceptibility to feeding intolerance due to poor absorption of formula or breast milk; low stomach capacity; increased transit time through the GI system and decreased absorption and metabolism of milk.

Renal status—delayed glomerular filtration with inability to concentrate urine in the first month of life; unable to compensate for increased water losses through the immature skin; immature renal function further compromises electrolyte balance since this is primarily determined by circulating fluid volume.

Hematologic status—increased turnover of red blood cells, in comparison to adult or older child, and decreased oxygen-carrying capacity in hemoglobin place infant at risk for hyperbilirubinemia, anemia, and hypoxemia; decreased rate of erythropoiesis further compromises infant red cell volume.

Immune status and infection prevention—immaturity of cellular and humoral immune system prevents rapid recognition of foreign viruses and bacteria and localization and phagocytosis of same; thus immature infants are susceptible to common pathogens; decreased skin maturity also contributes to infection susceptibility as does the immature gut mucosal barrier, making the neonate more susceptible to certain viruses and bacteria that enter the GI system; increased invasive procedures place the infant at higher risk for infection.

7. b, d, and e; Retractions, nasal flaring reflect increased effort and work to breathe; a, c, and f are all expected findings consistent with efficient respiratory effort in the preterm newborn.

8. b; Although a, c, and d are appropriate and important, respiration with adequate gas exchange takes precedence, especially because adequate surfactant is not produced before 32 weeks of gestation.

9. c; Fracture from trauma is more common in the upper body (e.g., humerus, clavicle); hypocalcemia is common; the newborn of a gestational diabetic mother is more likely to experience congenital anomalies such as heart defects.

III. Clinical Judgment and Next-Generation NCLEX® Examination-style Questions

1. See Nutrition and Gavage Feeding sections.
    a. Observe for the ability to suck and swallow and the coordination of each; signs of respiratory distress during the feeding; length of time for the feeding and the amount ingested; the presence of regurgitation, vomiting, or abdominal distention after feeding; daily weight gains and losses and elimination patterns.
    b. Emphasize tubing choice and measurement of tubing length, insertion without trauma and securing to maintain placement, checking placement.
    c. Imbalanced nutrition: less than body requirements related to weak suck associated with premature status.
    d. Initiate measures to prevent aspiration with proper tube insertion, removal, and position check techniques.
        • Instill breast milk or formula by gravity rather than pushing syringe barrel to expedite feeding.
        • Cuddle, swaddle infant during feedings; involve parents; use nonnutritive sucking.
        • Document assessment findings and specifics of the procedure.
    e. Proceed cautiously, checking for gastrointestinal, respiratory (signs of distress, decreased pulse oximetry), nutritional, and signs of tolerance or intolerance for advancement; decrease gavage feedings as the ability to suck improves; alternate oral feedings and gavage feedings according to infant tolerance.

2. See Gavage Feeding section. Current practice dictates a radiograph as the only certain way to determine nasogastric (NG) tube placement in the stomach. Methods such as auscultation of an air bubble, neck-ear-xiphoid (NEX) measurements for insertion depth, and pH measurements are considered imprecise when used as the only method for determination of placement. See also section on Gavage Feeding.

3. See Developmental Considerations section and Nursing Care Plan for High-Risk Infant.
    a. • Infant stressors: continuous exposure to light and noise; administration of sedatives and pain medications; invasive procedures and medications required for treatment
        • Family stressors: infant size and compromised and often fluctuating health status of their newborn; difficulty interacting with newborn and making eye contact; increased learning needs regarding status of newborn and care needs; concern regarding potential disabilities
    b. See Developmental Considerations section for a description of these behaviors.
    c. See Developmental Considerations section for many ideas, including waterbeds, kangaroo care, swaddling, coordinated plan of care to provide for period of interrupted rest and sleep, use pain medications and sedatives as needed, provide diurnal

299

light patterns, decrease noise level, and use stroking, talking, mobiles, decals, music, and windup toys for stimulation.

    d. Change position frequently, observing the effect of position change on breathing and oxygenation and preventing aspiration; consider boundaries, body alignment, sense of security and comfort when positioning; teach parents; use facilitated tucking and blanket swaddling.

4. See Postterm Infants section.

    a. Rationale for increased mortality: increased oxygen demands are not met and the likelihood for impaired gas exchange occurs, leading to hypoxia and passage of meconium into the amniotic fluid; risk for aspiration of meconium into lungs.

    b. Typical assessment findings: thin, emaciated appearance (dysmature) caused by loss of subcutaneous fat and muscle mass; peeling of skin; meconium staining on fingernails; long hair and nails; absence of vernix.

    c. Two major complications: meconium aspiration syndrome and persistent pulmonary hypertension of the newborn (PPHN); see the separate section that describes each complication.

5. See Nutrition section. Minimal enteral (trophic gastrointestinal priming) feedings have been shown to stimulate the infant's gastrointestinal tract, preventing mucosal atrophy and subsequent enteral feeding difficulties. Enteral feedings with as little as 0.1 to 4 mL/kg of breast milk or preterm formula may be given by gavage as soon as the infant is medically stable. These enteral feedings have been shown to simulate the infant's gastrointestinal tract, preventing mucosal atrophy and subsequent enteral feeding difficulties.

6. See Facilitating Parent-Infant Relationships section. 1. Physical separation; 2. Detached; 3. Anticipatory grief; 4. Normal responses.

CHAPTER 26

I. Learning Key Terms

1. e	2. j	3. a	4. b	5. g	6. c
7. i	8. f	9. l	10. h	11. d	12. k
13. n	14. o	15. m	16. p	17. r	18. q

II. Reviewing Key Concepts

1. a   2. d   3. b   4. d

5. Possible answers: homelessness; poverty; low birth weight; chronic illnesses; foreign-born adopted; day care centers

6. a   7. a

8. a   9. Congenital anomalies, disorders relating to short gestation and unspecified LBW, newborn affected by maternal complications of pregnancy, and sudden infant death syndrome.

10. c

11. Quality of care refers to the degree to which health services for individuals and populations increase the likelihood of desired health outcomes and are consistent with current professional knowledge (Institute of Medicine, 2000).

12. The six domains of the National Strategy for Improvements in Healthcare are: Patient and family engagement, patient safety, care coordination, population/public health, efficient use of health care resources, and clinical process/effectiveness.

III. Clinical Judgment and Next-Generation NCLEX® Examination-Style Questions

1. a, d, & f
2. b, e, f, & g
3. Answers could include:

Obesity- education and promotion of optimal nutrition beginning in infancy, encouraging physical activity at an early age, continuation of that physical activity. Education and promotion of lifestyle interventions to decrease the risk of childhood obesity.

Childhood injuries- implementation of developmentally appropriate accident prevention programs, as the type of injury and the circumstances surrounding it are usually related to normal growth and development. Education about pedestrian and bicycle safety, firearm safety, poisoning prevention, and water safety.

Violence – a thorough assessment and identification of individuals at risk, referral to qualified individuals.

Mental health illnesses – thorough assessment (being alert to signs/symptoms of depression or suicidal ideations) and identification of individuals at risk, referral to qualified individuals. Collaborate with interprofessional team members to identify mental health services which may be appropriate for the individual.

Infant and childhood mortality – thorough assessment of high-risk infants and children, education, and preventative strategies to reduce sudden infant death syndrome (SIDS). Continued firearm safety, screening for depression, and suicidal ideations. Reduce/ eliminate health disparities.

CHAPTER 27

I. Learning Key Terms

1. d	2. e	3. c	4. b	5. f	6. g
7. a	8. k	9. l	10. i	11. j	12. h
13. m	14. n	15. o	16. p	17. q	

II. Fill in the Blank

1. Family Stress Theory
2. Developmental Theory
3. Traditional nuclear family
4. Blended family
5. Binuclear family

6. Role structuring
7. Single parenting
8. Kinship care
9. Boundary
10. Family Systems Theory

II. Reviewing Key Concepts

1. c 2. b 3. b 4. e 5. c 6. d

7. a 8. a 9. c

10. Test their limits of control, achieve in areas appropriate for mastery at their level, channel undesirable feelings into constructive activity, protect themselves from danger, learn socially acceptable behavior.

11. Responses could include: children want and need limits, unrestricted freedom could be detrimental to their overall safety and well-being, children may gain reassurance there is someone to guide them and protect them from harm.

12. b 13. c 14. a

III. Clinical Judgment and Next-Generation NCLEX® Examination-Style Questions

Nursing Action	Indicated	Contraindicated	Non-Essential
Continue empowering this family through active participation in the child's care.	X		
Determine the type of parenting style used by these parents.			X
Offer the parents support and resources for possible future hospitalizations.	X		
Appreciate the family's strengths and uniqueness, use these to facilitate the discharge process.	X		

Rationale: Although the parents are not present in the hospital, they are still involved in their child's care by phoning in once or twice daily to discuss the plan of care with the healthcare providers. The type of parenting style is non-essential for the discharge process. Offering additional support and resources to assist the family with maintaining balance to cope with future hospitalizations would be appropriate. Even though the parents are unable to visit frequently, they are committed toward promoting the well-being of their child.

CHAPTER 28

I. Learning Key Terms

1. c 2. a 3. l 4. b 5. k 6. j

7. i 8. h 9. p 10. g 11. o 12. f

13. n 14. e 15. m 16. d

II. Reviewing Key Concepts

1. c 2. a 3. c 4. b 5. b 6. b

7. c 8. a 9. c 10. d 11. c 12. d

13. a 14. Difficult children 15. Slow to warm up children 16. Easy children

17. a 18. d

19. b 20. c 21. d 22. a 23. c 24. d

25. c 26. g 27. d 28. c 29. e 30. f

31. j 32. b 33. a 34. i 35. h 36. a

37. d 38. c 39. b 40. a

41. Using principles of family-centered care, treat the family with dignity and respect, provide open honest communication to allow the family to make informed decisions regarding their child's care, encourage expression of the feelings and concerns, promote participation in and collaboration of care by the family. Possible nursing interventions include:
- Recognizing multiple stressors, strains, and transitions in their lives (e.g., unmet family needs).
- Discuss and implement strategies for reducing family demands (e.g., setting realistic attainable expectations, setting priorities, and reducing the number of outside activities family members are involved in).
- Identify and use individual, family, and community resources (e.g., humor, family flexibility, supportive extended family, respite care, local support groups, and Internet resources).
- Expand the range and efficacy of their coping strategies (e.g., increase the use of active strategies such as reframing, mobilize their ability to acquire and accept help, and decrease the use of passive appraisal).
- Encourage the use of an affirming style of the family problem-solving communication (e.g., one that conveys support and caring and exerts a calming influence).

42. Malformations 43. Dysplasia 44. Disruptions 45. Deformations

III. Clinical Judgment and Next-Generation NCLEX® Examination-Style Questions

1. Option 1 – family health history, option 2 – major anomaly, option 3 – 3 or more
2. Parents of a 2-year-old child with Down syndrome are considering genetic testing before getting pregnant again.

Discuss information the nurse could provide to assist and instruct the family regarding genetic testing.

Possible answers include genetic testing may help provide early recognition of a disorder before signs and symptoms develop and early identification allows for anticipation of potential complications, implementation of preventive measures, and the ability for early interventions to promote the child's optimal well-being. Genetic testing may identify carriers of a genetic disorder for the purposed of preventing another unexpected birth of an affected child in the immediate or extended family. Genetic testing can occur at any point of life depending on the circumstances.

3. Identify and discuss the significance of nursing interventions to assist families with children with a genetic disorder.

Possible answers include nurses can direct individuals and families to needed services and encourage families to be active participants in the genetic evaluation and counseling process. Nurses are aware of special services that can help manage and support affected children and are familiar with facilities in their areas where these services are available and can refer families to these facilities. Nurses can help patients and families process and clarify the information they receive during a genetics clinical visit as the misunderstanding of information may occur, it may be difficult to absorb the information. Nurses can assess parental/family concerns or issues about any feelings they may be having about "giving their child a disease" to dispel any possible misconceptions. Nurses can play an important role in helping parents identify reliable, accurate resources for information about their child's disorder at whatever time they desire it as everything described for the genetic condition may not be relevant to their child and information on the Internet can be terrifying, overwhelming, and inaccurate or misleading.

CHAPTER 29

I. Learning Key Terms

1. e   2. a   3. b   4. c   5. d   6. m

7. o   8. v   9. k   10. u   11. n   12. t
13. h   14. l   15. s   16. j   17. r   18. g
19. q   20. f   21. p   22. i

II. Reviewing Key Concepts

1. b   2. d   3. d   4. T   5. T   6. T
7. b   8. a   9. c   10. d   11. d

12. Components of a pediatric health history: identifying information, chief complaint, present illness, past history, birth history (if applicable), previous illnesses, injuries, & surgeries, allergies, current medications, review of systems, growth & development, family medical history, psychosocial history, sexual history, nutritional/dietary history, and cultural considerations.

13. b   14. c   15. c   16. d   17. b   18. c
19. d   20. a   21. c   22. b   23. b   24. a
25. d
26. 0 and 2; 2 years old and older
27. a   28. T   29. T   30. T   31. b
32. apical, 1 full minute
33. d   34. c   35. d
36. Pupils Equal, Round, React to Light, and Accommodation
37. b   38. b   39. c   40. b   41. c   42. c
43. b

III. Clinical Judgment and Next-Generation NCLEX® Examination-Style Questions

1. a, c, e, & f
2. Growth measurements are essential in assessing children's health status. Linear growth is one of those measurements. Which of the following would be appropriate nursing actions for obtaining linear growth in children? Use an X for the nursing actions listed below which are Indicated (appropriate or necessary), Contraindicated (could be harmful), or Non-Essential (makes no difference or not necessary).

Nursing Actions	Indicated	Contraindicated	Non-Essential
All children should be measured at least twice, three times is preferred, using the mean value of measurements.	X		
Use a tape measure to measure the infant's length if a length board is unavailable.		X	
Children between 24 and 36 months of age can be measured using recumbent length or height with a stadiometer depending on the cooperation of the child.	X		
When using the stadiometer, it is important to place the headboard just above the crown of the head.		X	
The linear growth measurement should be read to the last completed millimeter or 1/16 inch.	X		

Rationale: The evidence supports all children should be measured at least twice if not three times using the mean value of the measurements, the measurements should agree within 0.5 cm (ideally 0.3 cm). Using a tape measure is not appropriate as it is inaccurate and unreliable. Children between the ages of 24–36 months can be measured either way depending on their ability to stand erect and on their cooperation. The stadiometer headboard should be positioned to the head of the crown, compressing the hair. Linear growth should be as accurate as possible, thus the measurement should be read at the last millimeter or 1/16 inch.

d. Mind-body techniques (mental healing, expressive treatments, spiritual healing, hypnosis, relaxation)
e. Alternative medical systems (homeopathy; naturopathy; ayurvedic; and traditional Chinese medicine, which includes acupuncture and moxibustion)

III. Fill in the Blank

21. Patient administered boluses
22. Continuous basal rate infusion
23. Nurse-administered boluses

IV. Clinical Judgment and Next-Generation NCLEX® Examination-Style Questions

1.

Health Teaching	Indicated	Contraindicated	Non-Essential
It is important to observe the infant for distress behaviors such as crying, changes in facial expressions, unexpected or unusual body movements.	X		
There are specific pain assessment tools that can be used to assess pain by examining various behaviors of infants.	X		
Infant do not really feel pain because their nerves and pain receptors are not fully developed yet.		X	
Healthcare personnel can use different techniques such as rocking infants or cuddling to relax them in addition to pain medication.	X		
There really is not a good way to determine if they are in pain or not, once they start crying hard, healthcare personnel can administer the ordered pain medication.		X	

CHAPTER 30

I. Learning Key Terms

1. c   2. e   3. a   4. l   5. m   6. f

7. h   8. i   9. g   10. j   11. k   12. d

13. b   14. p   15. o   16. n   17. q

II. Reviewing Key Concepts

1. a 2. d   3. a 4. b 5. d 6. T

7. T 8. T   9. T 10. T 11. T 12. F

13. T 14. Sleep disruption 15. T

16. 8
17. Functional Disability Inventory (FDI)
18. Cognitive impairment
19. Complex regional pain syndrome and daily headaches
20. a. Biologically based (foods, special diets, herbal or plant preparations, vitamins, other supplements)
    b. Manipulative treatments (chiropractic, osteopathy, massage)
    c. Energy-based (Reiki, bioelectric or magnetic treatments, pulsed fields, alternating and direct currents)

Rationale: Observing for distress behaviors such as crying, changes in facial expression, unexpected or unusual body movements would be indicated as these types of behavior are often associated with pain. If present, this would indicate a need for pain medication as ordered. Using Behavioral tools to measure pain in neonates is recommended as it provides a more complete picture of the total pain experience. Infants do feel pain, this is a misconception about the pain experienced by neonates/infants, there is the possibility of long-term consequences of untreated pain in infants. Nonpharmacologic strategies can also be effective in reducing pain.

2. Behavioral measures of pain such as the FLACC scale, are often used in children of any age who are unable to report pain due to neurocognitive or communication challenges. Behavioral pain assessment may provide a more complete picture of the total pain experience.

CHAPTER 31

I. Learning Key Terms

1. h	2. f	3. j	4. g	5. b	6. e
7. a	8. i	9. c	10. l	11. d	12. k
13. m					

II. Reviewing Key Concepts

1. c	2. b	3. c	4. c	5. b	6. d
7. b	8. a	9. b	10. c	11. c	12. c
13. c	14. F	15. T	16. F	17. F	18. T
19. T	20. T	21. e	22. b	23. c	24. d
25. f	26. a	27. h	28. l	29. j	30. g
31. k	32. i				

III. Clinical Judgment and Next-Generation NCLEX® Examination-Style Questions

1. Place the following social development milestones of an infant in the order in which they occur.

Developmental Milestone	Order of Occurrence (earliest to latest)
Object permanence.	3
Recognizes self in a mirror.	2
Develops a social smile.	1
Points to body parts.	4

2.

Preventive Teaching	Indicated	Contraindicated	Non-Essential
Room sharing is not indicated as long as the parents have a baby monitor/camera to observe the baby.		X	
The infant's head position can be alternated during sleep time to prevent plagiocephaly (flat spot on the infant's head).			X
Soft bedding, stuffed animals, and crib bumper pads should not be used.	X		
A pacifier is a SIDS protective factor and does not interfere with breastfeeding.	X		
All infants should be placed supine to sleep unless a medical condition prohibits this position of sleeping and places them at greater risk of death than the risk of death from SIDS.	X		

Rationale: According to the American Academy of Pediatrics (AAP) (2016), room sharing not bedsharing is recommended for at least the first 6 months of age and preferably the first year of life. The infant's head positioning is not related to SIDS but alternating the position may decrease the incidence of plagiocephaly. Per the AAP safe sleep practices, no soft bedding, stuffed animals, or bumper pads are recommended, they are considered a SIDS risk factor and all infants should be placed supine to sleep unless contraindicated.

3. Option 1 – 400 IU, Vitamin D, Option 2 – Iron, Option 3 – water, juice.

CHAPTER 32

I. Learning Key Terms

1. c	2. i	3. d	4. h	5. b	6. e
7. g	8. f	9. a	10. j		

II. Reviewing Key Concepts

1. b	2. d	3. c	4. a	5. a	6. c
7. d	8. d	9. d	10. a	11. a	12. b
13. b	14. b	15. 18 months of age	16. d		
17. a	18. Locomotion	19. Temper tantrums	20. Sibling rivalry		

III. Clinical Judgment and Next-Generation NCLEX® Examination-Style Questions

1.

Developmental Milestone	Order in which they occur (earliest to latest)
Uses a spoon well.	2
Turns pages of a book one at a time.	3
Scribbles spontaneously.	1
Draws/copies circles.	4

2. Signs of toilet-training readiness = b, d, f

3. a, b, c, d, e, f

CHAPTER 33

I. Learning Key Terms

1. h	2. m	3. g	4. p	5. t	6. f
7. e	8. q	9. l	10. d	11. k	12. u
13. s	14. c	15. r	16. j	17. b	18. o
19. a	20. n	21. i			

II. Reviewing Key Concepts

1. c
2. 2 to 3; 4.5 to 6.5
3. b   4. b   5. d
6. T   7. T   8. F   9. T
10. Telegraphic   11. d   12. c   13. b   14. b
    speech
15. c   16. A   17. b   18. b

III. Clinical Judgment and Next-Generation NCLEX® Examination-Style Questions

1.

Language Developmental Milestones of Preschoolers	Order in which they occurs (earliest to latest)
Uses sentences with 6–8 words, can follow 3 commands in succession.	3
Vocabulary of about 900 words. Uses sentences with 3–4 words.	1
Questioning is at its peak. Tells exaggerated stories, obeys prepositional phrases.	2

2. a, c, d

CHAPTER 34

I. Learning Key Terms

1. i   2. j   3. h   4. e   5. d   6. k
7. a   8. b   9. m   10. c   11. f   12. g
13. l

II. Reviewing Key Concepts

1. c
2. d
3. T   4. T   5. T   6. F   7. T   8. F
9. age 10, age 12, age 8
10. Concrete   11. b   12. a   13. d
    operations
14. d   15. b   16. b   17. T   18. T
19. Direct bullying, indirect bullying
20. T

III. Fill in the Blank with the School-Age Disorders with Behavioral Components

1. posttraumatic stress disorder
2. childhood schizophrenia
3. conversion reaction
4. anxiety
5. childhood depression
6. school phobia
7. attention-deficit hyperactivity disorder

IV. Clinical Judgment and Next-Generation NCLEX® Examination-Style Questions

1. a, b, c
2.

Nursing Action	Effective	Ineffective	Unrelated
Encouraging free time at a time of day that the child chooses.		X	
Providing structured responsibilities during the child's routine.	X		
Make organizational charts to allow for more choices and responsibility for actions.	X		
Children receiving medication for ADHD need regularly scheduled appointments for medication effectiveness, side effects, and to monitor development and health status.	X		
Attempt to provide a consistent routine for the child.	X		

Rationale: The nurse should review providing structured responsibilities, adhering to a consistent specific routine, and providing an organizational chart to promote more responsibility and choices for the child. The child with attention deficit hyperactivity disorder (ADHD) may not be able to choose an appropriate time during the day for free activities and will be more likely to exhibit developmentally appropriate behavior with a structured routine. The child needs to be reevaluated on a regular schedule to determine medication effectiveness, to monitor for side effects and if the medication is affecting the child's growth and development.

CHAPTER 35

I. Learning Key Terms

1. e   2. m   3. f   4. o   5. n   6. g
7. d   8. h   9. l   10. c   11. b   12. k
13. a   14. i   15. j

II. Reviewing Key Concepts

1. 10.5, 15; 12 years, 8 months; 12 years, 2 months
2. a   3. c
4. pubertal delay, 13
5. b   6. d
7.   2, 8; 15.5,
   55; 4, 12;
   15.5, 66
8. d   9. b   10. d   11. c   12. T   13. a
14. T   15. T   16. F   17. T   18. T   19. Fourteen

III. Clinical Judgment and Next-Generation NCLEX® Examination-Style Questions

1. a, b, c, d
2. a, b, c, d, e
3. a, c, f

CHAPTER 36

I. Learning Key Terms

1. b   2. h   3. e   4. g   5. i   6. c
7. d   8. f   9. k   10. a   11. j

II. Reviewing Key Concepts

1. c   2. b

3. Support the family's coping and/or promote the family's optimum functioning throughout the child's life.
4. The parent may be overwhelmed, stressed, and feel an enormous burden physically, psychosocially, and financially. Financial and supportive resources may already be strained thus it would be important to identify available resources to assist this single-parent family. It would be important to identify roles that could be delegated to relatives and friends to reduce some of the burdens.
5. a
6. Denial
7. Rejection
8. Overprotection
9. Gradual acceptance
10. Shock/denial, adjustment, and reintegration/acknowledgment

11. b   12. c

13. Possible answers include loss of senses, confusion, muscle weakness, loss of bowel and bladder control, difficulty swallowing, change in respiratory pattern, and weak/slow pulse.

14. b   15. a   16. d   17. d   18. c

III. Clinical Judgment and Next-Generation NCLEX® Examination-Style Questions

1. a, c, e
2.

Nursing Action	Effective	Ineffective	Unrelated
Provide the child with developmentally appropriate information about their condition.	X		
Encourage increased responsibility for own care and management of the disease or condition.		X	
Encourage socialization in clubs as appropriate.	X		
Encourage independence in as many areas as possible.		X	
Help with decision making and other skills necessary to manage personal plans.		X	

Rationale: School-age children are in the industry vs. inferiority stage of development, they are trying to achieve a sense of accomplishment. They may have limited opportunities to socialize with other children due to their chronic illness. They learn through concrete operations thus they need developmentally appropriate information.

3. c, d, e

CHAPTER 37

I. Learning Key Terms

1. i   2. p   3. j   4. h
5. g   6. f   7. o   8. e   9. k
10. d   11. n
12. c   13. l   14. b   15. m   16. a

II. Reviewing Key Concepts

1. c   2. c   3. b   4. Toddler, boys than girls
5. genetic counseling
7. b   8. b   9. a   10. a   11. d
12. b   13. 18 months
                and 24 months
14. Possible strategies include the following: Talk to the child about everything that is occurring; emphasize aspects of procedures that are felt/ heard; approach the child with identifying information; explain sounds; encourage parents to room in; encourage parents' participation; bring familiar objects from home; orient child to surroundings. (If the child has sight on admission but will lose sight during hospitalization [e.g., as a result of eye surgery], point out significant aspects of the room's layout and practice ambulation with eyes closed before the procedure.)

15. c   16. T

III. Clinical Judgment and Next-Generation NCLEX® Examination-Style Questions

1. a, b, c

2.

Health Teaching	Indicated	Contraindicated	Non-Essential
Encourage the need for play and exercise.	X		
Initially, it may be beneficial to avoid individuals who may not understand cognitive development.		X	
Focus should be on the development of verbal skills as physical skills are often delayed and require additional intervention.		X	
Limit-setting measures should be simple and consistent, with behavior modification as a very effective discipline strategy.	X		
Seek out opportunities for social interaction such as early intervention programs and appropriate preschool programs	X		

Rationale: Play is based on the child's developmental age. Parents should use every opportunity to expose the child to as many different sounds, sights, and sensations as possible. It is beneficial to the child to be exposed to various outings and have visitors who directly interact with the child. Discipline is important and should begin early, Behavior modification is an effective strategy for children with cognitive impairment. Verbal skills are often delayed and need further intervention.

CHAPTER 38

I. Learning Key Terms

1. f   2. b   3. e   4. a   5. c   6. d

II. Reviewing Key Concepts

1. Separation anxiety, 6 months to 30 months of age
2. b   3. c   4. a
5. T   6. T
7. c   8. a   9. a
10. Answers could include initial aloofness toward parents, followed by a tendency to cling to parents, demands for parents' attention, vigorous opposition to any separation. Other negative behaviors include new fears, resistance to going to bed, night waking, withdrawal and shyness, hyperactivity, temper tantrums, food finickiness, attachment to blanket or toy, regression in newly learned skills.

11. b   12. b   13. c   14. a   15. c   16. c

17. Factors include the seriousness of the threat to the child, previous experience with illness or hospitalization, medical procedures involved in diagnosis and treatment, available support systems, personal ego strengths, previous coping abilities, additional stresses on the family system, cultural and religious beliefs, and communication patterns among family members.

18. All ages: cognitively appropriate explanations regarding the procedure being aware of medical terminology used as children and most parents do not understand medical terminology, use of doll or drawing for the child to "explain" thoughts about the upcoming procedure, no rectal temperatures unless indicated, take axillary, oral, or tympanic temperatures. Use of Band-Aids to prevent "leaking" of bodily parts.

III. Clinical Judgment and Next-Generation NCLEX® Examination-Style Questions

1. b, c, e

2.

Nursing Actions	Indicated	Contraindicated	Non-Essential
Encourage parental participation in the child's care, during family-centered rounds, and visitation.	X		
Have the parents bring familiar objects from home to place in the child's hospital room.	X		
Refrain from having siblings visit as it may be upsetting to see their sibling ill, especially for younger siblings.		X	
Enabling independence and promoting self-care when appropriate for the child.	X		
Provide the family information about the disease, its treatment, prognosis, and home care	X		

Rationale: The family is considered a partner in the care of their children. It is important to offer developmentally appropriate information and hospital visits for siblings if possible to keep the family as a unit and recognize all members of the family. Providing the family with accurate information may help decrease parental stress and anxiety during the hospitalization. Familiar objects for the child also help decrease stress and anxiety for the child.

CHAPTER 39

I. Learning Key Terms

1. m 2. d 3. l 4. c 5. e
6. f 7. b 8. k 9. g 10. j
11. h 12. a 13. i

II. Reviewing Key Concepts

1. c 2. c 3. a

4. Infant: keep parent in infant's line of vision, include parents if desired, if unable to stay provide a familiar object. Toddler: similar to infants, include parents if desired, use firm, direct approach, tell child it is okay to cry, yell. Preschooler: include parents if desired, demonstrate use of equipment, explain procedure in simple terms and in relation to how it affects child. School-age: include parents if desired, explain procedures using correct scientific and medical terminology, explain procedure using simple diagrams and photographs., allow child to manipulate equipment. Adolescents: discuss why procedure is necessary or beneficial, encourage questioning regarding fears, options, and alternatives, provide privacy; describe how the body will be covered and what will be exposed, include parents if desired.
5. a. Give a toddler a push-pull toy.
   b. Touch or kick Mylar balloons.
   c. Make creative objects out of needleless syringes.
   d. Practice band instruments.
   e. Move the patient's bed to the playroom, activity room, or lobby (within reasonable expectations of child's condition).
   f. Put toys at the bottom of the bath container.
   g. Make freezer pops using the child's favorite juice.

6. T 7. T 8. T 9. a 10. b 11. a
12. b 13. d 14. d 15. b 16. d 17. d
18. a 19. T 20. c 21. d 22. eye drops, eye ointment 23. c
24. b 25. d 26. c 27. a 28. b 29. Down and back, up and back, room temperature.
30. c

III. Clinical Judgment and Next-Generation NCLEX® Examination-Style Questions

1. a, d, e
2. Option 1 – vastus lateralis muscle, Option 2 – ventrogluteal muscle, Option 3 – deltoid muscle, Option 4 – 1 ml

CHAPTER 40

I. Learning Key Terms

1. g 2. f 3. p 4. e 5. m 6. k
7. d 8. j 9. b 10. i 11. c 12. h
13. a 14. o 15. n 16. l

II. Reviewing Key Concepts

1. b 2. c 3. c 4. b 5. b 6. c
7. d 8. a 9. c 10. a 11. b 12. a
13. c 14. c 15. c 16. d 17. c 18. a
19. b 20. a 21. b 22. c 23. a 24. b
25. c 26. d 27. c 28. b 29. a 30. b
31. a 32. c 33. a 34. a 35. d 36. d
37. d 38. a
39. a 40. a
41. h 42. b 43. e 44. c 45. l 46. a
47. d 48. i 49. k 50. j 51. g 52. f

III. Clinical Judgment and Next-Generation NCLEX® Examination-Style Questions

1. a, d, e
2.

Health Teaching	Indicated	Contraindicated	Non essential
In certain strains of this disease, a characteristic erythematous sandpaper-like rash; known as Scarlet Fever may develop.	X		
A follow-up throat culture is recommended after completion of antibiotic therapy.			X
Children who experience a GABHS infection are at increased risk for the development of acute rheumatic fever and acute glomerulonephritis, thus it is imperative to complete the antibiotic therapy prescribed.	X		
Application of a warm or cold compress to the neck area may provide pain relief, anti-pyretics may also be administered for throat pain and to decrease fevers.	X		
Children should discard their toothbrushes after completion of antibiotic therapy.		X	
Children are considered contagious until they have received antibiotic therapy for a full 48- hour period of time.		X	

Rationale: Parents should be aware that certain strains of the organism may produce an erythematous sandpaper-like rash known as Scarlet Fever. A throat culture is not needed but completion of antibiotic therapy is imperative to reduce the risk of any sequelae. The child needs a full 24- hour period of antibiotics, once received is no longer considered contagious. Likewise, the child's toothbrush should be discarded after receiving antibiotics for a full 24-hour period. Warm or cold compresses along with anti-pyretics are appropriate for pain relief and fever reduction.

CHAPTER 41

I. Learning Key Terms

1. e   2. d   3. k   4. j   5. i   6. c
7. h   8. b   9. l   10. g   11. a   12. f

II. Reviewing Key Concepts

1. c   2. b   3. a   4. d   5. d
6. b   7. d
8. Isotonic
9. hypotonic, less
10. hypertonic; loss, intake; greater
11. b   12. c
13. Skin turgor, capillary refill, body weight, level of consciousness, activity level, respiratory pattern, status of the oral mucosa (dry), thirst (in older child), urine output in last 24 hours

14. c   15. c   16. a   17. a   18. a   19. c
20. a   21. d
22. handwashing
23. d
24. a   25. b   26. e   27. d
28. c   29. b   30. d
31. Pruritis
32. c   33. b   34. b   35. c   36. a   37. d
38. c   39. a   40. b   41. b   42. d   43. c
44. d   45. a
46. Phase 1 (initial phase)—expand ECF volume quickly and improve circulatory and renal function; an isotonic solution is used at a rate of 20 mL/kg, given as an IV bolus over 5–20 minutes and repeated as necessary after assessment of the child's response to therapy.
   a. Phase 2 (subsequent phase)—replace deficits, meet maintenance water and electrolyte requirements, and catch up with ongoing losses. Water and sodium requirements for the deficit, maintenance, and ongoing losses are calculated at 8-hour intervals, taking into consideration the amount of fluids given with the initial boluses and the amount administered during the first 24-hour period. With improved circulation during this phase, water and electrolyte deficits can be evaluated, and acid–base status can be corrected either directly through the administration

of fluids or indirectly through improved renal function. Potassium is withheld until kidney function is restored and assessed and circulation has improved.

b. Phase 3 (final phase)— patient to return to normal and begin oral feedings, with a gradual correction of total body deficits.

47. When the child is alert, awake, and not in danger, correction of dehydration may be attempted with oral fluid administration. Mild cases of dehydration can be managed at home or in the ED or urgent care by this method. Oral rehydration management consists of replacement of fluid loss over 4 to 6 hours, replacement of continuing losses, and provision for maintenance fluid requirements. Clear fluids are preferred initially; breastfeeding may be resumed, and the child tolerating clear fluids can be advanced to solid foods after tolerance is demonstrated. Avoid fatty foods like French fries and pizza during this phase. In general, a mildly dehydrated child may be given 50 mL/kg of oral rehydration solution (ORS), and a child with moderate dehydration may be given 100 mL/kg of ORS.

III. Clinical Judgment and Next-Generation NCLEX® Examination-Style Questions

1. a, b, d, e, f
2. Option 1 – Intussusception, Option 2 – crampy abdominal pain, Option 3 – currant jelly-like, Option 4 – brown.

CHAPTER 42

I. Learning Key Terms

1. o	2. r	3. n	4. p	5. m
6. l	7. q	8. k	9. t	10. e
11. d	12. u	13. f	14. c	15. j
16. a	17. g	18. s	19. b	20. h
21. i				

II. Reviewing Key Concepts

| 1. b | 2. b | 3. a | 4. c | 5. a |
| 6. c | 7. c | | | |

8. The most significant complications include stroke, seizures, tamponade, and death. The patient may also suffer the loss of circulation to the affected extremity, dysrhythmias, hemorrhage, cardiac perforation, hematoma, hypovolemia and dehydration, hypoglycemia in infants, and changes in the temperature and color of the affected extremity.

9. d	10. d	11. 90th, 130/80	12. d	13. a	14. b
15. c	16. b	17. c	18. c	19. c	20. d
21. a	22. b	23. c			
24. c	25. d	26. c	27. d	28. b	
29. c	30. d				
31. a	32. d	33. a	34. d	35. b	36. c
37. b					
38. c	39. b	40. a	41. b	42. a	43. d
44. a	45. d	46. b	47. a	48. a	49. d
50. a	51. a	52. b	53. c		
54. 3, annually					
55. b					

III. Clinical Judgment and Next-Generation NCLEX® Examination-Style Questions

1. a, b, c, d, e, f
2.

Defect (option 1)	Hemodynamic characteristics (option 2)	Effect on blood flow (option 3)
Tetralogy of Fallot	Usually a right-to-left shunt depends on the size of VSD and degree of pulmonary stenosis. Includes four defects	Decreased pulmonary blood flow.
Patent ductus arteriosus (PDA)	Continued patency of this vessel allows blood to flow from the higher-pressure aorta to the lower pressure pulmonary artery, which causes a left-to-right shunt.	Increased pulmonary blood flow.
Coarctation of the aorta	Localized narrowing near the insertion of the ductus arteriosus. Increased pressure proximal to the defect and decreased pressure distal to the obstruction	Obstructed blood flow.
Transposition of the great vessels	No communication between the systemic and pulmonary circulations.	Mixed pulmonary blood flow.

CHAPTER 43

I. Learning Key Terms

1. e   2. c   3. a   4. f   5. b   6. d

II. Reviewing Key Concepts

1. a
2. iron deficiency
3. a   4. c
5. b
6. a   7. d   8. a   9. d   10. b   11. c
12. immune thrombocytopenia
13. T
14. 9.5 gm/dl
15. d   16. c
17. *Pneumocystis carinii* pneumonia
18. d   19. d   20. a

III. Clinical Judgment and Next-Generation NCLEX® Examination-Style Questions

1.

Health Teaching	Indicated	Contraindicated	Non-Essential
The child needs to be taken to a physician/provider when seriously ill, not for a common cold.		X	
Offer genetic counseling.	X		
The infant needs to be well hydrated, observe for signs of dehydration (↓ number of wet diapers).	X		
Prophylactic penicillin	X		
Factor VIII will be given IV during a crisis.		X	
Encourage routine vaccine administration	X		

Rationale: Genetic counseling would be appropriate to offer in this situation. Sickle-cell anemia is an autosomal recessive disease, when both parents carry the trait, there is a 25% chance with each pregnancy child will have the disease. Adequate hydration to prevent sickling and delay the vaso-occlusion and hypoxia-ischemia cycle. Families should seek early intervention for problems, even the common cold to prevent sickling from developing. Oral penicillin prophylaxis is recommended by 2 months old to reduce the chance of pneumococcal sepsis. Routine vaccines are recommended for these children because of their susceptibility to infection as a result of functional asplenia. Factor VIII is used for those with Hemophilia A.

2. Apply pressure to the area of bleeding for 10 to 15 minutes to allow for clot formation. Immobilize and elevate the area above the level of the heart to decrease blood flow. Apply cold to promote vasoconstriction.

CHAPTER 44

I. Learning Key Terms

1. e   2. d   3. a   4. h   5. f   6. g
7. b   8. i   9. c   10. f   11. e   12. b
13. i   14. a   15. d   16. h   17. c   18. j
19. g

II. Reviewing Key Concepts

1. d
2. 0 and 4 years and 15 and 19 years
3. Cardinal symptoms: unusual mass or swelling, unexplained paleness and loss of energy, the sudden tendency to bruise, persistent localized pain or limping, prolonged unexplained fever/illness, frequent headaches often with vomiting, sudden eye or vision changes, excessive rapid weight loss
4. c   5. a   6. T
7. Superior vena cava syndrome (SVCS), airway, and respiratory
8. Back pain, MRI

9. Overwhelming infection, malaise, possible secondary infections
10. T
11. CSFs (colony-stimulating factor)
12. a   13. d
14. <100,00 mm^3
15. Administer anti-emetic 30 minutes before chemotherapy begins and continue with scheduled administration for at least 24 hours after chemotherapy has been completed.
16. Interventions for infants and children with mucosal ulcerations include bland, moist, soft diet; use of a "sponge" toothette instead of a regular toothbrush; frequent rinsing with chlorhexidine mouthwash, use of local anesthetics without alcohol; use of a gauze soaked in saline or plain water to cleanse the gums, palate, and inner cheeks. This should be done before and after feeding and every 2 to 4 hours as needed to cleanse the mouth of debris.

17. F
18. Post-irradiation somnolence may occur 5 to 8 weeks after CNS irradiation. It may last 4 to 15 days and is often characterized by somnolence with or without fever, anorexia, nausea, and vomiting.
19. Strategies to decrease hemorrhagic cystitis include liberal oral or IV fluid intake, frequent voiding, administration of the drug early in the day to allow for sufficient fluid intake and frequent voiding to occur, administration of Mesna.
20. d   21. F
22. The three main consequences of bone marrow infiltration are (1) anemia from decreased erythrocytes, (2) infection from neutropenia, and (3) bleeding from decreased platelet production.
23. d
24. Invasion of the CNS by leukemic cells; CNS prophylactic therapy (intrathecal chemotherapy)

25. a   26. T   27. b   28. c

29. Temperature—this vital sign is important to monitor because of possible hyperthermia as a result of the surgical procedure in the hypothalamus area or related to the anesthesia used during the procedure.
30. Nursing care would include frequent vital signs assessment, proper positioning, fluid regulation, pain and comfort measures, support for the family, and assisting in promoting optimal functioning of the child.
31. Location and extent of the disease
32. Due to metastasis of the cancer.
33. An abdominal neuroblastoma is usually firm, non-tender, and an irregular mass that crosses the midline in contrast to a nephroblastoma (Wilms tumor) which does not cross the midline, and it is usually confined to one side.
34. Characteristics of phantom limb pain include tingling, itching, and pain felt in the amputated limb.
35. Discovery of Wilms tumor often happens when parents are giving their child a bath or dressing them.
36. Do not palpate the abdominal mass as this may increase dissemination of cancer cells to adjacent and distant sites.
37. b

III. Clinical Judgment and Next-Generation NCLEX® Examination-Style Questions
1. b, c
2. a, c, d, f

CHAPTER 45

I. Learning Key Terms

1. q	2. a	3. j	4. i	5. l	6. h
7. b	8. p	9. k	10. c	11. o	12. f
13. d	14. n	15. g	16. m	17. e	

II. Reviewing Key Concepts
1. Urinary stasis
2. Uncircumcised

3. d	4. a	5. b	6. b

7. corticosteroid

8. a	9. c	10. c	11. d	12. b	13. a
14. c	15. b	16. b	17. b	18. b	

19. hemodialysis, peritoneal dialysis, hemofiltration
20. c
21. Peritoneal

III. Clinical Judgment and Next-Generation NCLEX® Examination-Style Questions
1. a, d, e, f
2. a, b, c, d

CHAPTER 46

I. Learning Key Terms

1. j	2. f	3. k	4. g	5. m
6. e	7. i	8. l	9. d	10. a
11. c	12. b	13. h		

II. Reviewing Key Concepts

1. b	2. b	3. b	4. c	5. d	6. c
7. a	8. b	9. c	10. c	11. a	

12. Meningococcal meningitis

13. a	14. d	15. a	16. c	17. d	18. d
19. a	20. c	21. a	22. d		

III. Clinical Judgment and Next-Generation NCLEX® Examination-Style Questions
1. a, c, e
2. Option 1 - 38°C, Option 2 – 6 to 60 months, Option 3 – 5 minutes.

CHAPTER 47

I Learning Key Words

1. e	2. j	3. d	4. n	5. i
6. m	7. k	8. c	9. l	10. g
11. b	12. h	13. a	14. f	

II. Reviewing Key Concepts

1. b   2. c

3. Constitutional growth
4. Acromegaly results from hypersecretion of growth hormone that occurs after epiphyseal closure. If hypersecretion occurs before epiphyseal closure, the disorder is called *pituitary hyperfunction*, and physical features do not become distorted as in acromegaly.

5. 7, 6; 9
6. c   7. a   8. b   9. b
10. d   11. b   12. c   13. b
14. insulin
15. c   16. b   17. b   18. d
19. Glucose spills into the urine which causes an osmotic diuresis of water (polyuria). The urinary fluid losses cause the excessive thirst (polydipsia) observed in diabetes. This water "washout" results in a depletion of other essential chemicals, especially potassium.
20. a
21. d
22. c

III. Clinical Judgment and Next-Generation NCLEX® Examination-Style Questions
1. a, c, d, e
2. a, b, e

CHAPTER 48

I. Learning Key Terms
1. g   2. f   3. h   4. m   5. e   6. d
7. i   8. l   9. c   10. k   11. j   12. a
13. c   14. o   15. q   16. r   17. p   18. n
19. s

II. Reviewing Key Concepts
1. d   2. d   3. b   4. h   5. i   6. a
7. c   8. b   9. d   10. e   11. f   12. g
13. b   14. d
15. lower extremities, tibia; cross country running and gymnastics
16. b   17. b   18. c   19. d
20. c   21. a   22. d
23. lordosis, kyphosis
24. d   25. a   26. b   27. a   28. limp; complaints of hip, thigh, groin, or knee pain.
29. c
30. a   31. d   32. a   33. c   34. d

III. Clinical Judgment and Next-Generation NCLEX® Examination-Style Questions
1. a, b, d, f
2. Option 1 = IV opioids on a regular schedule, option 2 = log rolled, option 3 = neurologic status to assess for any delayed paralysis or spinal column injury.

CHAPTER 49

I. Learning Key Terms
1. g   2. c   3. f   4. d
5. b   6. a   7. e

II. Reviewing Key Concepts
1. a   2. Anencephaly   3. b   4. d   5. d
6. b   7. b   8. a   9. a
10. latex allergy; latex sensitivity
11. b   12. b   13. b   14. c
15. a   16. c   17. a   18. b   19. c

III. Clinical Judgment and Next-Generation NCLEX® Examination-Style Questions
1. a, b, c, d, e
2. c, b, d, a

CHAPTER 50

I Learning Key Concepts
1. f   2. j   3. e   4. g   5. b
6. d   7. i   8. h   9. c   10. A
11. l   12. k   13. p   14. n   15. o
16. m

II. Reviewing Key Concepts
1. b   2. c   3. T   4. T   5. F
6. a   7. c   8. d   9. F   10. Amoxicillin, doxycycline; 14 to 21 days.
11. d   12. a   13. b   14. c   15. F   16. c
17. T   18. c   19. a   20. c   21. b   22. c

III. Fill in the Blank
1. Partial thickness burns (second-degree burns)
2. Minor burns
3. Fourth-degree burns
4. Total body surface area
5. Superficial burns (first-degree burns)
6. Full-thickness burns (third-degree burns)
7. Major burns
8. Allograft
9. Sheet graft
10. Synthetic skin coverings
11. Xenograft
12. Cultured epithelial autografts

1.

Health Teaching	Indicated	Contraindicated	Non-Essential
The infant's skin should be thoroughly dried before applying an acceptable emollient preparation.		X	
Fingernails and toenails are cut short, kept clean, and filed frequently to prevent sharp edges.	X		
An anti-seborrheic shampoo containing sulfur and salicylic acid maybe used.			X
Skinfolds and diaper areas need frequent cleansing with plain water.	X		
Colloid baths and cool wet compresses can be used as they are soothing to the skin and providing antiseptic protection.	X		
Occasional flare-ups may require the use of topical steroids to diminish inflammation.	X		
Bathing may need to be done four to five times per day to prevent skin drying depending on the child's status.		X	
Nonsedating antihistamines such as loratadine (Claritin) or fexofenadine (Allegra) may be prescribed for daytime pruritus relief. As pruritus increases at night, a mildly sedating antihistamine may be prescribed by the provider.	X		

Rationale: It is imperative an emollient preparation be applied immediately after bathing (while the skin is still slightly moist) to prevent drying. Acceptable emollients for skin hydration include but are not limited to Aquaphor, Cetaphil, and Eucerin. Use emollients as prescribed by the healthcare provider. Keeping finger and toenails short and clean helps decrease the risk of scratching and causing a secondary infection. An anti-seborrheic shampoo is not necessary for children with atopic dermatitis, a mild shampoo would be appropriate. Bathing may be necessary once or twice daily as excessive bathing without appropriate emollient preparation applied will result in drying out of the skin.

2. b, e, f
3. a, c, d, f, g